Women and Obesity

Guest Editor

RAUL ARTAL, MD

OBSTETRICS AND GYNECOLOGY CLINICS OF NORTH AMERICA

www.obgyn.theclinics.com

Consulting Editor
WILLIAM F. RAYBURN, MD, MBA

June 2009 • Volume 36 • Number 2

SAUNDERS an imprint of ELSEVIER, Inc.

W.B. SAUNDERS COMPANY

A Division of Elsevier Inc.

Elsevier, Inc. • 1600 John F. Kennedy Blvd. • Suite 1800 • Philadelphia, PA 19103-2899

http://www.theclinics.com

OBSTETRICS AND GYNECOLOGY CLINICS OF NORTH AMERICA Volume 36, Number 2
June 2009 ISSN 0889-8545, ISBN-13: 978-1-4377-1248-3, ISBN-10: 1-4377-1248-7

Editor: Carla Holloway
Developmental Editor: Theresa Collier

Obstetrics and Gynecology Clinics (ISSN 0889-8545) is published quarterly by Elsevier Inc., 360 Park Avenue South, New York, NY 10010-1710. Months of issue are March, June, September, and December. Business and Editorial Offices: 1600 John F. Kennedy Blvd., Suite 1800, Philadelphia, PA 19103-2899. Customer Service Office: 11830 Westline Industrial Drive, St. Louis, MO 63146. Periodicals postage paid at New York, NY, and additional mailing offices. Subscription price per year is $234.00 (US individuals), $399.00 (US institutions), $118.00 (US students), $281.00 (Canadian individuals), $504.00 (Canadian institutions), $174.00 (Canadian students), $342.00 (foreign individuals), $504.00 (foreign institutions), and $174.00 (foreign students). To receive student/resident rate, orders must be accompanied by name of affiliated institution, date of term, and the signature of program/residency coordinator on institution letterhead. Orders will be billed at individual rate until proof of status is received. Foreign air speed delivery is included in all *Clinics* subscription prices. All prices are subject to change without notice. POSTMASTER: Send address changes to *Obstetrics and Gynecology Clinics*, Elsevier Periodicals Customer Service, 11830 Westline Industrial Drive, St. Louis, MO 63146. **Customer Service: 1-800-654-2452 (US). From outside of the United States, call 314-453-7041. Fax: 314-453-5170. E-mail: JournalsCustomerService-usa@elsevier.com (for print support); JournalsOnlineSupport-usa@elsevier.com (for online support).**

Reprints. For copies of 100 or more of articles in this publication, please contact the Commercial Reprints Department, Elsevier Inc., 360 Park Avenue South, New York, New York 10010-1710. Tel.: 212-633-3818; Fax: 212-462-1935; E-mail: reprints@elsevier.com.

Obstetrics and Gynecology Clinics of North America is also published in Spanish by McGraw-Hill Interamericana Editores S.A., P.O. Box 5-237, 06500, Mexico; in Portuguese by Reichmann and Affonso Editores, Rio de Janeiro, Brazil; and in Greek by Paschalidis Medical Publications, Athens, Greece.

Obstetrics and Gynecology Clinics of North America is covered in MEDLINE/PubMed (Index Medicus), Excerpta Medica, Current Concepts/Clinical Medicine, Science Citation Index, BIOSIS, CINAHL, and ISI/BIOMED.

Printed and bound in the United Kingdom
Transferred to Digital Print 2011

GOAL STATEMENT
The goal of *Obstetrics and Gynecology Clinics of North America* is to keep practicing physicians up to date with current clinical practice in OB/GYN by providing timely articles reviewing the state of the art in patient care.

ACCREDITATION
The *Obstetrics and Gynecology Clinics of North America* is planned and implemented in accordance with the Essential Areas and Policies of the Accreditation Council for Continuing Medical Education (ACCME) through the joint sponsorship of the University of Virginia School of Medicine and Elsevier. The University of Virginia School of Medicine is accredited by the ACCME to provide continuing medical education for physicians.

The University of Virginia School of Medicine designates this educational activity for a maximum of 15 AMA PRA Category 1 Credits™ for each issue, 60 credits per year. Physicians should only claim credit commensurate with the extent of their participation in the activity.

The American Medical Association has determined that physicians not licensed in the US who participate in this CME activity are eligible for a maximum of 15 AMA PRA Category 1 Credits™ for each issue, 60 credits per year.

Category 1 credit can be earned by reading the text material, taking the CME examination online at: http://www.theclinics.com/home/cme, and completing the evaluation. After taking the test, you will be required to review any and all incorrect answers. Following completion of the test and evaluation, your credit will be awarded and you may print your certificate.

FACULTY DISCLOSURE/CONFLICT OF INTEREST
The University of Virginia School of Medicine, as an ACCME accredited provider, endorses and strives to comply with the Accreditation Council for Continuing Medical Education (ACCME) Standards of Commercial Support, Commonwealth of Virginia statutes, University of Virginia policies and procedures, and associated federal and private regulations and guidelines on the need for disclosure and monitoring of proprietary and financial interests that may affect the scientific integrity and balance of content delivered in continuing medical education activities under our auspices.

The University of Virginia School of Medicine requires that all CME activities accredited through this institution be developed independently and be scientifically rigorous, balanced and objective in the presentation/discussion of its content, theories and practices.

All authors/editors participating in an accredited CME activity are expected to disclose to the readers relevant financial relationships with commercial entities occurring within the past 12 months (such as grants or research support, employee, consultant, stock holder, member of speakers bureau, etc.). The University of Virginia School of Medicine will employ appropriate mechanisms to resolve potential conflicts of interest to maintain the standards of fair and balanced education to the reader. Questions about specific strategies can be directed to the Office of Continuing Medical Education, University of Virginia School of Medicine, Charlottesville, Virginia.

The faculty and staff of the University of Virginia Office of Continuing Medical Education have no financial affiliations to disclose.

The authors/editors listed below have identified no professional or financial affiliations for themselves or their spouse/partner:
Patrick M. Catalano, MD; John R.G. Challis, PhD, FRSC; J. Ricardo Loret de Mola, MD, FACOG, FACS; Jeffrey A. Gavard, PhD; Erica P. Gunderson, PhD; Carla Holloway (Acquisitions Editor); William Irvin, MD (Test Author); Stephen James Lye, PhD; Faidon Magkos, PhD; Bettina Mittendorfer, MS, PhD; Michelle F. Mottola, PhD, FACSM; John P. Newnham, MD, FRANZCOG; Emily Oken, MD, MPH; Craig E. Pennell, FRANZCOG, PhD; Sharon Theresa Phelan, MD, FACOG; William F. Rayburn, MD, MBA (Consulting Editor); Mitul B. Shah, MD; Yariv Yogev, MD; and Gerald S. Zavorsky, PhD.

The authors/editors listed below identified the following professional or financial affiliations for themselves or their spouse/partner:
Raul Artal, MD (Guest Editor) is an industry funded research/investigator for Xanodyne, Luitpold Pharmaceuticals, Columbia Labs, Ortho-Clinical Diagnostics, and Ottawa Health Research Institute.
Jonathan Rampono, MBBS, FRACP serves on the Advisory Board for Wyeth Pharmaceuticáls.

Disclosure of Discussion of non-FDA approved uses for pharmaceutical products and/or medical devices:
The University of Virginia School of Medicine, as an ACCME provider, requires that all faculty presenters identify and disclose any off-label uses for pharmaceutical and medical device products. The University of Virginia School of Medicine recommends that each physician fully review all the available data on new products or procedures prior to clinical use.

TO ENROLL
To enroll in the Obstetrics and Gynecology Clinics of North America Continuing Medical Education program, call customer service at 1-800-654-2452 or visit us online at: www.theclinics.com/home/cme. The CME program is available to subscribers for an additional fee of $195.00.

Contributors

CONSULTING EDITOR

WILLIAM F. RAYBURN, MD, MBA
Seligman Professor and Chair, Department of Obstetrics and Gynecology; Chief of Staff, University Hospital, University of New Mexico Health Science Center, Albuquerque, New Mexico

GUEST EDITOR

RAUL ARTAL, MD
Professor and Chairman, Department of Obstetrics, Gynecology and Women's Health, Saint Louis University School of Medicine, Saint Louis, Missouri

AUTHORS

PATRICK M. CATALANO, MD
Department of Reproductive Biology, Case Western Reserve University at Metro Health Medical Center, Cleveland, Ohio

JOHN R.G. CHALLIS, PhD, FRSC
Professor and President, Chief Executive Officer, Michael Smith Foundation for Health Research, Vancouver, British Columbia, Canada

JEFFREY A. GAVARD, PhD
Research Assistant Professor, Department of Obstetrics, Gynecology, and Women's Health, St. Louis University School of Medicine, St. Louis, Missouri

ERICA P. GUNDERSON, PhD
Epidemiologist and Research Scientist, Epidemiology and Prevention, Division of Research, Kaiser Permanente Northern California, Oakland, California

J. RICARDO LORET DE MOLA, MD, FACOG, FACS
Chairman, Department of Obstetrics and Gynecology, Southern Illinois University School of Medicine, Springfield; Medical Director, Carol Jo Vecchie Women's Health, Springfield, Illinois

STEPHEN J. LYE, PhD
Professor, Samuel Lunenfeld Research Institute, Mount Sinai Hospital, Toronto, Ontario, Canada

FAIDON MAGKOS, PhD
Center for Human Nutrition, Division of Geriatrics and Nutritional Science, Washington University School of Medicine, St. Louis, Missouri; Department of Nutrition and Dietetics, Harokopio University, Kallithea, Athens, Greece

BETTINA MITTENDORFER, MS, PhD
Center for Human Nutrition, Division of Geriatrics and Nutritional Science, Washington University School of Medicine, St. Louis, Missouri

MICHELLE F. MOTTOLA, PhD, FACSM
Associate Professor, School of Kinesiology, Faculty of Health Sciences, Department of Anatomy and Cell Biology, Schulich School of Medicine and Dentistry, London, Ontario; Associate Scientist, Child Health Research Institute, Lawson Health Research Institute, London, Ontario; Director, R. Samuel McLaughlin Foundation-Exercise and Pregnancy Laboratory, The University of Western Ontario, London, Ontario, Canada

JOHN P. NEWNHAM, MD, FRANZCOG
Professor, Head, School of Women's and Infants' Health, The University of Western Australia, Perth, Australia

EMILY OKEN, MD, MPH
Assistant Professor, Department of Ambulatory Care and Prevention, Harvard Medical School and Harvard Pilgrim Health Care, Boston, Massachusetts

CRAIG E. PENNELL, FRANZCOG, PhD
Senior Lecturer, School of Women's and Infants' Health, The University of Western Australia, Perth, Australia

SHARON T. PHELAN, MD, FACOG
Professor, Department of Obstetrics and Gynecology, School of Medicine, University of New Mexico, Albuquerque, New Mexico

JONATHAN RAMPONO, MBBS, FRACP
Head, Department of Psychological Medicine, King Edward Memorial Hospital, Perth, Australia

MITUL B. SHAH, MD
Assistant Professor, Department of Obstetrics and Gynecology and Women's Health, Saint Louis University, Saint Louis, Missouri

YARIV YOGEV, MD
Perinatal Division, Helen Schneider Hospital for Women, Rabin Medical Center, Sackler Faculty of Medicine, Tel Aviv University, Petah-Tiqva, Israel

GERALD S. ZAVORSKY, PhD
Associate Professor, Department of Obstetrics, Gynecology and Women's Health, School of Medicine, Saint Louis University, Saint Mary's Health Center, St. Louis; Department of Pharmacological and Physiological Science, School of Medicine, Saint Louis University, St. Louis, Missouri

Contents

Foreword **xiii**

William F. Rayburn

Preface **xv**

Raul Artal

Health Care Costs of Obesity in Women **213**

Jeffrey A. Gavard

This article summarizes and critically evaluates the scientific literature for the annual and lifetime medical care costs of obesity in women in the United States. Studies involving actual and projected costs are reviewed. Studies were favored that included large, nationally representative samples; accounted for the influence of potential confounding factors; and adjusted for decreased survival in obese women when comparing costs with women of normal weight. Despite a wide variety of methodology in model cost estimation and projection in the studies published, the evidence suggests significant costs attributable to overweight and obesity in women that vary throughout the lifespan and by specific racial and obesity categories.

Early Life Origins of Obesity **227**

John P. Newnham, Craig E. Pennell, Stephen J. Lye, Jonathan Rampono, and John R.G. Challis

There is increasing evidence that obesity has its origins in early life. Predisposition is based on interactions between the genome and environmental influences acting through epigenetic modifications. Individuals most at risk are those whose ancestral line has made a rapid transition from a traditional to a Westernized style of life. The process involves not only metabolism, but also behavior. As a result, those people who are most at risk of obesity may be those least likely to respond to educational programs based on lifestyle modification. Understanding the mechanisms and pathways that underpin the early origins of obesity is vital if we are to make progress in addressing this major problem of modern life.

Gender Differences in Lipid Metabolism and the Effect of Obesity **245**

Faidon Magkos and Bettina Mittendorfer

There are many differences between men and women, and between lean and obese subjects, in fatty acid and very low-density lipoprotein triglyceride and apolipoprotein B-100 metabolism. Currently, observations in this area are predominantly descriptive. The mechanisms responsible for sexual dimorphism in lipid metabolism are largely unknown.

Cardiopulmonary Aspects of Obesity in Women 267

Gerald S. Zavorsky

This review discusses the cardiopulmonary aspects of obesity in nonpregnant women. The effects of obesity on pulmonary diffusing capacity and pulmonary gas exchange are related to the waist-to-hip ratio. Obese women have an increased risk for heart failure compared with normal-weight women, a risk that progressively worsens with increasing body mass index. They also have poor cardiac accommodation and possess a lower oxygen pulse at peak exercise. Cardiac output, heart rate, and total blood volume are higher in obese women whereas ejection fraction is lower compared with normal-weight women; substantial weight loss normalizes these parameters.

Pregnancy and Obesity 285

Yariv Yogev and Patrick M. Catalano

Obesity has become a worldwide epidemic: it is associated with increased rate of infertility and with many pregnancy complications. Moreover, it is associated with gestational diabetes mellitus, which increases the risk of these complications. As the prevalence of obesity is increasing, so is the number of women in the reproductive age who are overweight and obese. This article addresses issues concerning pregravid obesity and weight gain during pregnancy and their implication on gestational diabetes and pregnancy outcome.

Exercise Prescription for Overweight and Obese Women: Pregnancy and Postpartum 301

Michelle F. Mottola

Once a low-risk pregnancy has been established, walking in combination with nutritional control may be effective in preventing excessive weight gain in overweight and obese women. Maternal exercise prescription should use the Frequency, Intensity, Time spent and Type of exercise principle, with a frequency of three to four sessions per week as ideal. Intensity based on a target heart-rate zone of 110 to 131 beats per minute for women 20 to 29 years of age and 108 to 127 beats per minute for women 30 to 39 years of age, coupled with use of the rating of perceived exertion scale and the "Talk Test" is suggested. Dieting and exercise together are most effective in reducing weight retention after childbirth and compliance may be improved by incorporating child-care and children into the exercise routine. After medical consultation, postpartum women should begin exercise slowly, starting from 15 minutes, and building to at least 150 minutes of aerobic activity per week, with this activity spread throughout the week.

Childbearing and Obesity in Women: Weight Before, During, and After Pregnancy 317

Erica P. Gunderson

Weight gain and the development of obesity during midlife are strong independent predictors of cardiovascular disease, particularly among women, as well as the metabolic syndrome, type 2 diabetes, and early mortality. Primiparity and maternal body size before pregnancy affect long-term postpartum weight retention and the development of obesity among women of reproductive age. As a modifiable risk factor, body weight during the preconception, prenatal, and postpartum periods may present critical windows to implement interventions to prevent weight retention and the development of overweight and obesity in women of childbearing age.

Obesity and Its Relationship to Infertility in Men and Women 333

J. Ricardo Loret de Mola

This review focuses on the negative impact of obesity in reproduction by considering the pathophysiology of obesity and infertility in men and women, the influence of obesity on the prevalence of polycystic ovary syndrome, and the benefits of weight loss on reproduction and on menstruation, ovulation, semen parameters, and reproductive outcomes.

Obesity and Sexuality in Women 347

Mitul B. Shah

Sexual health is an important part of an individual's overall health. This article presents the definitions and classifications of female sexual dysfunction (FSD), emphasizes the importance of obtaining a sexual health assessment, and describes the tools that can be used for this assessment. The impact of obesity on reproductive health over a women's entire life span (in the family-planning years, reproductive years, and menopause years) is described. The treatment of obesity will have a positive effect on a woman's sexual health, with a likely improvement in FSD and a decrease in risk factors related to contraception, pregnancy, infertility, and menopause.

Maternal and Child Obesity: The Causal Link 361

Emily Oken

Studies have found that higher maternal weight entering pregnancy increases risk for obesity and its cardiometabolic complications among offspring. Epidemiologic studies have found that higher maternal gestational weight gain is associated with higher weight and consequent risk for obesity, and elevated blood pressure among children. While these associations are partly mediated by shared genes and behaviors, the abundance of human evidence, supported by extensive data from experimental animal studies, suggests that intrauterine exposure to an obese intrauterine environment programs offspring obesity risk by influencing appetite, metabolism, and activity levels. Efforts to interrupt this cycle of obesity are important for public health and economical, as a successful intervention could benefit the child, the mother, her future pregnancies, and subsequent generations.

Obesity in Minority Women: Calories, Commerce, and Culture **379**

Sharon T. Phelan

Obesity is increasing at epidemic rates in all women, but especially in minority women and children. Factors that contribute to this include changes in caloric intake and expenditure (calories), cost and ease of acquiring food along with pressures from the marketplace and media (commerce) and the community response to the increasing prevalence of obesity and sedentary lifestyle (culture).

Index **393**

FORTHCOMING ISSUES

September 2009
Pelvic Floor Dysfunction
Joseph Schaffer, MD, *Guest Editor*

December 2009
Genetic Screening and Counseling
Anthony Gregg, MD
and Joe Leigh Simpson, MD,
Guest Editors

RECENT ISSUES

March 2009
Pediatric and Adolescent Gynecology
S. Paige Hertweck, MD, *Guest Editor*

December 2008
Colposcopy, Cervical Screening, and HPV
Alan G. Waxman, MD, MPH,
Guest Editor

September 2008
Office Obstetrics
Sharon T. Phelan, MD, FACOG,
Guest Editor

RELATED INTEREST

Primary Care: Clinics in Office Practice June 2009 (Vol. 36, Issue 2)
Obesity Management
Ann Rodden, MD and Vanessa Diaz, MD, *Guest Editors*
www.primarycare.theclinics.com

Child and Adolescent Psychiatric Clinics of North America January 2009 (Vol. 18, Issue 1)
Eating Disorders and Obesity
B. Herpertz-Dahlmann, MD and J. Hebebrand, MD, *Guest Editors*
www.childpsych.theclinics.com

Endocrinology and Metabolism Clinics of North America September and December 2008 (Vol. 37, Issues 3 and 4)
Obesity: Brain-Gut and Inflammation Connection: Parts I and II
Eddy Karnieli, MD, *Guest Editor*
www.endo.theclinics.com

Psychiatric Clinics of North America March 2005 (Vol. 28, Issue 1)
Obesity
Thomas A. Wadden, PhD, Albert J. Stunkard, MD, and Robert I. Berkowitz, MD, *Guest Editors*
www.psych.theclinics.com

Foreword

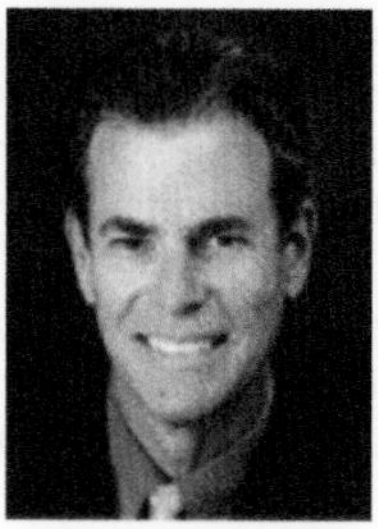

William F. Rayburn, MD, MBA
Consulting Editor

This issue of the *Obstetrics and Gynecology Clinics of North America*, with Dr. Raul Artal as Guest Editor, provides a timely update on the assessment and management of obese women. Obesity is the fastest growing health problem in the United States, especially among minority women, and approximately one third of all US women are obese. This issue describes how obesity is associated with increased healthcare costs and such morbid conditions as type 2 diabetes, infertility, gallbladder disease, and several cancers, including breast, colon, and uterine malignancies. Endometrial cancer, the most common gynecologic malignancy, is nearly five times more common in obese than in nonobese women. Obesity and being overweight are also associated with hypertension and an increased risk for heart disease, the leading cause of death of American women.

As described in this issue, the lipid metabolic consequences of obesity are influenced by fat distribution. Women with abdominal obesity have higher levels of male hormones than do women with lower body fat. Visceral obesity is associated with hyperinsulinemia, hypertriglyceridemia, and glucose intolerance. Furthermore, polycystic ovary syndrome is characterized by obesity with insulin resistance, dysmenorrhea, and hirsutism.

The patient's medical, social, and family history should be reviewed for weight-related conditions. The clinician should inform the patient in a sensitive manner that her weight is a health concern and assist her in developing a weight loss and exercise plan. Clinicians should offer patients appropriate interventions or referrals to promote a healthy weight and lifestyle. Educational handouts for the patient to read can be discussed at a follow-up visit. Contact information for community resources, support groups, and weight loss programs may be provided. Certain insurance carriers provide coverage for weight loss interventions.

For many women, achieving and maintaining a healthy weight is a difficult and life-long process. Setting an initial goal of losing 5-10% of total body weight over a 6-month period is realistic and achievable. The initial approach should reinforce the

Obstet Gynecol Clin N Am 36 (2009) xiii–xiv
doi:10.1016/j.ogc.2009.05.001
0889-8545/09/$ – see front matter

importance of weight loss and exercise, and include the assessment of the patient's readiness to make behavioral changes. Drug therapy may be appropriate for some women. For example, orlistat and sibutramine hydrochloride monohydrate are approved by the US Food and Drug Administration for patients with a body mass index (BMI) of 30 or greater and for those with a BMI of 27 or greater with other risk factors. Orlistat is a gastrointestinal lipase inhibitor that limits fat absorption while sibutramine is a dopamine, norepinephrine, and serotonin reuptake inhibitor. Discontinuation of any pharmacotherapy may lead to rapid weight regain.

Gastric surgery can be used to achieve a weight loss of more than 100 pounds for patients with a BMI of 35-40 and sleep apnea or other significant morbidity, or for patients with a BMI of greater than 40. Results may be best at experienced centers with a combined medical and surgical approach, to ensure fewer complications. Patients using drugs or undergoing surgery should use guidelines for diet, exercise, and lifestyle modifications as recommended for milder forms of obesity. It should be stressed that pharmacotherapy and surgery are only adjuncts to diet and lifestyle changes when it comes to treating obesity.

This issue focuses on obesity during pregnancy. Obese women are at increased risk for several adverse perinatal outcomes, including anesthetic, perioperative, and other maternal and fetal complications. Ideally, obstetricians should provide preconception counseling and education about these complications and encourage a weight reduction program before attempting conception. Prenatal and peripartum care considerations are especially relevant for obese patients, including those who have undergone bariatric surgery. Of particular interest is the article pertaining to the casual link between maternal and child obesity.

It is our desire for this issue to attract the attention of obstetricians and gynecologists caring for the many women who are obese. Practical information provided herein by this distinguished panel of contributors will hopefully aid in the development and implementation of more specific and individualized treatment plans.

William F. Rayburn, MD, MBA
Department of Obstetrics and Gynecology
University of New Mexico School of Medicine
MSC10 5580; 1 University of New Mexico
Albuquerque, NM 87131-0001, USA

E-mail address:
wrayburn@salud.unm.edu (W.F. Rayburn)

Preface

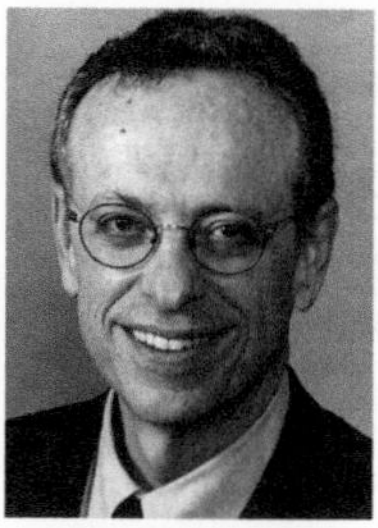

Raul Artal, MD
Guest Editor

This issue of the *Obstetrics and Gynecology Clinics of North America* is devoted to women and obesity. An overview of up to date and relevant information on this topic is provided by well recognized experts in the field who have contributed to this issue. Articles include information that will be useful to clinicians and researchers alike.

The obesity pandemic remains unabated and has been frequently in the forefront of medical news for the past two decades. Particularly relevant is the fact that obesity is more prevalent in women, 33.4% compared with 27.5% in men, and affects significantly quality of life and longevity. The gender differences are now better understood. Some aspects of gender related findings are addressed in an article by Drs. Magkos and Mittendorfer.

Healthcare costs of obesity in women is reviewed in an article by Dr. Gavard who summarizes the pertinent literature; included are the projected prevalence and related attributable future annual costs of obesity.

Obesity related co-morbidities and mortality are on the rise as is healthcare cost. The increase in prevalence for Diabetes and Metabolic Syndrome are of significant concern.

It has been widely recognized that obesity is a chronic relapsing disease that manifests itself at different life stages in women: childhood, reproductive years, and menopausal/post menopausal years and in the elderly. The ethnical aspects of obesity in minorities are addressed in an article by Dr. Phelan.

Several articles address the roots and evolution of obesity in our society. The early life origins of obesity and the Barker and Hales "thrifty phenotype hypothesis" along with environmental influences are described by Dr. Newnham and colleagues. The generational link in maternal and child obesity is explored in detail from another angle by Dr. Oken.

For years, infertility has been frequently encountered among overweight/obese women. Dr. Loret de Mola details the etiology and management of infertility in obese women. Another aspect of quality of life and potential related infertility is addressed in Dr. Shah's article on sexuality.

Obstet Gynecol Clin N Am 36 (2009) xv–xvi
doi:10.1016/j.ogc.2009.05.002

The causes for obesity closely relate to lifestyle factors, and several of the articles cover different aspects, pathophysiology and managing strategies. The cardiovascular and pulmonary aspects of obesity are being described in an article by Dr. Zavorsky.

Exercise prescription for overweight/obese subjects is the focus of Dr. Mottola's article. Pregnancy, obesity and related complications are now a common clinical occurrence and the focus of an article by Dr. Yogev and Dr. Catalano. Of particular concern is the increase in prevalence of gestational diabetes and weight retention in the post partum period and beyond. Weight retention after excessive weight gain in pregnancy is addressed in an article by Dr. Gunderson.

I wish to express my gratitude to the co-authors of this issue of *Obstetrics and Gynecology Clinics of North America* for their outstanding and up to date contributions. Many thanks also to Carla Holloway, Senior Managing Editor and her assistants for their support and professionalism.

Raul Artal, MD
Professor and Chairman
Department of Obstetrics
Gynecology and Women's Health
Saint Louis University School of Medicine
6420 Clayton Road Ste. 290
Saint Louis, MO 63117

E-mail address:
artalr@slu.edu (R. Artal)

Health Care Costs of Obesity in Women

Jeffrey A. Gavard, PhD

KEYWORDS

- Obesity • Health care costs • Direct medical costs
- Annual costs • Cumulative lifetime costs

The prevalence of obesity has increased in the United States over the past several decades, from 15% of the adult population in 1980 to approximately 32% of the adult population in 2003 to 2004.[1] Direct medical costs of obesity in 2000 were estimated to be $61 billion, whereas indirect costs of absenteeism, lowered productivity, and premature death were estimated to be $56 billion.[2] The rising prevalence of obesity carries an increased cost burden. Many studies have quantified annual and lifetime medical costs of obesity and have dealt with actual and projected costs. Such estimates have not been without controversy. The nature of the populations examined, how measurements of body mass index (BMI) are obtained, the influence of confounding factors, if a gradient of increased costs exists for different obesity classes or racial groups, and differential survival between obese and normal-weight individuals all may impact cost estimates of obesity. The latter is especially important when estimating lifetime costs attributable to obesity. Although annual costs allow for a direct comparison between obese and normal-weight women, lifetime costs must account for the shorter life expectancy in obese women.[3–5]

This article summarizes and critically evaluates the scientific literature for annual and lifetime medical care costs of obesity in women.

RESEARCH DESIGN AND METHODS

A computer-generated literature review published in English of all available existing studies on the annual and lifetime medical care costs of obesity in women in the United States was undertaken. No time constraints were imposed on when the papers had to have been published or presented.

Articles were cited that could provide the best evidence for estimating actual and projected costs. Articles were favored having large sample sizes that were nationally representative; accounted for the influence of potential confounding factors; adjusted for decreased survival in obese women when comparing costs with women of normal weight; and provided contrasts in costs between gender, racial, and obesity class

Department of Obstetrics, Gynecology, and Women's Health, St. Louis University School of Medicine, 6420 Clayton Road, Suite 290, St. Louis, MO 63117, USA
E-mail address: gavardja@slu.edu

Obstet Gynecol Clin N Am 36 (2009) 213–226
doi:10.1016/j.ogc.2009.04.002
obgyn.theclinics.com

groups. Review articles of annual and lifetime costs of obesity in women also were considered.

A review of earlier studies and their methodologic strengths and weaknesses is initially provided followed by a summary and critical evaluation of more recent studies that address these concerns.

EARLIER STUDIES ON THE ANNUAL AND LIFETIME MEDICAL CARE COSTS OF OBESITY IN WOMEN

Annual and Lifetime Costs of Obesity Characterized by Prevalence-Attributable Fraction Approaches

One of the earliest studies of the medical care costs of obesity was performed by Wolf and Colditz.[6] Relative risk estimates for obese (BMI ≥29) versus nonobese (BMI <29) persons for coronary heart disease, hypertension, type II diabetes mellitus, gallbladder disease, musculoskeletal disease, and breast, endometrial, and colon cancer were applied to cost estimates of the diseases from the Nurses Health Study and the Health Professionals Follow-up Study to obtain aggregate medical spending attributable to obesity. This prevalence-based approach does not account for differential mortality between obese and nonobese persons and is equivalent to calculating cost savings if obese persons were replaced with the same number of nonobese persons at any particular time period that costs are being estimated. The estimated health care costs attributable to obesity were $52 billion in 1995, representing 5.7% of direct health care costs in the United States. Because some of the data used in this study were collected as early as 1985, however, this aggregate estimate may be unrealistic for the present day.

The analyses of Wolf and Colditz[6] were expanded in a later study by Allison and colleagues.[7] The percentages of age-specific and cumulative lifetime costs attributable to obesity from 20 to 85 years of age were calculated taking the higher mortality of obesity into account. Age-specific prevalences of obesity were estimated using data from the National Health and Nutrition Examination Survey (NHANES) III (1988–1994). Age-specific relative risks of mortality for obese (BMI ≥29) versus nonobese (BMI <29) persons were obtained from a recently published study involving a national sample.[8] The health care costs of an obese person versus a nonobese person were based on the 5.7% of direct health care costs attributable to obesity estimated by Wolf and Colditz[6] and the overall adult prevalence of obesity (BMI ≥29) of 27% that was estimated by NHANES III. The percentage of age-specific costs attributable to obesity rose until approximately 52 years of age and declined thereafter, becoming negative at about 79 years of age. The implication is that elimination of obesity would result in potential cost savings until 79 years of age, after which elimination of obesity would result in increased health care costs because of the greater number of persons living past that age. The percentage of cumulative lifetime health care costs attributable to obesity was reduced from 5.7% to 4.3% when higher mortality of obesity was taken into account. Although documenting that costs of obesity remain positive for virtually the entire lifespan even after accounting for differential mortality, many methodologic issues make interpretation of findings difficult. Costs were calculated using only a limited number of obesity-related diseases; obesity was defined as a BMI ≥ 29 to be compatible with the Wolf and Colditz[6] study rather than the more conventional BMI ≥ 30; the cost differential was calculated using nonobese (BMI <29) persons as the reference group rather than normal-weight individuals; age-specific relative risks of mortality were estimated from an averaging of the gender-specific relative risks provided in the reference paper;[8] no adjustment for confounding factors occurred; no cost estimates were provided for different gender, racial, or obesity classes; and costs were calculated assuming that obese and nonobese individuals remained in their respective groups throughout the lifespan.

An attributable fraction approach to lifetime medical costs of obesity also was followed by Thompson and colleagues.[9] Costs were estimated according to the risks of five obesity-related diseases: (1) hypertension, (2) hypercholesterolemia, (3) type II diabetes mellitus, (4) coronary heart disease (CHD), and (5) stroke. The first three were viewed as risk factors for the last two, and hence, cost modeling occurred in two stages. The first stage predicted age-specific risks of hypertension, hypercholesterolemia, and type II diabetes mellitus through 99 years of age separately for men and women according to the midpoints of four BMI classes: (1) 22.5 (nonobese); (2) 27.5 (mildly obese); (3) 32.5 (moderately obese); and (4) 37.5 (severely obese). The second stage predicted age-specific risks of CHD, stroke, and death through 99 years of age separately for men and women according to BMI level and the predicted risks of hypertension, hypercholesterolemia, and type II diabetes mellitus obtained from the first stage of the model. Age-specific risks of hypertension, hypercholesterolemia, and type II diabetes mellitus were estimated using data from NHANES III (1988–1994). Age-specific risks of CHD and stroke were estimated using data from the Framingham Heart Study. Annual costs of hypertension, hypercholesterolemia, type II diabetes mellitus, CHD, and stroke were obtained from recently published studies and the CHD Policy Research Institute.[9–13] The final model generated annual BMI-specific disease risks and costs beginning at the current age of 35 to 64 years through 99 years. Lifetime costs according to each of the four BMI levels were calculated by summing the annual costs after adjustment for survival to each future year. Results were expressed according to three groups of starting ages: (1) 35 to 44, (2) 45 to 54, and (3) 55 to 64. A gradient of increasing lifetime medical costs by increasing BMI was found for both men and women for each of the three starting age groups. The lifetime costs for men 45 to 54 years of age for the four BMI categories of 22.5, 27.5, 32.5, and 37.5 were $19,600, $24,000, $29,600, and $36,500, respectively; the corresponding lifetime costs for women 45 to 54 years of age were $18,800, $23,200, $28,700, and $35,300, respectively. Using nonobesity as the reference group, mild obesity increases lifetime medical costs by approximately 20%, moderate obesity increases costs by approximately 50%, and severe obesity increases costs by almost 100%. Although documenting that lifetime medical care costs increase with increasing BMI, numerous methodologic issues remain with model assumptions that were made to expedite cost estimation. The view of hypertension, hypercholesterolemia, and type II diabetes mellitus as risk factors for CHD and stroke assumed that obesity-related mortality could only result from CHD and stroke but not from the other three. Age-specific probabilities of survival were calculated as the sum of three conditional probabilities: (1) survival given previous onset of CHD, (2) survival given previous onset of stroke, and (3) survival free of CHD and stroke. Persons were assumed to be able to develop either CHD or stroke but not both in the same year or in different years. It was assumed that CHD and stroke would impact medical care costs and mortality only for a 10-year period after onset. Although costs were estimated for major diseases where obesity is a risk factor, the models omitted inclusion of other obesity-related diseases of lower incidence, such as gallbladder disease, sleep apnea, and some cancers. Potential confounding factors that could influence costs were not included in the models. Costs also were calculated assuming that individuals remained in their respective BMI groups throughout life.

Annual Medical Costs of Obesity in the Workplace

Obesity in the workplace may result in higher health insurance premiums that may be borne by both employer and employee, diminished productivity, and increased absenteeism.[14] Studies of obesity in the workplace can provide valuable information to employers on decisions regarding the implementation of intervention strategies to reduce the higher medical expenditures of obesity among their employees. Annual medical costs of overweight and obesity were estimated for fulltime employed adults 18 to 64 years of age in the United States.[15] The study included cost and demographic data supplied from 2000 to 2001 by the Medical Expenditure Panel Survey (MEPS), a nationally representative survey of the civilian noninstitutionalized population of the United States that quantifies the type, frequency, cost, and source of payment of health care expenditures. The sample included 14,179 men and 8480 women. Annual medical expenditures were predicted separately for men and women through regression modeling for five self-reported BMI classes: (1) normal weight (BMI 20–24.9); (2) overweight (BMI 25–29.9); (3) obesity class I (BMI 30–34.9); (4) obesity class II (BMI 35–39.9); and (5) obesity class III (BMI ≥40). Annual medical costs attributable to each overweight and obesity class were achieved through comparison with normal-weight individuals of the same gender. All analyses were adjusted for age, race, education, income, smoking, and region of the country. Annual medical costs attributable to overweight, obesity class I, obesity class II, and obesity class III in men were $169, $392, $569, and $1591, respectively. Corresponding annual medical expenditures in women were higher for all BMI classes except for obesity class III. Annual medical costs attributable to overweight, obesity class I, obesity class II, and obesity class III in women were $495, $1071, $1549, and $1359, respectively. This study provides evidence of how increasing obesity could have deleterious consequences for working individuals. Questions remain on how to translate this information to preventive strategies. Self-reported BMI may be inaccurate and costs attributable to overweight and obesity may not represent actual savings because of costs of the intervention programs and the irreversibility of some of the health effects of obesity.

RECENT STUDIES ON THE ANNUAL AND LIFETIME MEDICAL CARE COSTS OF OBESITY IN WOMEN

Annual Costs of Overweight and Obesity and Lifetime Costs Attributable to Obesity

Obesity prevention efforts are formulated with the belief that reduction of obesity translates to savings in medical costs of obesity-related diseases. Although obesity certainly increases the risk for many diseases and their accompanying annual medical costs, obesity also shortens the lifespan, which may actually result in reduced lifetime medical spending. It is unknown if the lifetime medical costs of obesity result in greater expenditures or savings compared with normal-weight individuals.

A very recent study investigated annual medical expenditures by BMI class from 20 to 85 years of age.[16] The study included cost and demographic data supplied from 2001 to 2004 by the MEPS. The sample included 26,114 white men, 5385 black men, 27,334 white women, and 7328 black women. Annual medical expenditures were initially examined for each of the four race-gender groups by four BMI classes: (1) normal weight (BMI 20–24.9); (2) overweight (BMI 25–29.9); (3) obesity class I (BMI 30–34.9); and (4) obesity classes II-III (BMI ≥35). Lifetime medical costs for obese individuals relative to normal-weight individuals were estimated for obesity class I and obesity classes II-III from two starting ages: 20 and 65. The former quantifies medical costs attributable to obesity that largely encompass the time in life characterized by employment, whereas the latter quantifies medical costs attributable to obesity when a person becomes eligible for Medicare. Earlier studies addressing costs from the perspective of Medicare did not provide estimates by race[17,18] or by obesity class.[18]

Costs were initially estimated through linear regression analysis where annual age-specific expenditures using the MEPS data were multiplied by the probability of survival to that age. Survival probabilities to certain ages were obtained for each race-gender group and BMI class from estimates calculated from linked data from the 1986 to 2000 National Health Interview Survey (NHIS) and the 1986 to 2002 National Death Index (NDI).[19] The NHIS is the principal source of information on the health of the civilian noninstitutionalized population of the United States; the MEPS is a subset of households taken from the NHIS. Cost estimates were adjusted for education, smoking, insurance, marital status, region of the country, and population density. The age-specific costs adjusted for survival for obese individuals were then summed from either age 20 or age 65 through 85 years of age and compared with the summation of similar age-specific rates adjusted for survival in normal-weight individuals of the same race-gender group. The differences in lifetime costs between the obese group and normal-weight group was the lifetime medical costs attributable to obesity starting from age 20 or age 65.

The annual medical costs from 20 to 85 years of age by BMI class and race-gender group adjusted for survival are shown in **Fig. 1**. Costs were generally higher throughout the lifespan with increasing BMI for all race-gender groups. White men

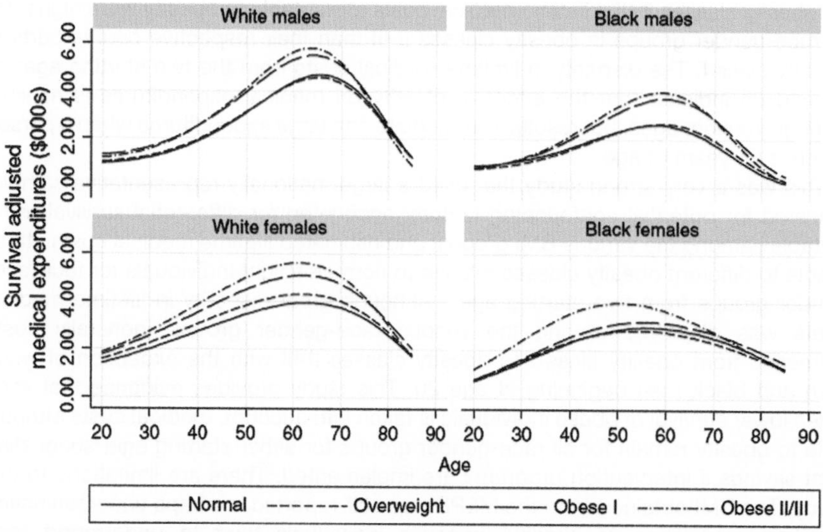

Fig. 1. Survival-adjusted annual costs from the perspective of a 20 year old. All estimates are presented in 2007 dollars. Normal weight (BMI 20–24.9); overweight (BMI 25–29.9); obesity class I (BMI 30–34.9); obesity classes II-III (BMI ≥35). BMI, body mass index. (*From* Finkelstein EA, Trogdon JG, Brown DS, et al. The lifetime medical cost burden of overweight and obesity: implications for obesity prevention. Obesity (Silver Spring) 2008;16:1843–8; with permission.)

and white women had annual costs increase throughout life until they peaked during their early 60s regardless of BMI. The annual costs were lower for black men and black women, perhaps because of lack of accessibility of care, higher mortality, or both. The costs rose during life for black men, peaking at about 60 years of age for all BMI classes. The annual cost distributions shifted to younger ages for black women, where the peak costs were reached during their mid 50s for the three lower BMI classes; the annual costs peaked at $3950 during their upper 40s for black women in obesity classes II-III. The latter finding reflects increased and earlier mortality in black women in obesity classes II-III.

Lifetime medical costs through 85 years of age attributable to obesity are shown in **Table 1** from the perspective of starting from age 20 or age 65. When lifetime costs were estimated beginning at 20 years of age, white men and black men who were obesity class I had similar respective lifetime costs ($16,490 and $12,290) and white men and black men who were obesity classes II-III had similar respective lifetime costs ($16,720 and $14,580). The worsening of obesity apparently did not significantly impact lifetime costs among men from the perspective of a 20 year old. The highest lifetime costs were found in white women, which were over four times higher ($21,550) than those of black women ($5340) who were obesity class I. The disparity in lifetime costs between white women and black women was less pronounced for obesity classes II-III ($29,460 and $23,750, respectively). The worsening of obesity significantly impacted lifetime costs among women, especially black women. Black men had the highest percentage of lifetime medical costs occurring after age 65 for obesity class I (28%) and for obesity classes II-III (21%); black women who were obesity classes II-III had only 3% of their lifetime costs occurring after age 65. When lifetime medical costs were estimated beginning at 65 years of age, the lifetime costs attributable to obesity ranged from $4660 for black women to $19,270 for black men for obesity class I, and from $7590 for black women to $25,300 for white women for obesity classes II-III. Lifetime medical costs attributable to obesity were higher for all race-gender groups in obesity classes II-III than their respective counterparts in obesity class I. The disparity in lifetime medical costs from the two starting ages of 20 and 65 indicate that the effect of obesity on medical expenditures is minimal through younger ages, but results in immediate and large expenditures when a person reaches 65 years of age.

This was a very strong study that used a large, nationally representative sample; adjusted for potential confounding factors; accounted for differential survival using lifetables among the various BMI groups; and estimated lifetime medical costs attributable to different obesity classes relative to normal-weight individuals for four race-gender groups from two starting ages. Although great disparity in lifetime medical costs was displayed among the various race-gender groups, generally costs increased from obesity class I to obesity classes II-III with the exception of white men and black men beginning at age 20. This study provides evidence that even when lower survival of obese individuals is taken into account, medical costs attributable to obesity remain for all race-gender groups for either starting age, suggesting cost savings if intervention programs are implemented. There are limitations to this study. The BMI obtained from the MEPS was self-reported, perhaps underestimating the true prevalence of obesity, because individuals tend to underreport their weight.[20,21] All cost estimates were calculated under the assumption that obesity class I and obesity classes II-III individuals relative to normal-weight individuals remained in those BMI classes for life, never transitioning to other BMI categories. The survival estimates based on the NDI from 1986 to 2002 may not be accurate when applied to data collected during 2001 to 2004. Future costs of obese individuals

Table 1
Lifetime attributable costs of obesity by starting age and obesity class: United States

	Obesity Class I[a]				Obesity Classes II-III[b]			
	Cost Total		Cost After 65[c]		Cost Total		Cost After 65[c]	
Race and Gender	**$**	**95% CI**	**%**	**95% CI**	**$**	**95% CI**	**%**	**95% CI**
Starting at age 20								
White men	16,490	(14,790–18,170)	10	(7–14)	16,720	(13,070–20,410)	9	(3–15)
Black men	12,290	(8160–16,330)	28	(20–44)	14,580	(9320–19,730)	21	(14–33)
White women	21,550	(19,280–23,740)	16	(13–18)	29,460	(26,390–32,460)	13	(11–16)
Black women	5340	(3130–7570)	16	(10–27)	23,750	(22,300–25,140)	3	(2–3)
Starting at age 65								
White men	9940	(7080–12,760)	—	—	20,510	(15,510–25,380)	—	—
Black men	19,270	(15,610–23,030)	—	—	24,830	(19,210–30,500)	—	—
White women	17,640	(15,990–19,230)	—	—	25,300	(22,720–27,860)	—	—
Black women	4660	(3140–6180)	—	—	7590	(6700–8520)	—	—

All figures represent 2007 dollars.
Abbreviation: CI, confidence interval.
[a] Body mass index (kg/m^2) $\geq$30 and <35.
[b] Body mass index (kg/m^2) $\geq$35.
[c] The percentage of lifetime costs attributable to obesity that occur for a 20 year old after the age of 65.
Modified from Finkelstein EA, Trogdon JG, Brown DS, et al. The lifetime medical cost burden of overweight and obesity: implications for obesity prevention. Obesity (Silver Spring) 2008;16:1843–8; with permission.

versus normal-weight individuals also could dramatically worsen with a greater prevalence of morbid obesity and more costly technologic treatments. Lastly, this study only involved noninstitutionalized populations as represented by the MEPS. Lifetime costs attributable to obesity could markedly change with the inclusion of prisoners, nursing homes, and other institutionalized populations.

Projected Prevalence of Overweight and Obesity and Related Attributable Annual Costs

Annual health care costs attributable to overweight and obesity also may be projected for the future. Such predictions can be an impetus not only to prepare for the greater cost burden of overweight and obesity, but to plan intervention efforts to curtail the rising prevalence of obesity and its related costs. A very recent study projected overweight and obesity prevalences in the United States and their related health care costs among adults ≥20 years of age if current trends in this country continued.[22] Prevalence data from NHANES II (1976–1980), NHANES III (1988–1994), and NHANES data collected annually from 1999 to 2004 were used to estimate the mean annual percentage increase in overweight and obesity from 1976 to 2004 through linear regression modeling and then to estimate the projected prevalence of overweight and obesity in future years were such an annual increase to continue. A second methodology used for comparison purposes involved applying observed shifts in the BMI distribution among adults ≥20 years of age from 1976 to 2004 to predict future shifts in the BMI distribution and then to predict the future prevalence of overweight and obesity based on these projected BMI distributions. Estimates of projected health care costs attributable to overweight and obesity were calculated from two recently published studies using data from the MEPS. The respective per capita excess health care costs of overweight and obesity in United States adults relative to normal-weight individuals were $340 and $1069 in a study conducted in 2001.[23] These amounts were higher than their respective estimates of $247 and $732 in a study conducted in 1998.[24] The latter study also made use of 1998 estimates from the National Health Expenditure Account (NHEA), which provides aggregate measures of health care expenditures in the United States and their source of payment for institutionalized populations, such as prisoners and nursing homes, and noninstitutionalized populations. The per capita excess health care costs of overweight and obesity were estimated annually for 2000 to 2030, assuming that these excess costs grew at the same rate as the overall personal health care cost projections in the NHEA, which have been projected to 2016.[25] To calculate the total health care costs attributable to overweight and obesity, the projected prevalences of overweight and obesity were applied to total population projections provided by the Census Bureau and expressed as a percentage of the total estimated projected health care costs of the NHEA and the MEPS.

Observed and projected prevalence estimates for overweight and obesity are given in **Fig. 2**. When overweight and obesity were considered together (see **Fig. 2**A), men always had higher rates than women during the observed period from 1976 to 2004. The estimates increased and gradually converged until approximately 85% of both men and women would become overweight or obese by 2030. When obesity was considered alone (see **Fig. 2**B), women always had higher rates than men throughout both the observed and projected periods, gradually increasing and diverging until 42.5% of adult women in the United States would be obese by 2010, 50.3% obese by 2020, and 58% obese by 2030. This higher rate of obesity in women is primarily caused by the higher rate found in black women (**Table 2**). The mean annual rate of increase in obesity in black women was estimated to be 0.878%, which means that

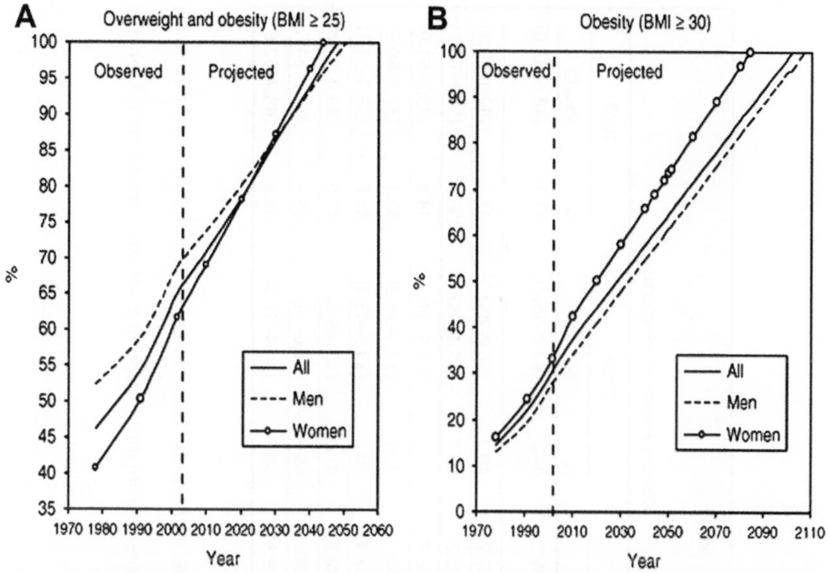

Fig. 2. Prevalence of overweight and obesity combined (*A*) and obesity alone (*B*) among United States adults for observed period from 1976–2004 and projected period after 2004. The observed period was based on data from the National Health and Nutrition Examination Survey (NHANES) II (1976–1980), NHANES III (1988–1994), and NHANES data collected annually from 1999–2004. Projected prevalence estimates were calculated based on linear regression modeling. BMI, body mass index. (*From* Wang Y, Beydoun MA, Liang L, et al. Will all Americans become overweight or obese? Estimating the progression and cost of the U.S. obesity epidemic. Obesity (Silver Spring) 2008;16:2323–30; with permission.)

58.1% would be obese in 2010, 66.9% would be obese in 2020, and 75.6% would be obese in 2030. The projected health care costs attributable to overweight and obesity are provided in **Table 3**, which are based on their per capita excess health care costs relative to normal-weight individuals from the studies of Thorpe and colleagues[23] and Finkelstein and colleagues.[24] Both sets of projections indicate more than a doubling of health care costs attributable to overweight and obesity every decade until the projected costs for both overweight and obesity in 2030 range from $861 to $957 billion, representing 9.8% to 10.9% of all health care costs according to NHEA projected estimates and 15.8% to 17.6% of all health care costs according to MEPS projected estimates. When obesity was considered alone, the 2030 projected expenditures ranged from $698 to $785 billion, representing 8% to 9% of all health care costs according to NHEA projected estimates and 12.8% to 14.4% of all health care costs according to MEPS projected estimates. The prevalence estimates of obesity achieved by mean annual increase in linear regression modeling projections and linear increase in BMI to projected BMI distributions were consistent in that the former predicted the prevalence of obesity in adult men and women by 2030 to be 51.1% (see **Table 2**), whereas the latter predicted the prevalence of obesity in adult men and women by 2030 to be 49.9%.

This was a thorough study using a large nationally representative sample from NHANES over a 28-year period to estimate future projections of overweight and obesity and their accompanying excess health care costs relative to normal-weight individuals. The projected estimates were further verified by two different

Table 2
Mean annual increase in prevalence of obesity[a] and future projections in U.S. adults ≥20 years[b]

				Obesity Prevalence Projections					
				2010		2020		2030	
Gender	Ethnicity	Current Prevalence 1999–2004 (%)	Mean Annual Increase (%)	%	95% CI	%	95% CI	%	95% CI
Men and women	All	32.2	0.68	37.4	(35.6–39.2)	44.2	(42.2–46.2)	51.1	(48.5–53.6)
Men	All	27.7	0.69	33.9	(30.6–37.2)	40.7	(36.4–45)	47.6	(42.1–53.1)
Women	All	34	0.78	42.5	(38.8–46.2)	50.3	(45.4–55)	58	(51.9–64.1)
Men	Non-Hispanic white	31.1	0.73	34.3	(32.3–36.3)	41.5	(38.9–44)	48.8	(45.7–51.9)
	Non-Hispanic black	34	0.64	36.4	(28.7–44)	42.7	(33.1–52.3)	49.1	(37.3–60.9)
	Mexican American	31.6	0.58	33.3	(29.2–37.4)	39	(33.9–43.3)	44.8	(38.5–51.1)
Women	Non-Hispanic white	30.2	0.62	35.6	(32.7–38.5)	41.7	(38–45.4)	47.9	(43.4–52.4)
	Non-Hispanic black	53.9	0.88	58.1	(52.2–64)	66.9	(59.6–74.1)	75.6	(66.6–84.6)
	Mexican American	42.3	0.57	44.4	(39.9–48.9)	50.1	(44.4–57.8)	55.8	(48.7–62.8)

Abbreviation: CI, confidence interval.

[a] Body mass index (kg/m^2) ≥30.

[b] Estimates based on National Health and Nutrition Examination Survey (NHANES) II (1976–1980); NHANES III (1988–1994); and NHANES conducted annually from 1999–2004.

Modified from Wang Y, Beydoun MA, Liang L, et al. Will all Americans become overweight or obese? Estimating the progression and cost of the U.S. obesity epidemic. Obesity (Silver Spring) 2008;16:2323–30; with permission.

Table 3
Projected direct health care costs caused by overweight and obesity in United States adults ≥20 years

	Overweight and Obesity[a]				Obesity[b]			
Year	Billions ($)	Billions of $2000	% NHEA	% MEPS	Billions ($)	Billions of $2000	% NHEA	% MEPS
Projection A[c]								
2000	81.5	81.5	7.1	13	60.9	60.9	5.3	9.7
2010	194.3	151.1	8.4	13.5	151.3	117.7	6.5	10.5
2020	437.6	276	9.7	15.6	351.1	221.4	7.8	12.5
2030	956.9	507.5	10.9	17.6	784.8	416.2	9	14.4
Projection B[d]								
2000	72.2	72.2	6.3	11.5	53.2	53.2	4.7	8.5
2010	175.2	136.3	7.6	12.2	114.6	104.7	5.8	9.4
2020	394	248.5	8.8	14.1	312.3	197	6.9	11.2
2030	860.7	456.4	9.8	15.8	698.3	370.3	8	12.8

Abbreviations: MEPS, Medical Expenditure Panel Survey; NHEA, National Health Expenditure Account.

[a] Body mass index (kg/m^2) ≥25.

[b] Body mass index (kg/m^2) ≥30.

[c] Projections based on per capita excess health care costs attributable to overweight and obesity as estimated by Thorpe et al.[23]

[d] Projections based on per capita excess health care costs attributable to overweight and obesity as estimated by Finkelstein et al.[24]

Modified from Wang Y, Beydoun MA, Liang L, et al. Will all Americans become overweight or obese? Estimating the progression and cost of the U.S. obesity epidemic. Obesity (Silver Spring) 2008;16:2323–30; with permission.

methodologies of mean annual linear increase in overweight and obesity prevalence and shifts in BMI distributions. BMI was measured by direct physical examination in NHANES rather than by self-report.[26] The study was not without potential methodologic shortcomings. The prevalence projections of overweight and obesity were calculated assuming no changes in the population distribution of age, gender, and ethnicity after the end of the observed period in 2004. It also was assumed that the per capita excess health care costs of overweight and obesity that were estimated annually to 2030 grew at the same rate as the per capita total health care costs. This may actually have underestimated the future costs of obesity, because the disparity in health care costs for obese and nonobese persons may become wider because of greater obesity in younger adults; a greater prevalence and accompanying complications of morbidly obese individuals (BMI $\geq$35); and development of more costly technologic treatments for obesity. The models also did not take into account any future potential changes in policy, environment, or behavior that could impact overweight and obesity.[22] Inclusion of such factors, however, is largely based on conjecture.

SUMMARY

This article summarizes and critically evaluates the scientific literature for the annual and lifetime medical care costs of obesity in women in the United States. Actual and projected costs are reviewed. A wide variety of study designs and statistical models are presented to estimate costs including a prevalence-based approach where costs attributable to obesity are estimated by the simple replacement of obese individuals with an equal number of nonobese individuals; an attributable fraction approach where costs attributable to obesity are estimated through the risk and costs associated with a certain number of obesity-related diseases adjusting for differential mortality between obese and comparison groups; and the use of nationally representative samples, such as NHANES and MEPS, to determine the prevalence of obesity and medical costs associated with obesity relative to normal-weight individuals. Despite differences in the populations examined, the comparison populations used, if BMI was self-reported or physically measured, and whether potential confounding factors were adjusted for in the models, virtually all annual and lifetime costs supported higher medical expenditures for obese persons relative to their comparison groups. An especially important revelation was that lifetime costs attributable to obesity remained after accounting for the higher mortality in obese individuals. The rising prevalence of obesity should serve as an impetus for intervention programs to reduce obesity and its increased cost burden. Future research is needed to examine how lifetime medical costs are affected by individuals transitioning to different BMI categories throughout life, increasing annual and lifetime costs attributable to obesity as the prevalence of morbid obesity increases and more costly technologic treatments for obesity are developed, how cost estimates are affected if obesity is reduced and greater numbers of individuals live through older ages as life expectancy continues to increase, the cost of implementing intervention programs to reduce obesity, the age when such implementation results in greater immediate and lifetime cost savings of obesity, and if specific intervention programs should be tailored to various race-gender groups at different periods of life.

REFERENCES

1. Centers for Disease Control. Prevalence of overweight and obesity among adults: United States, 2003–2004. Available at: http://www.cdc.gov/nchs/products/pubs/pubd/hestats/overweight/overwght_adult_03.htm. January 27, 2009.

2. Centers for Disease Control. Chronic disease prevention and health promotion: preventing obesity and chronic diseases through good nutrition and physical activity. Available at: http://www.cdc.gov/nccdphp/publications/factsheets/prevention/obesity.htm. Accessed January 27, 2009.
3. Peeters A, Bonneux L, Barendregt J, et al. Methods of estimating years of life lost due to obesity. JAMA 2003;289:2941.
4. Fontaine KR, Redden DT, Wang C, et al. Years of life lost due to obesity. JAMA 2003;289:187–93.
5. Flegal KM, Graubard BI, Williamson DF, et al. Excess deaths associated with underweight, overweight, and obesity. JAMA 2005;293:1861–7.
6. Wolf AM, Colditz GA. Current estimates of the economic cost of obesity in the United States. Obes Res 1998;6:97–106.
7. Allison D, Zannolli R, Narayan K. The direct health care costs of obesity in the United States. Am J Public Health 1999;89:1194–9.
8. Stevens J, Cai J, Pamuk ER, et al. The effect of age on the association between body mass index and mortality. N Engl J Med 1998;338:1–7.
9. Thompson D, Edelsberg J, Colditz G, et al. Lifetime health and economic consequences of obesity. Arch Intern Med 1999;159:2177–83.
10. Odell TW, Gregory MC. Cost of hypertension treatment. J Gen Intern Med 1995; 10:686–8.
11. Oster G, Borok GM, Menzin J, et al. Cholesterol-Reduction Intervention Study (CRIS): a randomized trial to assess effectiveness and costs in clinical practice. Arch Intern Med 1996;156:731–9.
12. Huse DM, Oster G, Killen AR, et al. The economic costs of non-insulin-dependent diabetes mellitus. JAMA 1989;262:2708–13.
13. Oster G, Huse DM, Lacey MJ, et al. Cost-effectiveness of ticlopidine in preventing stroke in high-risk patients. Stroke 1994;25:1149–56.
14. Thompson D, Edelsberg J, Kinsey K, et al. Estimated economic costs of obesity to U.S. business. Am J Health Promot 1998;13:120–7.
15. Finkelstein E, Fiebelkorn IC, Wang G. The costs of obesity among fulltime employees. Am J Health Promot 2005;20:45–51.
16. Finkelstein EA, Trogdon JG, Brown DS, et al. The lifetime medical cost burden of overweight and obesity: implications for obesity prevention. Obesity (Silver Spring) 2008;16:1843–8.
17. Lakdawalla D, Goldman D, Shang B. The health and cost consequences of obesity among the future elderly. Health Affairs Millwood (VA) 2005;24(Suppl 2): W5R30–41.
18. Daviglus M, Liu K, Yan L, et al. Relation of body mass index in young adulthood and middle age to Medicare expenditures in older age. JAMA 2004;292:2743–9.
19. Finkelstein E, Brown D, Wrage L, et al. Individual and aggregate years of life lost associated with overweight and obesity. RTI, submitted for publication.
20. Rowland ML. Self-reported weight and height. Am J Clin Nutr 1990;52:1125–33.
21. Palta M, Prineas RJ, Berman R, et al. Comparison of self-reported and measured height and weight. Am J Epidemiol 1982;115:223–30.
22. Wang Y, Beydoun MA, Liang L, et al. Will all Americans become overweight or obese? Estimating the progression and cost of the U.S. obesity epidemic. Obesity (Silver Spring) 2008;16:2323–30.
23. Thorpe KE, Florence CS, Howard DH, et al. The impact of obesity on rising medical spending. Millwood (VA): Health Aff; 2004. (Suppl) (Web Exclusives): W4-480.

24. Finkelstein E, Fiebelkorn I, Wang G. National medical expenditures attributable to overweight and obesity: how much and who's paying? Health Aff 2003;(Suppl) (Web Exclusives). W3–W219–26.
25. Poisal JA, Truffer C, Smith S, et al. Health spending projections through 2016: modest changes obscure part D's impact. Health Aff (Millwood) 2007;26:242–53.
26. Centers for Disease Control. National Health and Nutrition Examination Survey. Available at: http://www.cdc.gov/nchs/nhanes.htm. Accessed January 28, 2009.

Early Life Origins of Obesity

John P. Newnham, MD, FRANZCOG[a,*], Craig E. Pennell, FRANZCOG, PhD[a], Stephen J. Lye, PhD[b], Jonathan Rampono, MBBS, FRACP[c], John R.G. Challis, PhD, FRSC[d]

KEYWORDS

• Obesity • Diabetes • Early origins • Fetus • Epigenetics

In numerical terms, we are now in the midst of the greatest epidemic ever experienced by humans. Rates of obesity and diabetes, together with a host of their related disorders, are increasing rapidly throughout much of the world. The increasing burden of people suffering from these conditions is generally believed to result from increased population numbers, aging, urbanization, plentiful supplies of food, and physical inactivity.[1] In 2000, about 171 million adults had diabetes. Conservative estimates predict that this number will double by 2030. In India alone, the number of diabetic adults is expected to increase from 31 million in 2000 to 79 million in 2030. In Australia, the prevalence of childhood obesity has trebled in little more than a decade.[2] It has been estimated the combined annual cost of obesity, diabetes, and cardiovascular disease in the United States is nearly half a trillion dollars.[3] Tackling the epidemic of obesity and diabetes must be one of our highest priorities in health care, both in our local environment and globally.

WE MAY KNOW THE ANSWER

We may already know how to tackle the worldwide epidemic of obesity and diabetes. Eating better and exercising more will prevent the problem. Our ancestors did this, although their behavior resulted from necessity rather than an awareness of health promotion. What we do not know however is how to apply this answer to the ever-increasing proportion of the world's population so much in need of the cure. Arguably,

This work was supported by Grant No. 527613 from the National Health and Medical Research Council of Australia and the Raine Foundation of Western Australia.

[a] School of Women's and Infants' Health, The University of Western Australia, 374 Bagot Road, Subiaco, Perth, Western Australia 6008, Australia

[b] Samuel Lunenfeld Research Institute, Mount Sinai Hospital, Toronto, Ontario M5G 1X5, Canada

[c] Department of Psychological Medicine, King Edward Memorial Hospital, 374 Bagot Road, Subiaco, Perth, Western Australia 6008, Australia

[d] Michael Smith Foundation for Health Research, Suite 200, 1285 West Broadway Vancouver, BC V6H 3X8, Canada

* Corresponding author.

E-mail address: john.newnham@uwa.edu.au (J.P. Newnham).

Obstet Gynecol Clin N Am 36 (2009) 227–244
doi:10.1016/j.ogc.2009.03.004
obgyn.theclinics.com
0889-8545/09/$ – see front matter.

we cannot effectively implement the answer because we do not fully understand how to address the problem of varying risks of obesity and why many of those who need most to alter their lifestyle are most resistant to changing their behavior.

OUR SUCCESS SO FAR

The early stages of this epidemic did not pass unnoticed. Public health campaigns aimed at altering behavior to prevent obesity and diabetes in the general community may have had some successes, but have not turned the tide of the epidemic.[1] There is now widespread support for the view that effective prevention of these chronic human conditions requires us to tackle the conditions at their origins, and many of the origins are traced to early life. Evidence for these early origins has been accumulating for several decades, but our understanding of the probable mechanisms and their role before birth has come about only recently.

THE EARLY ORIGINS OF ADULT DISEASE

Environmental influences that alter development before birth can be categorized into one of two groups.[4] In the first group are those influences that may disrupt development, resulting in structural changes, such as teratogens. In the second group are those influences that may be aimed at altering development to optimize the offspring's future chances of surviving and reproducing, a process known as *developmental plasticity*. The field encompassing these two groups of influences is termed *developmental origins of health and disease*.[5] Both categories of altered development may be involved in predisposing individuals to subsequent ill-health, but most attention recently has focused on the latter, the influences related to developmental plasticity.

DEVELOPMENTAL PLASTICITY

In 1992, Barker and Hales[6] described the "thrifty phenotype hypothesis." Their proposal essentially states that, in pregnancies in which the woman's environment is poor, or in which the fetal environment is less than optimal, the fetus makes metabolic adaptations to ensure that it will maximize its chances of survival in a postnatal world assumed to be equally compromised. For individuals living in traditional lifestyles, characterized by low levels of nutrition and high levels of physical activity, their subsequent health in a similar environment would benefit from such adaptations. However, where there is a difference between the expected postnatal life and that which actually ensues, such as for those making a rapid transition from a "world of thrift" to a "world of plenty," the metabolic adaptations now act against the individual and predispose the person to obesity and diabetes. Such a rapid transition from a world of thrift to a world of plenty is being experienced by millions of people, either because of increasing prosperity in their local environment or from migration to more affluent communities. The concept of developmental plasticity has been advanced by the work of Gluckman and Hanson and colleagues,[4,7] who use the term *predictive adaptive response* for changes in the womb in response to the environment of the pregnant mother. Gluckman and Hanson assert that the predictive adaptive response probably evolved because it normally bestowed evolutionary advantages to offspring. That is, predictive adaptive response made offspring better equipped to face challenges of the environment they were likely to live in. Gluckman and Hanson also noted how problems arise when there is a "mismatch" between the expected and actual postnatal environments. The predictive adaptive response may shape both metabolic and behavioral characteristics.

THE MECHANISMS UNDERLYING THE PREDICTIVE ADAPTIVE RESPONSE

The classic illustration of the predictive adaptive response describes a fetus that adapts to its mother's poor environment by restricting its growth and undergoing a series of metabolic and behavioral adaptations that would be beneficial in its expected postnatal world of thrift. These adaptations center on insulin and leptin resistance.[4,8] Leptin, a hormone made by adipose tissue, has many functions, one of which is to influence appetite centrally. Central leptin resistance increases appetite while peripheral resistance to insulin enhances fat deposition. Together, these hormonal adaptations are beneficial in a world of thrift, but, in a world of plenty, may predispose the individual to obesity and diabetes. After such prenatal programming, a child born into an environment of plentiful nutrition may experience excessive "catch-up growth," which may then lead to obesity, diabetes, and a host of related conditions.[9,10] The mechanisms by which an individual may be predisposed by prenatal events to later obesity appear to be quite distinct from those of diet-induced obesity, which may have its origins at later ages.[11] Early research in this area focused simply on the relationships between birth weight and adult health outcomes,[12] but it is now clear the process involves interactions between the prenatal and postnatal environments, together with other influences passed down from previous generations. It is also clear that the process involves both metabolic and behavioral components, ensuring that effective interventions need to account for the many factors that are operative.

TACKLING THE CONSEQUENCES OF THE PREDICTIVE ADAPTIVE RESPONSE

The most effective strategy to tackle the consequences of developmental plasticity as described by this hypothesis would be to ensure that those individuals programmed to live in a world of thrift continue to live in such an environment. However, this would mean blocking paths to prosperity, which would be ethically, socially, and politically immoral and probably impossible as well. We therefore need to find ways in which people can make the transition from traditional to Westernized lifestyles without suffering the curses that may accompany such new-found affluence. At the heart of this challenge lies the fundamental principle that those individuals most at risk have behavioral adaptations that make them least sensitive to public health programs aimed at influencing their behavior. Those whose prenatal experiences have resulted in behavioral and metabolic patterns that increase appetite and lead to fat deposition may be those least able to change their lifestyle practices.[13] There is evidence from animal studies that such prenatal programming may also involve a general decrease in locomotion, aimed at conserving energy, rendering these individuals most resistant to campaigns aiming to encourage exercise.[14] Strategies that are most likely to be effective need to begin at earlier times of life.

TACKLING THE INTRAUTERINE ORIGINS

Fetal growth restriction may be part of an adaptation to a poor intrauterine environment that results from the circumstances of the mother's life. Growth restriction may also result from placental insufficiency, a cause that is more common in developed countries. We do not understand if the fetus responds to placental insufficiency with the same metabolic adaptations as those described by the thrifty phenotype hypothesis, but it is reasonable to suppose that similar pathways may be operating. If so, improving placental function may have great potential to prevent chronic adult disease. However, our current inability to fundamentally alter placental health leaves us severely compromised as practitioners. Clearly, our newfound understanding of the early origins of some of the major diseases affecting humans demands further research to understand the placenta and to discover strategies to improve its function.

For those women living in adverse environments, public health campaigns aimed at improving their immediate health and nutrition may have great potential for future generations. Recent debate on the "French paradox" could contain important lessons.[15] The term *French paradox* was coined after data from France and Britain showed differences in relative rates of coronary heart disease despite similar major risk factors in the two populations. Death from ischemic heart disease in France is about one quarter that in Britain, yet rates of animal fat consumption, exercise, and smoking are similar. It has been suggested the French are protected by their common practice of drinking alcohol on a daily basis. According to one hypothesis, the antioxidant properties in red wine provide specific protection.[16] However, a host of studies have provided evidence countering the view that alcohol provides such protection. Thus, the difference in cardiac mortality between the two countries remains a paradox. An explanation may be found in study of the nutrition of girls and pregnant women several generations ago.

The general populations of France and Britain in the 1800s were chronically malnourished.[17,18] In the latter part of that century, the French introduced widespread nutritional support for infants and children. The impetus for the various French programs did not result from lobbying by health professionals, but from the military. After the devastating defeat of the French army in the Franco-Prussian War of 1871, nutritional support programs were introduced to improve the nation's future military potential by improving infant survival and child health. Three decades later, the English adopted similar initiatives after finding poor health in their young men enlisted to fight in the Boer War. It has been suggested this 3-decade advantage of the French in terms of infant and child nutrition is now manifest as lower rates of cardiac mortality several generations later. Regardless of the relative contributions of the various hypotheses aiming to explain the French paradox, some role of improved health of young women seems likely. The possible influence of intergenerational effects, however, suggests that the task of tackling the current epidemic of obesity and diabetes may need to extend over many generations.

CAN IT BE EXPLAINED BY GENERAL MATERNAL NUTRITION?

Perhaps surprisingly, maternal macronutrient intake bears little correlation with newborn size. Indeed, attempts to improve fetal growth with improved maternal nutrition have been disappointing. Extensive reviews of the evidence regarding nutritional advice and supplementation in pregnancy have shown that such strategies may alter maternal behavior, but there is little evidence of benefit from providing nutritional advice,[19] or from supplementation with high-protein[20] or isocaloric balanced protein[21] diets. Attempting to enhance fetal growth may also increase risk to the mother by leading to obstructed labor[19] and possibly infant mortality.[20] Neither of these possibilities has been evaluated adequately. Tackling the epidemic of obesity and diabetes at its origins will not be achieved by simply providing more food to pregnant women.

COULD IT BE SIMPLE MICRONUTRIENTS?

The rate of diabetes is rising faster in South Asia than anywhere in the world.[1] Indian babies are amongst the smallest in the world.[22] In their population, low birth-weight predicts adiposity and insulin resistance in childhood.[22] However, when compared with white babies, these small Indian babies are relatively obese with more central fat and a higher percentage of adipose tissue, and are hyperinsulinemic and hyperleptinemic.[23] In childhood, these individuals become shorter and thinner, but with a higher percentage of body fat and are more likely to develop type 2 diabetes.[24]

The most extensive evaluation of these relationships in Indian children has come from the Pune Maternal Nutrition Study, which is a prospective population-based rural study designed to investigate the relationships between maternal nutrition and cardiovascular risk factors.[23,25] Maternal macronutritional intake was found to be unrelated to adiposity and insulin resistance in the children, consistent with the findings from other studies showing a lack of influence of general maternal food intake on fetal growth.[23] However, higher maternal folate levels predicted adiposity and insulin resistance in the offspring and lower vitamin B_{12} levels predicted insulin resistance. The highest insulin resistance was found in children of mothers who had the highest folate levels and the lowest vitamin B_{12} levels. This combination of high levels of folate in the face of vitamin B_{12} deficiency is common in India, where high rates of lactovegetarianism result in a high consumption of green leafy vegetables containing folate but with inadequate supplies of vitamin B_{12}. Eating patterns of this type featured in about 40% of Indian households and about 10% of the world's population. This observation suggests that nutritional disturbances in one-carbon metabolism resulting from vegetarianism, perhaps interacting with other features of modernization, may underpin much of the epidemic in obesity and diabetes afflicting South Asia. These observations are recent, and similar data from other regions are urgently required. In the meantime, it is clear that nutritional supplementation to overcome maternal malnutrition is a more complex issue than just replacement of calories.

IS THE THRIFTY PHENOTYPE HYPOTHESIS TRUE?

People from the Indian subcontinent are highly prone to central obesity and diabetes either within those countries of the subcontinent or after migration to the United Kingdom,[26] but recent evidence suggests that not all groups of people are equally vulnerable.[27] According to the general thrust of the thrifty phenotype hypothesis, the most important measure for determining risk of metabolic syndrome should be the speed of transition from a life of thrift to a life of plenty. However, this part of the hypothesis does not always hold true. It is not true, for example, in the case of Tibetans who have migrated to India. Coming from a life-of-thrift environment in Tibet to a more life-of-plenty environment in India, the Tibetans in India would, according to the thrifty phenotype hypothesis, be expected to be more prone to diabetes than peninsular Indians. That is not the case, however. Tibetans who have migrated to India are less prone to diabetes that peninsular Indians.[28] Similarly, Japanese who migrate to Hawaii and Los Angeles might be expected to be more prone to diabetes than people who have lived in Hawaii or Los Angeles for generations. Data show otherwise, however. Japanese migrants to those two places are less prone to obesity and diabetes than the established populations.[29] These observations have led to the hypothesis that another key factor in determining risk is climate: Risk may be lower for groups whose ancestors lived in cold harsh climates. In an environment in which agriculture and hunting is not possible for much of the year, reliance on limited quantities of stored food may be expected to result in insulin resistance. The principles that underpin the thrifty phenotype hypothesis would suggest that such descendents would be more at risk of diabetes, rather than less. This leads to the possibility that different groups of people may have different genetic predispositions to obesity and diabetes.

CAN IT BE EXPLAINED BY GENE-ENVIRONMENT INTERACTIONS?

It is now widely accepted that genetic and epigenetic pathways mediate much of the relationship between the environment and the developmental origins of health and disease paradigm (**Fig. 1**). Sequence variation within the genetic code can modify the effect an adverse environment has on the risk of adult disease, while the environment can in turn induce epigenetic modifications of the genome, which can influence an individual's risk of health and disease. Both mechanisms likely contribute to the variation seen in an individual's response to the environment, though their relative contributions and the extent of interactions between the pathways remain to be determined.

INTERACTION BETWEEN VARIATIONS IN GENETIC SEQUENCE, THE ENVIRONMENT, AND DEVELOPMENTAL ORIGINS OF HEALTH AND DISEASE

There is growing evidence in the literature attributing DNA sequence variation (particularly single nucleotide polymorphisms [SNPs]) within genes as primary factors in determining an individual's risk of disease. Initial research in this area has identified associations between polymorphisms in genes regulating energy metabolism and population differences in risk of adult metabolic disease. For example, polymorphisms in the peroxisome proliferator-activated receptor (PPAR)–γ2 gene modify the relationship between size at birth and adult diseases, such as insulin sensitivity and altered metabolism,[30,31] hypertension,[32] obesity,[33] and dyslipidemia.[34] Only individuals carrying the high-risk Pro12Pro allele within the PPAR-γ2 gene (and not the Pro12Ala variant) demonstrate an association between small body size at birth and insulin resistance or hypertension in later life.

Polymorphisms in genes within the hypothalamic-pituitary-adrenal (HPA) axis appear to play a significant role in influencing intrauterine glucocorticoid exposure during fetal growth and, perhaps, glucocorticoid metabolism and disease later in life. For example, polymorphisms in the glucocorticoid receptor have been causally linked to obesity,[35,36] hypertension,[37] hypercholesterolemia,[37] and responses to

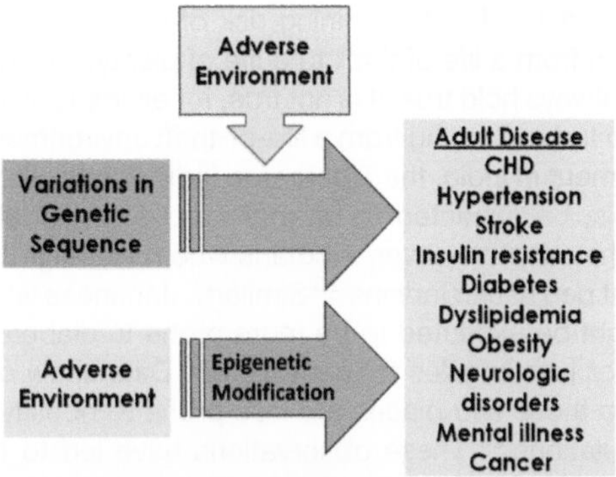

Fig. 1. Variations in genetic sequence can determine how the prenatal environment shapes an individual's vulnerability to disease outside the womb. Furthermore, the environment can induce epigenetic prenatal modification of the genome, which can influence an individual's postnatal health and risk of disease. The interactions of the genetic sequence and environmental factors are likely responsible for the variation seen in an individual's postnatal response to an adverse prenatal environment. How precisely those factors interact and the relative contributions of each have yet to be clearly determined. CHD, coronary heart disease.

psychosocial stress in adults.[36] Analysis of the haplotype structure of common variations within the glucocorticoid receptor gene locus has identified further genetic combinations linking birth weight to adult disease in the Helsinki Birth Cohort.[38] One such haplotype was associated with lower birth weight, shorter birth length, and higher fasting plasma and mean 24-hour salivary cortisol, supporting a link between body size at birth and HPA axis function in later life. Moreover, individuals carrying another haplotype exhibited an increased association between body size at birth and impaired glucose tolerance or diabetes as adults compared with noncarriers.[38] Other studies show gene-environment interactions linked to behavior. For example, in nonhuman primates,[39] polymorphisms within serotonin transporter (5-HTTLPR, also present in humans[40]) can alter behavioral vulnerability to modified early-rearing environment. These observations suggest that complex interactions between genes and the early environment modulate developmental programming of adult disease.

Genetic differences not only regulate gene-environment interactions underlying disease onset but also regulate disease susceptibility following environmental alterations. Ghrelin (a gastrointestinal-brain regulatory peptide), which plays a role in energy balance, contains a polymorphism (Leu72Met) that has been associated with impaired glucose tolerance and type 2 diabetes through defective first-phase insulin secretion.[41] In the Finnish Diabetes Prevention Study, where subjects with impaired glucose tolerance were randomized into either an intervention group (intensive diet and exercise intervention) or a control group, subjects with impaired glucose tolerance and the common Leu72Leu genotype developed type 2 diabetes less frequently under intervention circumstances (odds ratio 0.28, 95% CI 0.10–0.79; $P = .016$) than subjects with the Leu72Met allele.[41] Thus, polymorphic variation can convey differential response to therapies in multifunctional diseases, such as diabetes, in addition to predisposing individuals to disease risk.

INTERACTION BETWEEN THE ENVIRONMENT, THE EPIGENOME, AND DEVELOPMENTAL ORIGINS OF HEALTH AND DISEASE

Emerging evidence suggests that epigenetic modification of genes is an important mechanism by which environmental exposures in early life can induce alterations in gene expression, which may persist throughout life. Nutritional[42] and behavioral cues[43] during pregnancy and early postnatal life have been shown to influence the epigenomic state of a gene. Epigenetic changes can also be induced by exposure to tobacco smoke, alcohol, chemical carcinogens, infectious agents, UV radiation, and other factors in the environment or related to lifesyle.[44] Significantly, increasing evidence shows that some of these epigenetic-mediated changes in gene expression can persist across multiple generations.[45] In mice, for example, modulation of the methyl content of the maternal diet during pregnancy results in altered DNA methylation patterns in offspring and altered gene expression.[46] In rats, persistent changes in DNA methylation and expression of the glucocorticoid receptor and PPAR-γ can be induced by an unbalanced prenatal diet.[47] Furthermore, recent evidence demonstrates that in utero dietary manipulation affects gene expression and alters susceptibility to obesity in adulthood as a result of modifications to the epigenome.[48] Epigenetic regulation of 11β-hydroxysteroid dehydrogenase type 2 expression by DNA methylation has been demonstrated in vitro, providing a potential mechanism for programming of hypertension.[49] Studies in humans have shown that manipulation of dietary folate causes detectable changes in global genomic DNA methylation status,[50,51] providing potential mechanisms to explain the possibility of long-term modifications in gene expression in response to diet.

Maternal behavioral cues have also been shown to induce epigenetic modifications. Using a rat model, Weaver and colleagues[43] demonstrated that high levels of maternal care-giving behavior (pup nursing, licking, and grooming) in the early postnatal period induce increased glucocorticoid receptor transcription through a permanent hypomethylation of the glucocorticoid receptor promoter. The mechanism mediating this interaction between behavior and gene expression involved (1) an altered CpG methylation pattern within the I_7 glucocorticoid receptor promoter, which modified a transcription factor binding site, and (2) the subsequent long-term change in the level of transcription of the glucocorticoid receptor gene. Through this mechanism, maternal behavior induced a permanent increase in hippocampal glucocorticoid receptor, although changes to the offspring hippocampal transcriptome could subsequently be reversed in adulthood by histone deacetylase administration.[52]

Thus, nutritional manipulations can epigenetically mark the genome and affect gene expression over the life course. The dietary factors involved, the genes that are susceptible, and the developmental plasticity of the effects remain to be determined. Variable penetrance is a recognized feature of disease-associated SNPs. It is conceivable that epigenetic regulation of SNP-containing genes or the occurrence of SNPs that alter epigenetic targets may explain a proportion of such variable penetrance. Thus, genetic variation and epigenetic variation may act in concert to modulate disease risk.

THE U-SHAPED CURVE OF BIRTH WEIGHT

Most of the early research in the developmental origins of health and disease field centered on the causes and consequences of low birth weight. The risks of obesity and diabetes are increased at the lower end of the birth-weight curve, but they may also be increased at the upper end of the curve. Among individuals of high birth weight, the risk is especially high for those from pregnancies complicated by poorly controlled diabetes. Glucose can cross the placenta, but insulin cannot. In the face of maternal hyperglycemia, high circulating levels of glucose in the fetus lead to increased production of insulin from the fetal pancreas, causing macrosomia.[53] This sequence of events may predispose the child to insulin resistance in later life. There may also be lasting injury to the insulin-producing islets of the pancreas. The mechanism underpinning how poorly controlled diabetes may cause fetal overgrowth has been known for many years, but the U-shaped relationship between birth weight and future glucose intolerance has only been described more recently.

The observation was first made in Pima Indians[54] and in Taiwan,[55] but the relationship may also occur in Westernized communities. Researchers in Western Australia have described a U-shaped relationship between percentage of expected birth weight and high-risk cluster of metabolic syndrome features at 8 years of age.[56] These children were enrolled into a longitudinal cohort study at 18 weeks' gestation and remain under frequent follow-up.[57] In contrast to many of the populations studied in this regard, the children in the Western Australian study were generally of European descent with no recent family history of migration to a more affluent environment. Also, they enjoyed a relatively high standard of living and consumed a contemporary Western diet. The analysis was restricted to those born at term gestation, precluding a role of preterm birth or growth restriction that warranted early delivery. Previous studies did not involve accurate estimation of gestational age by ultrasound biometry, a calculation that was routine in the Western Australian study.[57]

In contrast to reports from other communities, the Western Australian curve for birth weight plotted against subsequent metabolic syndrome risk extended further to the right.[56] Indeed, the mean birth weight was 3501 g, much greater than the mean of 2600 g and 2800 g in girls and boys respectively in contemporary India.[58] In such a Westernized and affluent community, a rightward shift in the birth-weight curve may indicate that the life-long consequences of fetal hyperglycemia at the upper end of the birth-weight curve will be of greater importance for public health than the consequences of fetal growth restriction in the lower birth-weight ranges. In such a developed community, fetal growth restriction resulting from maternal deprivation is uncommon, and is more likely to result from specific pathology, such as placental insufficiency. Many of the cohorts underpinning the concepts in this field came from developing countries or European communities during periods of deprivation. For those populations, the consequences of fetal growth restriction at the left end of the birth-weight curve may have held greater relevance.

Only 1.1% of pregnancies in the Western Australian cohort had received a diagnosis of gestational diabetes.[56] At the time, routine testing for gestational diabetes was not well established. It remains possible that the cohort included many cases of undiagnosed diabetes, or that maternal obesity or unknown lifestyle factors predispose the offspring to obesity, diabetes, and metabolic syndrome through other pathways. One contributing variable was clearly evident. Maternal smoking during the pregnancy modified the relationship between birth weight and metabolic syndrome cluster. Smoking is known to consistently reduce fetal growth, but the highest risk of metabolic syndrome cluster was observed in those babies in the highest birth-weight ranges who had come from pregnancies in which the mother had smoked. It is likely that the combination of maternal hyperglycemia and smoking yields the greatest future risk for the offspring.

The importance of risk associated with birth weight at the right end of the curve has clear implications for health care during pregnancy. Vigilance is required to ensure early diagnosis of gestational diabetes. Blood glucose levels must be rigorously controlled in those women found to be glucose intolerant.

COULD IT BE EXPLAINED BY LACTATION?

Breast-feeding, which confers a variety of benefits for the child,[59] may also play a key role in preventing obesity. A systematic review of the effects of breast-feeding on childhood obesity supported the protective effect, but also highlighted inconsistencies in the association.[60] Studies in this field have been confounded by the observation that shorter duration of breast-feeding is associated with maternal obesity, lower socioeconomic status, smoking, and other familial factors. In a study of adolescents in the United States, Gillman and colleagues[61] observed a reduction in obesity in those who had been breast-fed for at least 7 months, when compared with those breast-fed for 3 months or less. In the Western Australian Pregnancy Cohort (Raine) Study, being overweight at 8 years of age was associated with breast-feeding for less than 4 months.[62] In this prospective study, a shorter duration of breast-feeding was also observed in women who were overweight or of lower socioeconomic status. Together, these studies provide strong evidence that the duration of breast-feeding may play an important role in the future health of the child, and that a variety of maternal factors influence the duration of breast-feeding.

Diabetes may also influence the duration and quality of breast-feeding. Being overweight at 2 years of age has been associated with a greater volume of breast milk in diabetic mothers[63] and the breast milk of diabetic women has been shown to have a higher energy content.[64]

In experimental conditions, induction of uteroplacental insufficiency has been shown to diminish mammary development and subsequent lactation.[65] The fetal growth restriction induced by reduced placental function may be further influenced by the adequacy of postnatal lactation. Wlodek and colleagues[66] have shown that induction of uteroplacental insufficiency in the rat impairs mammary development, which is associated with impaired postnatal growth and nephron deficit in the offspring, followed by an increase in the offspring's blood pressure. The effects of diminished lactation following uteroplacental insufficiency on postnatal nephron development and blood pressure were investigated by cross-fostering experiments in which the growth-restricted newborns were placed either with control mothers or with those with restricted mammary development. These studies showed that the effects of fetal growth restriction could be reversed by providing the newborn with a normal breast-feeding experience.

In clinical practice, exposure of the pregnancy to glucocortocoid treatment has also been shown to affect lactation. Maternal intramuscular glucocorticoid injections are given to pregnant women at risk of early preterm birth to enhance fetal maturation.[67] This treatment is highly effective and significantly reduces the risk of lung disease and death in the preterm newborn. In a prospective study, Henderson and colleagues[68] observed that this glucocorticoid treatment impaired the onset of lactogenesis if delivery occurred between 3 and 9 days after treatment. The effect was on quantity, with no changes observed in levels of citrate or lactose. This study has shown that pharmacologic treatment acting on the HPA axis during pregnancy can influence mammary function after birth.

Despite the key importance of breast-feeding, most of the studies linking pre- and postnatal factors with subsequent health have bypassed this important stage in human nutrition. This omission has resulted from an absence of necessary data in most retrospective cohorts and perhaps a general lack of appreciation by many researchers of the potential importance of this aspect of biology. It remains possible that much of the relationship between maternal nutrition and lifestyle in pregnancy and subsequent health of the offspring is strongly influenced by the duration and adequacy of breast-feeding. If so, strategies to improve the quantity and quality of infant nutrition are well within our reach.

PHYSICAL ACTIVITY

Physical inactivity is a major contributor to our epidemic of obesity and diabetes.[3] The human genome evolved in an environment of physical activity and the sedentary behavior that is a feature of modern life is relatively new. There has been much research demonstrating the benefits of physical activity in preventing or reducing obesity and type II diabetes.[69,70] During pregnancy, evidence suggests the benefits of physical activity may include a reduction in risk of gestational diabetes,[71] reduced maternal weight-gain,[72] and improved self-esteem and mental health.[73] For the child, there may be improved morphometric and developmental outcomes at 5 years of age.[74]

Despite the clear benefits of physical exercise in preventing or ameliorating obesity and diabetes, public health campaigns aimed at encouraging physical activity have not achieved the success that should be expected.[3] This lack of success may be partially due to inadequate commitment by politicians, health care planners, and research funding agencies. However, it is also possible that those individuals who need most to increase their physical activity are "programmed " to remain inactive.

Vickers and colleagues[14] have shown that lifestyle choices may have a prenatal origin. In rats, maternal undernutrition during pregnancy leads to offspring that display hyperphagia, hyperinsulinemia, and hyperleptinemia.[13,75] These features are likely to represent adaptations by the fetus in preparation for its expected postnatal life of "thrift." Such features would confer a survival advantage if the postnatal reality were an environment that required adaptation to a low plane of nutrition. When exposed to a postnatal life in which food is plentiful, the augmented appetite and insulin and leptin resistance act together to produce obesity. These offspring also display a reduction in physical activity independent of postnatal nutrition.[14] It is proposed that programming for a reduction in physical activity may also be a survival strategy, as long periods of inactivity would be an advantage if food were scarce.

Based on the animal experiments, it may be that those people most prone to develop obesity are also programmed to be inactive. In such a case, public health campaigns aimed at encouraging people to exercise may be most effective in those who need it the least. Those people who would benefit most from physical activity—those with insulin and leptin resistance—may be the ones least likely to respond positively to calls to increase their exercise. By observing developmental disturbances that affect subsequent behavior through epigenetic mechanisms, we may gain some insights into the origins of these responses and find keys in the search for possible biomarkers (genetic or epigenetic) that might predict at birth the risk of metabolic disease later in life.

Thus, our challenge is to not only encourage physical activity, but also to make sure that those least likely to respond receive the message and take up a more active lifestyle. In pregnant women who declare themselves to be sedentary, we have shown that a structured exercise program based on swimming can be highly effective in improving fitness.[76] Women who could swim little more than 10 m at commencement of the program were able to swim a kilometer or more by the third trimester. The program appeared safe, with no untoward effects demonstrable on maternal or fetal testing. Swimming has many advantages over other forms of activity because the pregnant woman has the comfort of being virtually weightless and not at risk of hyperthermia. However, many obese women are reluctant to join a program that involves exposing themselves in a swimming costume in a public place. Exercise programs tailored specifically for obese pregnant women are required, and the programs need to include incentives that overcome any programmed reluctance to be physically active.

BEHAVIOR

The basis of many concepts in this field has come from study of people who have been involved in war and famine. These events have included the Dutch winter famine during the occupation of The Netherlands in World War II.[77] The majority of analyses have been based on evaluation of the consequences of nutritional deficiency in the women who were pregnant at the time. These studies have shown that nutritional deprivation at different times in pregnancy results in various cardiovascular and neuropsychiatric sequelae for the offspring. Because of insufficient data, a possible role for anxiety and depression, which must have been prominent in many of these pregnant women, has been incompletely evaluated. Recent studies have provided strong evidence that anxiety during pregnancy may have lasting effects on behavior in the child.

Pregnant women near the World Trade Center during the terrorist attacks of September 11, 2001, were nearly twice as likely to give birth to a growth-restricted newborn.[78] Furthermore, infants of women who developed posttraumatic stress disorder following this attack had lower cortisol levels than infants of women who were in the vicinity but did not develop posttraumatic stress disorder.[79] The effect was greatest for those in the third trimester at the time of the event. Young children of mothers pregnant at the time of the 1998 ice storm in Quebec, which resulted in a 5-week disruption to basic services, have been shown to have had lower scores on the Bayley Mental Development Index test.[80] Together these studies demonstrate that major traumatic events during pregnancy may have lasting consequences for the child.

In normal daily life, high levels of anxiety during pregnancy have been shown to predict neuro-behavioral outcomes in infancy. Anxiety appears to have a greater capacity than depression to affect the developing infant.[81] It has been estimated that the attributable load in behavioral problems in childhood due to maternal anxiety in pregnancy is of the order of 15%.[82]

A key feature of the childhood behavioral consequence of maternal anxiety during pregnancy appears to be attentional deficit.[83,84] Some components of attention deficit hyperactivity disorder arising from intrauterine experiences may be adaptive. According to the predictive adaptive responses concept, a pregnant woman who perceives her world to be threatening may "program" her child for that world, and survival in such an environment may benefit from hyperactivity and a short attention span. Behavioral features such as these may confer survival advantage in a world of great danger. When viewed in this light, the child does not have a disorder, but has been adapted positively for a different environment.

Experimental insights into the consequences of stimulating the fetal HPA axis during pregnancy have followed the discovery that maternal injection of glucocorticoids enhances maturation of the fetal lungs and other organs.[67] Unlike cortisol, synthetic glucocorticoids can freely cross the placenta.[85] Studies with sheep have shown that intramuscular injections given to the pregnant ewe each week for 3 or 4 weeks restrict fetal growth[86,87] and inhibit myelination of the developing brain.[88] The offspring's HPA axis is also altered.[89–93] From early postnatal life through to adulthood in sheep, the fetal HPA axis after repeated prenatal corticosteroid treatments has patterns of responsiveness that evolve through the spectrum of being increased, to levels similar to controls, and then to being diminished.[94] In a cohort of more than 500 children born with very low birth weight, three or more antenatal courses of glucocorticoids were associated with a significant increase in externalizing behavioral scores.[95]

The scientific literature contains plenty of evidence linking activation of the maternal HPA axis during pregnancy with altered behavior in childhood.[82,95] As people move from a world of thrift to a world of plenty, as described by the thrifty phenotype hypothesis, or are exposed to war or famine, there are likely to be many changes other than just alterations in nutrition and physical activity. Moving from one such environment to another may be associated with considerable anxiety carrying potential consequences for child development. As a result, interventions in pregnancy based only on changes to nutrition and exercise, and failing to account for the psychological well-being of the woman, may have limited effectiveness.

SUMMARY

As a world community, we find ourselves in the unusual position of facing the greatest epidemic in our history, with perhaps knowledge of the cure, but a limited ability to implement the solution. Research has taught us much about the mechanisms that underpin the early-life development of obesity and diabetes, but the information has not yet translated into an effective strategy to address the problem.

Preventing obesity and diabetes is especially difficult because it involves not just interrupting a standard pathologic pathway, but requires changing human behavior. Furthermore, those people whose behavior needs most to be changed may be programmed through their genome to continue their lifestyle pattern adapted for an environment different from the one they now inhabit.[4,96] Exposure of humans to a plentiful food supply coupled with physical inactivity is a feature of our contemporary civilization and affluence. For many people, this lifestyle represents modernity and privilege. To advocate retreat from such a life is a difficult message to sell. Development of programs that encourage physical activity and dietary changes requires innovation and an understanding of the culture and developmental biology of those whose behavior we are trying to change.

The solution requires a multitude of interventions. It could be that alterations to micronutrient intake will be effective in communities with high rates of vegetarianism,[23] and that treatment with leptin or a similar compound may alter the propensity to disease in some at risk.[8] We know already that rigorous control of blood glucose levels in women with gestational diabetes is vital for the future health of the offspring. Others have called for a declaration of war on physical inactivity.[3] Perhaps we need to start by admitting that we humans are not as adaptable to a changing environment as we may once have presumed. Our challenges now are to expand our research efforts and to ensure the science benefits from involvement of the many disciplines in health care and the community that together may make a difference. Inherent in the solution is a clear understanding that the future health of our community requires that we not only treat established illnesses, but we also put greater attention on preventing disease at its origins.

REFERENCES

1. Wild S, Roglic G, Green A, et al. Global prevalence of diabetes: estimates for the year 2000 and projections for 2030. Diabetes Care 2004;27:1047–53.
2. Booth ML, Chey T, Wake M, et al. Change in the prevalence of overweight and obesity among young Australians, 1969–1997. Am J Clin Nutr 2003;77:29–36.
3. Booth FW, Gordon SE, Carlson CJ, et al. Waging war on modern chronic diseases: primary prevention through exercise biology. J Appl Physiol 2000;88: 774–87.
4. Gluckman PD, Lillycrop KA, Vickers MH, et al. Metabolic plasticity during mammalian development is directionally dependent on early nutritional status. Proc Natl Acad Sci U S A 2007;104:12796–800.
5. Gluckman PD, Hanson MA. Developmental origins of health and disease. Cambridge (UK): Cambridge University Press; 2006.
6. Hales CN, Barker DJ. Type 2 (non-insulin-dependent) diabetes mellitus: the thrifty phenotype hypothesis. Diabetologia 1992;35:595–601.
7. Gluckman PD, Hanson MA. The fetal matrix. Cambridge (UK): Cambridge University Press; 2005.
8. Vickers MH. Developmental programming and adult obesity: the role of leptin. Curr Opin Endocrinol Diabetes Obes 2007;14:17–22.
9. Hales CN, Ozanne SE. The dangerous road of catch-up growth. J Physiol 2003; 547:5–10.

10. Ozanne SE, Nicholas Hales C. Poor fetal growth followed by rapid postnatal catch-up growth leads to premature death. Mech Ageing Dev 2005;126:852–4.
11. Thompson NM, Norman AM, Donkin SS, et al. Prenatal and postnatal pathways to obesity: different underlying mechanisms, different metabolic outcomes. Endocrinology 2007;148:2345–54.
12. Barker D. Fetal and infant origins of adult disease. London: British Medical Journal; 1992.
13. Vickers MH, Breier BH, Cutfield WS, et al. Fetal origins of hyperphagia, obesity, and hypertension and postnatal amplification by hypercaloric nutrition. Am J Physiol Endocrinol Metab 2000;279:E83–7.
14. Vickers MH, Breier BH, McCarthy D, et al. Sedentary behavior during postnatal life is determined by the prenatal environment and exacerbated by postnatal hypercaloric nutrition. Am J Physiol Regul Integr Comp Physiol 2003;285:R271–3.
15. Law M, Wald N. Why heart disease mortality is low in France: the time lag explanation. BMJ 1999;318:1471–6.
16. Frankel EN, Kanner J, German JB, et al. Inhibition of oxidation of human low-density lipoprotein by phenolic substances in red wine. Lancet 1993;341: 454–7.
17. Barker DJ. Why heart disease mortality is low in France. Commentary: intrauterine nutrition may be important. BMJ 1999;318:1477–8.
18. Dwork D. War is good for babies and other young children. London: Tavistock Publications; 1987.
19. Kramer M. WITHDRAWN: Nutritional advice in pregnancy. Cochrane Database Syst Rev 2007;18(4):CD000149.
20. Kramer M. WITHDRAWN: High protein supplementation in pregnancy. Cochrane Database Syst Rev 2007;18(4):CD000105.
21. Kramer M. WITHDRAWN: Isocaloric protein supplementation in pregnancy. Cochrane Database Syst Rev 2007;18(4):CD000118.
22. Bavdekar A, Yajnik CS, Fall CH, et al. Insulin resistance syndrome in 8-year-old Indian children: small at birth, big at 8 years, or both? Diabetes 1999;48: 2422–9.
23. Yajnik CS, Deshpande SS, Jackson AA, et al. Vitamin B(12) and folate concentrations during pregnancy and insulin resistance in the offspring: the Pune Maternal Nutrition Study. Diabetologia 2008;51:29–38.
24. Yajnik CS. The insulin resistance epidemic in India: fetal origins, later lifestyle, or both? Nutr Rev 2001;59:1–9.
25. Rao S, Kanade A, Margetts BM, et al. Maternal activity in relation to birth size in rural India. The Pune Maternal Nutrition Study. Eur J Clin Nutr 2003;57:531–42.
26. Yudkin JS. Non-insulin-dependent diabetes mellitus (NIDDM) in Asians in the UK. Diabet Med 1996;13:S16–8.
27. Watve MG, Yajnik CS. Evolutionary origins of insulin resistance: a behavioral switch hypothesis. BMC Evol Biol 2007;7:61.
28. Vaz M, Ukyab TT, Padmavathi R, et al. Body fat topography in Indian and Tibetan males of low and normal body mass index. Indian J Physiol Pharmacol 1999;43: 179–85.
29. Hara H, Egusa G, Yamakido M. Incidence of non-insulin-dependent diabetes mellitus and its risk factors in Japanese-Americans living in Hawaii and Los Angeles. Diabet Med 1996;13:S133–42.
30. Eriksson JG, Lindi V, Uusitupa M, et al. The effects of the Pro12Ala polymorphism of the peroxisome proliferator-activated receptor-gamma2 gene on insulin sensitivity and insulin metabolism interact with size at birth. Diabetes 2002;51:2321–4.

31. Laakso M. Gene variants, insulin resistance, and dyslipidaemia. Curr Opin Lipidol 2004;15:115–20.
32. Yliharsila H, Eriksson JG, Forsen T, et al. Interactions between peroxisome proliferator-activated receptor-gamma 2 gene polymorphisms and size at birth on blood pressure and the use of antihypertensive medication. J Hypertens 2004; 22:1283–7.
33. Pihlajamaki J, Vanhala M, Vanhala P, et al. The Pro12Ala polymorphism of the PPAR gamma 2 gene regulates weight from birth to adulthood. Obes Res 2004;12:187–90.
34. Eriksson JG, Forsen TJ, Osmond C, et al. Pathways of infant and childhood growth that lead to type 2 diabetes. Diabetes Care 2003;26:3006–10.
35. Rosmond R. Association studies of genetic polymorphisms in central obesity: a critical review. Int J Obes Relat Metab Disord 2003;27:1141–51.
36. Wust S, Van Rossum EF, Federenko IS, et al. Common polymorphisms in the glucocorticoid receptor gene are associated with adrenocortical responses to psychosocial stress. J Clin Endocrinol Metab 2004;89:565–73.
37. Di Blasio AM, van Rossum EF, Maestrini S, et al. The relation between two polymorphisms in the glucocorticoid receptor gene and body mass index, blood pressure and cholesterol in obese patients. Clin Endocrinol (Oxf) 2003;59: 68–74.
38. Rautanen A, Eriksson JG, Kere J, et al. Associations of body size at birth with late-life cortisol concentrations and glucose tolerance are modified by haplotypes of the glucocorticoid receptor gene. J Clin Endocrinol Metab 2006;91: 4544–51.
39. Champoux M, Bennett A, Shannon C, et al. Serotonin transporter gene polymorphism, differential early rearing, and behavior in rhesus monkey neonates. Mol Psychiatry 2002;7:1058–63.
40. Arbelle S, Benjamin J, Golin M, et al. Relation of shyness in grade school children to the genotype for the long form of the serotonin transporter promoter region polymorphism. Am J Psychiatry 2003;160:671–6.
41. Mager U, Lindi V, Lindstrom J, et al. Association of the Leu72Met polymorphism of the ghrelin gene with the risk of type 2 diabetes in subjects with impaired glucose tolerance in the Finnish Diabetes Prevention Study. Diabet Med 2006; 23:685–9.
42. Waterland RA, Dolinoy DC, Lin JR, et al. Maternal methyl supplements increase offspring DNA methylation at Axin Fused. Genesis 2006;44:401–6.
43. Weaver IC, Cervoni N, Champagne FA, et al. Epigenetic programming by maternal behavior. Nat Neurosci 2004;7:847–54.
44. Herceg Z. Epigenetics and cancer: towards an evaluation of the impact of environmental and dietary factors. Mutagenesis 2007;22:91–103.
45. Bertram C, Khan O, Ohri S, et al. Transgenerational effects of prenatal nutrient restriction on cardiovascular and hypothalamic-pituitary-adrenal function. J Physiol 2008;586:2217–29.
46. Waterland RA. Do maternal methyl supplements in mice affect DNA methylation of offspring? J Nutr 2003;133(1):238 [author reply 239].
47. Lillycrop KA, Phillips ES, Jackson AA, et al. Dietary protein restriction of pregnant rats induces and folic acid supplementation prevents epigenetic modification of hepatic gene expression in the offspring. J Nutr 2005;135:1382–6.
48. Dolinoy DC, Weidman JR, Waterland RA, et al. Maternal genistein alters coat color and protects Avy mouse offspring from obesity by modifying the fetal epigenome. Environ Health Perspect 2006;114:567–72.

49. Alikhani-Koopaei R, Fouladkou F, Frey FJ, et al. Epigenetic regulation of 11 beta-hydroxysteroid dehydrogenase type 2 expression. J Clin Invest 2004;114: 1146–57.
50. Friso S, Choi SW, Girelli D, et al. A common mutation in the 5,10-methylenetetrahydrofolate reductase gene affects genomic DNA methylation through an interaction with folate status. Proc Natl Acad Sci U S A 2002;99:5606–11.
51. Mathers JC. Reversal of DNA hypomethylation by folic acid supplements: possible role in colorectal cancer prevention. Gut 2005;54:579–81.
52. Weaver IC, Meaney MJ, Szyf M. Maternal care effects on the hippocampal transcriptome and anxiety-mediated behaviors in the offspring that are reversible in adulthood. Proc Natl Acad Sci U S A 2006;103:3480–5.
53. Silverman BL, Metzger BE, Cho NH, et al. Impaired glucose tolerance in adolescent offspring of diabetic mothers. Relationship to fetal hyperinsulinism. Diabetes Care 1995;18:611–7.
54. McCance DR, Pettitt DJ, Hanson RL, et al. Birth weight and non-insulin dependent diabetes: thrifty genotype, thrifty phenotype, or surviving small baby genotype? BMJ 1994;308:942–5.
55. Wei JN, Sung FC, Li CY, et al. Low birth weight and high birth weight infants are both at an increased risk to have type 2 diabetes among schoolchildren in Taiwan. Diabetes Care 2003;26:343–8.
56. Huang RC, Burke V, Newnham JP, et al. Perinatal and childhood origins of cardiovascular disease. Int J Obes (Lond) 2007;31:236–44.
57. Newnham JP, Evans SF, Michael CA, et al. Effects of frequent ultrasound during pregnancy: a randomised controlled trial. Lancet 1993;342:887–91.
58. Yajnik CS, Fall CH, Coyaji KJ, et al. Neonatal anthropometry: the thin-fat Indian baby. The Pune Maternal Nutrition Study. Int J Obes Relat Metab Disord 2003; 27:173–80.
59. Gartner LM, Morton J, Lawrence RA, et al. Breastfeeding and the use of human milk. Pediatrics 2005;115:496–506.
60. Arenz S, Ruckerl R, Koletzko B, et al. Breast-feeding and childhood obesity—a systematic review. Int J Obes Relat Metab Disord 2004;28:1247–56.
61. Gillman MW, Rifas-Shiman SL, Camargo CA Jr, et al. Risk of overweight among adolescents who were breastfed as infants. JAMA 2001;285:2461–7.
62. Burke V, Beilin LJ, Simmer K, et al. Breastfeeding and overweight: longitudinal analysis in an Australian birth cohort. J Pediatr 2005;147:56–61.
63. Plagemann A, Harder T, Franke K, et al. Long-term impact of neonatal breastfeeding on body weight and glucose tolerance in children of diabetic mothers. Diabetes Care 2002;25:16–22.
64. Jovanovic-Peterson L, Fuhrmann K, Hedden K, et al. Maternal milk and plasma glucose and insulin levels: studies in normal and diabetic subjects. J Am Coll Nutr 1989;8:125–31.
65. O'Dowd R, Kent JC, Moseley JM, et al. Effects of uteroplacental insufficiency and reducing litter size on maternal mammary function and postnatal offspring growth. Am J Physiol Regul Integr Comp Physiol 2008;294:R539–48.
66. Wlodek ME, Mibus A, Tan A, et al. Normal lactational environment restores nephron endowment and prevents hypertension after placental restriction in the rat. J Am Soc Nephrol 2007;18:1688–96.
67. Liggins GC, Howie RN. A controlled trial of antepartum glucocorticoid treatment for prevention of the respiratory distress syndrome in premature infants. Pediatrics 1972;50:515–25.

68. Henderson JJ, Hartmann PE, Newnham JP, et al. Effect of preterm birth and antenatal corticosteroid treatment on lactogenesis II in women. Pediatrics 2008;121: e92–100.
69. Brown WJ, Burton NW, Rowan PJ. Updating the evidence on physical activity and health in women. Am J Prev Med 2007;33:404–11.
70. Kavookjian J, Elswick BM, Whetsel T. Interventions for being active among individuals with diabetes: a systematic review of the literature. Diabetes Educ 2007;33:962–88 [discussion: 989–90].
71. Dempsey JC, Butler CL, Williams MA. No need for a pregnant pause: physical activity may reduce the occurrence of gestational diabetes mellitus and preeclampsia. Exerc Sport Sci Rev 2005;33:141–9.
72. Clapp JF 3rd, Little KD. Effect of recreational exercise on pregnancy weight gain and subcutaneous fat deposition. Med Sci Sports Exerc 1995;27:170–7.
73. Lederman RP. Treatment strategies for anxiety, stress, and developmental conflict during reproduction. Behav Med 1995;21:113–22.
74. Clapp JF 3rd. Morphometric and neurodevelopmental outcome at age five years of the offspring of women who continued to exercise regularly throughout pregnancy. J Pediatr 1996;129:856–63.
75. Breier BH, Vickers MH, Ikenasio BA, et al. Fetal programming of appetite and obesity. Mol Cell Endocrinol 2001;185:73–9.
76. Lynch AM, McDonald S, Magann EF, et al. Effectiveness and safety of a structured swimming program in previously sedentary women during pregnancy. J Matern Fetal Neonatal Med 2003;14:163–9.
77. Roseboom TJ, van der Meulen JH, Ravelli AC, et al. Effects of prenatal exposure to the Dutch famine on adult disease in later life: an overview. Twin Res 2001;4: 293–8.
78. Berkowitz GS, Wolff MS, Janevic TM, et al. The World Trade Center disaster and intrauterine growth restriction. JAMA 2003;290:595–6.
79. Yehuda R, Engel SM, Brand SR, et al. Transgenerational effects of posttraumatic stress disorder in babies of mothers exposed to the World Trade Center attacks during pregnancy. J Clin Endocrinol Metab 2005;90:4115–8.
80. Laplante DP, Barr RG, Brunet A, et al. Stress during pregnancy affects general intellectual and language functioning in human toddlers. Pediatr Res 2004;56: 400–10.
81. O'Connor TG, Heron J, Glover V, Alspac Study Team. Antenatal anxiety predicts child behavioural/emotional problems independently of postnatal depression. J Am Acad Child Adolesc Psychiatry 2002;41:1470–7.
82. Talge NM, Neal C, Glover V. Antenatal maternal stress and long-term effects on child neurodevelopment: how and why? J Child Psychol Psychiatry 2007;48: 245–61.
83. Van den Bergh BR, Mennes M, Oosterlaan J, et al. High antenatal maternal anxiety is related to impulsivity during performance on cognitive tasks in 14- and 15-year-olds. Neurosci Biobehav Rev 2005;29:259–69.
84. Van den Bergh BR, Mulder EJ, Mennes M, et al. Antenatal maternal anxiety and stress and the neurobehavioural development of the fetus and child: links and possible mechanisms. A review. Neurosci Biobehav Rev 2005;29: 237–58.
85. Sloboda DM, Challis JR, Moss TJ, et al. Synthetic glucocorticoids: antenatal administration and long-term implications. Curr Pharm Des 2005;11: 1459–72.

86. Ikegami M, Jobe AH, Newnham J, et al. Repetitive prenatal glucocorticoids improve lung function and decrease growth in preterm lambs. Am J Respir Crit Care Med 1997;156:178–84.
87. Moss TJ, Doherty DA, Nitsos I, et al. Effects into adulthood of single or repeated antenatal corticosteroids in sheep. Am J Obstet Gynecol 2005;192:146–52.
88. Dunlop SA, Archer MA, Quinlivan JA, et al. Repeated prenatal corticosteroids delay myelination in the ovine central nervous system. J Matern Fetal Med 1997;6:309–13.
89. Sloboda DM, Moss T, Nitsos I, et al. Antenatal glucocorticoid treatment in sheep results in adrenal suppression in adulthood. J Soc Gynecol Investig 2003;10: 435.
90. Sloboda DM, Moss TJ, Gurrin LC, et al. The effect of prenatal betamethasone administration on postnatal ovine hypothalamic-pituitary-adrenal function. J Endocrinol 2002;172:71–81.
91. Sloboda DM, Moss TJ, Li S, et al. Hepatic glucose regulation and metabolism in adult sheep: effects of prenatal betamethasone. Am J Physiol Endocrinol Metab 2005;289:E721–8.
92. Sloboda DM, Newnham JP, Challis JR. Effects of repeated maternal betamethasone administration on growth and hypothalamic-pituitary-adrenal function of the ovine fetus at term. J Endocrinol 2000;165:79–91.
93. Sloboda DM, Newnham JP, Challis JR. Repeated maternal glucocorticoid administration and the developing liver in fetal sheep. J Endocrinol 2002;175:535–43.
94. Sloboda DM, Moss TJ, Li S, et al. Prenatal betamethasone exposure results in pituitary-adrenal hyporesponsiveness in adult sheep. Am J Physiol Endocrinol Metab 2007;292:E61–70.
95. French NP, Hagan R, Evans SF, et al. Repeated antenatal corticosteroids: effects on cerebral palsy and childhood behavior. Am J Obstet Gynecol 2004;190: 588–95.
96. Gluckman PD, Hanson MA. Developmental origins of disease paradigm: a mechanistic and evolutionary perspective. Pediatr Res 2004;56:311–7.

Gender Differences in Lipid Metabolism and the Effect of Obesity

Faidon Magkos, PhD[a,b], Bettina Mittendorfer, MS, PhD[a,*]

KEYWORDS

- Fatty acid • Triglyceride • Substrate flux • Lipolysis
- Lipoprotein

Until recently, it was assumed that gender differences in physiology and metabolism do not occur, or are not relevant beyond the reproductive system. However, there is growing scientific evidence for sexual dimorphism in physiology and metabolism, which likely has important implications for developing new approaches to prevention, diagnosis, and treatment. Indeed, we now know that there are gender differences in the pathophysiology, diagnosis, prognosis, treatment, and prevention of a wide spectrum of diseases and organ dysfunctions, not limited to those typically considered to affect either men or women only (eg, those affecting the prostate or mammary glands). To discover the nature and extent of fundamental biologic differences in metabolism between men and women is a difficult task. Aside from ovarian cyclicity and menopause, there are numerous factors (eg, body composition, regional fat distribution, aerobic fitness, and so forth, all of which are known to affect substrate metabolism in persons of the same gender) that might complicate the interpretation of the results. Therefore, there are two general approaches when evaluating differences in substrate metabolism between males and females. One, which is clinically probably the most relevant, is to accept the differences in phenotype between men and women and acknowledge that the observed differences in metabolism may be secondary to those characteristics. The other strives to eliminate as many as practically feasible potentially confounding variables to determine if gender per se (ie, sexual genotype) affects the control of metabolism. The aim of this article is to review the literature regarding gender differences in human lipid metabolism and how obesity affects lipid metabolism in men and women. The authors present the major findings on differences in free fatty acid (FFA) and very low-density lipoprotein (VLDL) triglyceride, and apolipoprotein B-100 (apoB-100) metabolism between lean and obese men and women,

[a] Center for Human Nutrition, Division of Geriatrics & Nutritional Science, Washington University School of Medicine, 660 South Euclid Avenue, St. Louis, MO 63110, USA
[b] Department of Nutrition and Dietetics, Harokopio University, 70 El. Venizelou Avenue, Kallithea, Athens 17671, Greece
* Corresponding author.
E-mail address: mittendb@dom.wustl.edu (B. Mittendorfer).

Obstet Gynecol Clin N Am 36 (2009) 245–265
doi:10.1016/j.ogc.2009.03.001
obgyn.theclinics.com

predominantly in the basal, overnight-fasted state, as well as in response to physiologic challenges that affect lipid metabolism, such as prolonged fasting and exercise, food intake and conditions that mimic the postprandial state (hyperinsulinemia-hyperglycemia), and weight loss. The majority of data presented was drawn from studies that relied on tracer techniques to evaluate lipid transport and utilization in the body.[1] Reference to women in the following sections refers to premenopausal women unless specifically pointed out otherwise.

EFFECTS OF GENDER AND OBESITY ON FATTY ACID AND TRIGLYCERIDE METABOLISM IN THE POSTABSORPTIVE STATE

Circulating FFAs, which are mainly derived from the breakdown of endogenous triglyceride stored in adipose tissue, are an important source of fuel. FFA release from adipose tissue is well regulated by the coordinated action of many endocrine, paracrine, and other factors,[2,3] allowing appropriate availability of FFA to meet the energy requirements of tissues. FFA release in excess of metabolic demand leads to elevated plasma FFA availability, which is thought to be responsible for many of the metabolic abnormalities associated with obesity, including hypertriglyceridemia and insulin resistance.[4,5]

In the postabsorptive state (ie, after an overnight fast), the rate of FFA release (rate of appearance or Ra) into the circulation at the whole-body level (in μmol/min) is not different between men and women matched for body mass index (BMI), whether lean or obese.[6–11] However, this comparison, although often made, does not take into account differences in body size between men and women. In fact, FFA release relative to lean mass (in μmol/kg fat-free mass × min)—an index of FFA released into plasma in relationship to the tissues that consume FFA for use as a fuel (eg, skeletal muscle) or for other purposes (eg, synthesis of triglyceride in the liver)—is greater in women than men, whereas FFA release relative to the size of adipose tissue (in μmol/kg fat mass × min)—an index of FFA released into plasma with respect to the size of endogenous fat stores—is less in women than men.[6–12] The authors have recently found that the differences in FFA release between men and women present in lean, overweight, and obese individuals and are largely a result of differences in fat mass between men and women.[12] Specifically, the authors found that total FFA Ra increased linearly with increasing fat mass and there were no differences between men and women in the relationship between fat mass and total FFA Ra.[12] Consequently, FFA Ra in relationship to fat-free mass is greater in obese than lean subjects (both men and women) and greater in women than in men.[12–15] Very similar observations have been made for FFA Ra in relation to resting energy expenditure (greater in women than in men),[9,16] most likely because of the close relationship between resting energy expenditure and fat-free mass.[9,17] Despite the considerable lipolytic heterogeneity between different adipose tissue regions (eg, FFA release from upper-body adipose tissue is greater than that from lower-body adipose tissue) and the different patterns of fat storage in the body between genders, there are no major differences between men and women in the contribution of leg (lower-body), splanchnic, and upper-body nonsplanchnic subcutaneous adipose tissue beds to whole-body FFA Ra.[6,8,10,18,19] Increased release of FFA in obese compared with lean subjects (regardless of gender) is predominantly because of increased FFA release rates from splanchnic and lower-body (leg) adipose tissues (approximately two to three times higher in obese than lean subjects), but not from upper-body nonsplanchnic adipose tissue.[10]

In summary, FFA release into plasma appears to be tightly associated with energy requirements of lean tissues; however, for any given amount of fat-free tissues or energy expenditure, plasma FFA availability is greater in women than in men and in obese than lean subjects because women and obese subjects have more body fat than men and lean subjects, respectively.

The majority (50%–70%) of plasma triglyceride in the fasting state circulates in the core of VLDLs,[20–22] which are produced and secreted by the liver, thereby providing energy-dense substrates to peripheral tissues, while at the same time buffering excess amounts of plasma FFA that would otherwise be cytotoxic.[23] VLDL is assembled in hepatocytes in a two-step process that involves the partial lipidation of a newly synthesized apoB-100 molecule and the fusion of this small and dense precursor with a large triglyceride droplet to form mature VLDL.[24] Each VLDL contains a single molecule of apoB-100, which is an essential structural component and does not participate in the subsequent intravascular remodeling of the lipoprotein particle, whereas the availability of core triglyceride varies considerably and determines the size and possibly also the metabolic fate of VLDL.[25] Fatty acids used for hepatic triglyceride synthesis originate primarily from the systemic plasma FFA pool, as well as from several other, nonsystemic fatty acid sources, such as hepatic de novo lipogenesis, and lipolysis of intrahepatic and visceral fat triglyceride.[26] Dysregulation of VLDL metabolism can lead to increased plasma VLDL-triglyceride concentration, greater number of circulating VLDL particles (ie, VLDL-apoB-100 concentration), and large, triglyceride-rich VLDL, all of which are associated with increased risk for cardiovascular disease.[27–29]

It is well-known that obese compared with lean subjects,[30,31] and men compared with women,[32–34] have greater fasting plasma concentrations of total triglyceride and apoB-100 and greater concentrations of VLDL-triglyceride and VLDL-apoB-100.[20,21,35,36] The first studies examining the mechanisms responsible for differences in plasma triglyceride concentration between men and women indicated that lower plasma triglyceride concentrations in women as opposed to men are a result of increased efficiency of plasma triglyceride removal from the circulation in women.[37,38] Similarly, it was later reported that VLDL-apoB-100 removal efficiency is greater in women than in men.[39,40] The authors have recently examined differences between lean men and lean women in basal plasma VLDL-triglyceride kinetics,[7,41] and found that the plasma clearance rate of VLDL-triglyceride is much greater in women than in men; however, the secretion rate of VLDL-triglyceride from the liver is also greater in women than in men. Thus, the more efficient removal of VLDL-triglyceride in women offsets their greater secretion rates and maintains lower plasma VLDL-triglyceride concentrations.

In contrast, it has been found that the lower plasma VLDL-apoB-100 concentrations (ie, fewer VLDL particles) in lean women than in lean men is caused by a reduced hepatic secretion rate of VLDL-apoB-100 combined with shorter VLDL-apoB-100 residence time in the circulation in women when compared with men.[7] By analyzing the relationship between VLDL-triglyceride and VLDL-apoB-100 secretion, the authors observed that newly secreted VLDL particles in women are more triglyceride-rich than those in men.[7] Secretion of fewer but more triglyceride-rich VLDL is likely responsible, at least in part, for the more efficient removal of VLDL-triglyceride and apoB-100 in women,[7,37,38,41] because evidence from several in vivo studies in humans[7,42] and animals[43,44] suggests that the removal of triglyceride from the core of triglyceride-rich, large VLDL particles is more efficient than that from triglyceride-poor, small VLDL, possibly because increasing triglyceride content (and size) of lipoprotein particles enhances their susceptibility to hydrolysis by lipoprotein lipase.[45,46]

Until recently, hypertriglyceridemia in obese subjects was considered to be the result of increased hepatic triglyceride[47–51] and VLDL-apoB-100[47,49,50,52,53] secretion rates, with no major differences in respective removal rates (fractional turnover rates or plasma clearance rates). However, most of these studies were conducted in men[47,49,51–53] or in small groups of men and women,[39,49,50] which made it difficult if not impossible to detect differences between genders, if they existed. Only one study examined men and women separately and found increased VLDL-triglyceride secretion in obese men but not in obese women.[54] The authors have recently confirmed this phenomenon[41] and found that obesity is associated with increased hepatic secretion rates of VLDL-triglyceride and VLDL-apoB-100 in men but not in women, and with decreased plasma clearance rates of VLDL-triglyceride and VLDL-apoB-100 in women but not in men (B. Mittendorfer and colleagues, unpublished observations). Furthermore, the authors found that intra abdominal fat mass is an important regulator of hepatic VLDL-triglyceride secretion, presumably through the availability of nonsystemic fatty acids derived from lipolysis of intra abdominal and intrahepatic fat for VLDL-triglyceride production (B. Mittendorfer and colleagues, unpublished observations). This is consistent with the observation that the contribution from nonsystemic plasma FFA to total VLDL-triglyceride secretion is greater in obese compared with lean men and women,[14,55] indicating that a significant proportion of VLDL-triglyceride secreted by the liver in obesity is derived from fatty acids from lipolysis of visceral and intrahepatic fat and de novo lipogenesis in the liver. Furthermore, Gormsen and colleagues[56] recently reported that intra abdominal fat accumulation—but not obesity per se—is associated with increased VLDL-triglyceride secretion rates in women.

EFFECTS OF GENDER AND OBESITY ON FATTY ACID METABOLISM IN RESPONSE TO LIPOLYTIC AND ANTILIPOLYTIC STIMULI

Exercise and fasting are the most potent physiologic lipolytic stimuli. The initial response to fasting is characterized by a decrease in plasma insulin and glucose concentrations, and an increase in plasma catecholamine, glucagon, and FFA concentrations, as well as a shift toward fat as opposed to carbohydrate oxidation.[57] The available evidence indicates that adipose tissue lipolysis in women and lean subjects, compared to men and obese subjects, respectively, is more responsive to physiologic stimuli favoring FFA mobilization during conditions of metabolic stress (prolonged fasting and exercise); furthermore, FFA mobilization returns to baseline values more readily in women than men and in lean than obese subjects after removal of the lipolytic stimulus (ie, termination of exercise or administration of insulin after prolonged fasting). For example, the increase in glycerol and FFA Ra during the transition from overnight fasting conditions to prolonged (22 hour) fasting are reported to be greater in women than men[58] and less in obese than lean[59] subjects. Similarly, the relative increase in FFA Ra and glycerol Ra in plasma during moderate-intensity endurance exercise is greater in women than in men[60–62] and in lean than obese subjects,[63,64] whereas increased postexercise lipolysis rates and plasma FFA concentrations are not observed or return to baseline more readily in women than in men[65–67] and in lean than obese subjects.[68–70] The mechanisms responsible for sexual dimorphism in the stimulation of FFA release are unknown.

Insulin is probably the most potent physiologic inhibitor of adipose tissue lipolysis and FFA release into the circulation.[71–73] Despite a lot of studies, it is unclear whether the insulin-mediated suppression of FFA release is different in men and women. Some studies suggest that the suppression of plasma FFA concentration following a standard oral glucose load or mixed meal is greater in women than in men.[18,74–77] This gender difference was attributed to a more insulin-resistant upper-body subcutaneous adipose tissue in men as opposed to women.[18] Some investigators, however, failed to observe a consistently greater meal-induced suppression of plasma FFA concentration in nonobese women than men,[78] whereas others found that the fatty acid composition of the meal affected the response differently in men and women.[79,80] Recently, a large group of lean, overweight, and obese men and women was studied, and no differences between the genders in insulin-induced suppression of plasma FFA concentrations and whole-body FFA flux rates were found.[16] A lot of the discrepancy might be because of the degree of hyperinsulinemia. FFA Ra is very sensitive to insulin and almost completely suppressed at low postprandial insulin concentrations; although there might be differences between men and women in the sensitivity of FFA Ra to insulin, the maximal response (ie, the degree of suppression at relatively high plasma insulin concentrations) appears to be comparable in men and women.[16,76,81–84] Unfortunately, dose-response studies performed in men and women simultaneously are missing.

Obesity is associated with reduced sensitivity of adipose tissue to the effects of insulin,[15,16] and there is evidence, for reasons that are not entirely clear, that this effect is more pronounced in men than in women.[75,77] The differences appear to manifest only in response to insulin concentrations that result in submaximal suppression of FFA Ra and are absent at higher plasma insulin availability.[56,75,85–88]

EFFECT OF GENDER AND OBESITY ON PLASMA TRIGLYCERIDE METABOLISM IN RESPONSE TO EXERCISE, MEALS, AND INSULIN

The plasma triglyceride-lowering potential of exercise was first recognized some 40 years ago. The authors[89] and others[90–93] have shown that exercise reduces plasma triglyceride concentration through greater VLDL-triglyceride removal from the circulation. Few studies have contrasted the effects of exercise on plasma triglyceride concentration and metabolism in men and women. To date, there is no evidence that the response is different in men and women or lean and obese subjects.[94,95] However, the available data is limited and further investigations in this area are needed to draw firm conclusions.

Postprandial triglyceride metabolism is characterized by an increase in total plasma triglyceride concentration in response to dietary fat intake, which is predominately a result of the entry of triglyceride-rich chylomicrons in the circulation, with no major changes in the concentration of VLDL particles.[96] The postprandial rise in plasma triglyceride concentration is directly related to the fat content of the meal,[97] is influenced by the type of dietary fat,[98,99] prior diet,[100] and physical activity,[101] and is significantly attenuated by simultaneous consumption of carbohydrate.[102] The difference in plasma triglyceride concentration after a fatty meal with and without carbohydrate is because of reduced VLDL concentration,[103] probably as a result of the carbohydrate-induced rise in plasma insulin concentration. Insulin inhibits hepatic VLDL-triglyceride and VLDL-apoB-100 production.[86,104,105] The insulin-mediated reduction of plasma FFA availability is only partly responsible for the inhibitory effect of insulin on hepatic VLDL-triglyceride secretion, but appears to fully account for its inhibitory effect on VLDL-apoB-100 secretion.[106]

Women exhibit significantly lower postprandial triglyceride responses following ingestion of high-fat meals that are adjusted with regard to their energy content to subjects' body size (ie, when the test meal is allocated per kg of body weight).[18,19,78,107–109] This is most likely because of enhanced postprandial clearance of triglyceride-rich particles in women when compared with men,[40,110] much like the lower basal plasma triglyceride concentrations in women are because of increased

VLDL-triglyceride clearance.[7,37,38,41] Obesity, on the other hand, is associated with considerably greater postprandial plasma triglyceride concentrations because of both intestinal (chylomicrons) and hepatic (VLDL) triglyceride-rich lipoproteins in both men and women.[111–118] Results from studies measuring plasma triglyceride concentrations in response to insulin and glucose alone are conflicting. A reduction after an oral glucose load in women but not in men (mixed groups of lean, overweight, and obese),[74] a reduction of similar magnitude in both genders (nonobese) in response to glucose-induced hyperinsulinemia,[119] and no changes in either gender (obese) in response to insulin infusion[83] have been reported. Obesity has been associated with a blunted (but not absent) insulin-mediated reduction in plasma-triglyceride concentration[87] and VLDL concentration[120] in mixed groups of men and women. However, in a recent study no major changes in VLDL-triglyceride concentrations in response to insulin infusion were observed among lean, upper-body obese, and lower-body obese women.[56]

Few studies have examined differences between lean and obese men and women in the effect of insulin on VLDL kinetics, and the results are inconclusive. The authors have reported that moderate hyperinsulinemia induced by glucose infusion reduces hepatic VLDL-triglyceride secretion rate to the same extent in lean men, obese men, and lean women, whereas the insulin-mediated suppression of VLDL-triglyceride secretion was absent in obese women.[84] In another study it was found that hyperinsulinemia achieved via insulin infusion, reduced hepatic VLDL-triglyceride secretion to the same extent in both lean and obese women; however, contrary to lean women, obese women did not experience a decrease in VLDL-apoB-100 secretion.[86]

GENDER DIFFERENCES IN FATTY ACID AND TRIGLYCERIDE METABOLISM IN RESPONSE TO WEIGHT LOSS

Diet-induced moderate weight loss (10%–15% of initial body weight) reduces basal whole-body FFA and glycerol release rates into plasma by 10% to 35%;[14,121] the reduction persists when FFA Ra and glycerol Ra are expressed relative to fat-free mass, but not relative to fat mass.[121] Similar results have been obtained after greater weight loss (20%–30% of initial body weight) induced by calorie restriction or bariatric surgery.[122–124] These findings suggest that reduced-obese men and women have FFA release rates that are appropriate for their new, reduced total body fat mass. However, insulin-mediated suppression of plasma FFA concentrations[88,124] and glycerol Ra relative to fat mass[124] are augmented after weight loss, indicative of enhanced insulin sensitivity of adipose tissue lipolysis. There are no studies evaluating gender differences in lipid metabolism in response to weight loss and comparisons of the responses in men and women are likely complicated by differences in body composition as a result of weight loss. There is evidence that men lose more body weight (both in absolute terms and as a percent of initial body weight) and fat-free mass than women, whether in response to the same energy-reduced diet,[125] the same decrease in energy balance,[126] and bariatric surgery.[127] Men also lose more visceral fat than women during weight loss, in part because they have more visceral fat to begin with.[125,128–130]

Weight loss reduces plasma triglyceride and VLDL-triglyceride concentrations, predominantly by lowering hepatic VLDL-triglyceride secretion rates without affecting or even decreasing plasma VLDL-triglyceride clearance rates.[14,123,131,132] Although no study has directly evaluated the response to weight loss in men and women separately, suppression of hepatic VLDL-triglyceride production after weight loss has been observed in both men[131] and women[14,123] and mixed groups of men and women.[132] The majority of this reduction is because of reduced contribution of nonsystemic fatty acids to VLDL-triglyceride production (ie, fatty acids derived from lipolysis of visceral and liver fat and de novo lipogenesis).[14,123] These findings are in strong agreement with visceral fat being a determinant of VLDL-triglyceride secretion (see above). In addition, weight loss has been associated with a reduction in liver (and muscle) FFA uptake from the systemic circulation,[88,133] which could further limit intrahepatic availability for VLDL-triglyceride synthesis and secretion. On the other hand, weight loss apparently also lowers hepatic VLDL-apoB-100 secretion in men[53,131] but not in women.[14,123] However, direct comparison of men and women by the same investigators in the same study is missing.

EFFECTS OF SEX HORMONES ON FATTY ACID AND TRIGLYCERIDE METABOLISM

Physiologic fluctuations in endogenous sex hormone concentrations, such as those during the normal menstrual cycle in women, have not been associated with any significant changes in basal plasma FFA availability.[134–136] Likewise, in response to hypoinsulinemia, there are no differences in the degree of stimulation of adipose tissue lipolysis between the follicular and luteal phases.[134] These findings are consistent with the absence of differences in ex vivo basal and norepinephrine-stimulated lipolysis from femoral and abdominal subcutaneous adipocytes obtained from healthy women at different phases of the menstrual cycle.[137] Cross-sectional studies also indicate that use of exogenous female sex steroids, whether estrogen alone, progesterone alone, or estrogen and progesterone in combination, is not associated with any major changes in basal plasma FFA concentration and flux rates,[138,139] nor with any differences in glucose-induced suppression and epinephrine-induced stimulation of adipose tissue lipolysis rates.[139] There is only one study where estrogen administration was reported to suppress whole-body FFA Ra;[140] however, the effect was very small (10%–20%) and likely not physiologically important, considering that it falls within the intraindividual day-to-day variability in postabsorptive FFA kinetics (15%–30%).[9,141,142] Taken together, these data suggest that variations in plasma female sex hormone concentrations do not affect systemic plasma FFA availability.

In contrast to FFA metabolism, sex steroids appear to be major regulators of plasma triglyceride and apoB-100 metabolism. It is generally thought that the ovarian steroid hormones estrogen and progesterone have beneficial effects on plasma triglyceride metabolism because premenopausal women have lower plasma triglyceride concentrations than age- and BMI-matched men,[21] and this difference between genders is abolished after menopause.[143] Studies in which hormones were administered to pre- and postmenopausal women to evaluate the effects of various types of hormonal birth control and hormone-replacement therapy, however, indicate that estrogens have adverse and only progestins have beneficial effects on plasma triglyceride concentration. Hormone-replacement therapy providing estrogens alone to postmenopausal women increases fasting plasma triglyceride concentration, whereas progestins administered alone decrease fasting plasma triglyceride concentration;[144–148] and progestins administered in combination with estrogens blunt or completely abolish the increase in plasma triglyceride concentration that occurs when estrogen is given alone.[146,148] Furthermore, estrogen-rich oral contraceptives induce hypertriglyceridemia, whereas those containing both estrogens and progestins do not.[149] Progestins most likely exert their beneficial effect by stimulating plasma triglyceride removal by peripheral tissues to counteract high, estrogen-mediated hepatic triglyceride secretion rates. Estrogens have been found to increase VLDL-triglyceride secretion rate with no effect on triglyceride plasma clearance,[150,151] whereas progestins were found to increase endogenous and exogenous triglyceride removal from plasma without an

Box 1
Summary of the effects of gender and obesity on lipid metabolism

Fatty acid metabolism in the postabsorptive state

FFA Ra in plasma at the whole-body level is not different between men and women matched for BMI; however, it is greater in women than men relative to fat-free mass and energy requirements, and less in women than men relative to fat mass.

The contribution of leg (lower-body), splanchnic, and upper-body nonsplanchnic subcutaneous adipose tissue beds to whole-body FFA Ra in plasma is not different between men and women, despite the sexually dimorphic pattern of fat storage in the body.

Obese subjects (regardless of gender) have greater FFA Ra than lean subjects, predominantly because of increased FFA release rates from splanchnic and lower-body (leg) adipose tissues, but not from upper-body nonsplanchnic adipose tissue.

Triglyceride metabolism in the postabsorptive state

Lean women have lower plasma VLDL-triglyceride concentrations than lean men because of increased removal efficiency of VLDL-triglyceride from the circulation, which more than offsets their greater hepatic VLDL-triglyceride secretion rate.

Lean women have lower plasma VLDL-apoB-100 concentrations than lean men, because of decreased hepatic secretion of VLDL particles (which are more triglyceride-rich than those in men) and more efficient removal of VLDL particles from the circulation.

Obesity is associated with increased hepatic secretion rates of VLDL-triglyceride and VLDL-apoB-100 in men but not in women, and with decreased plasma clearance rates of VLDL-triglyceride and VLDL-apoB-100 in women but not in men.

Accumulation of intra abdominal fat is strongly related with hepatic VLDL-triglyceride secretion and thus, at least in part, responsible for the increased VLDL-triglyceride secretion rate in obese compared with lean individuals.

Fatty acid metabolism in response to lipolytic (exercise and fasting) and antilipolytic (insulin, glucose, and food intake) stimuli

In response to short-term fasting and exercise, FFA mobilization increases to a greater extent in women than in men and in lean than in obese subjects. Similarly, FFA mobilization rates return to baseline values more readily in women than in men and in lean than in obese subjects.

The suppression of plasma FFA concentrations following a standard oral glucose load or mixed meal is greater in women than in men; however, FFA suppression is not different in men and women in response to insulin infusion (typically low dose). The differences in response are likely because of differences in the extent of hyperinsulinemia during insulin clamp, oral glucose tolerance test, or meals.

Obesity is associated with reduced sensitivity of adipose tissue to the effects of insulin.

Plasma triglyceride metabolism in response to exercise, meals and insulin

There is no data available on the comparative effects of exercise on triglyceride metabolism in men and women or lean and obese subjects.

Women and lean subjects exhibit much lower postprandial plasma triglyceride concentrations after ingestion of a high-fat meal compared with men and obese subjects, respectively.

Studies evaluating VLDL metabolism in response to insulin and glucose infusion in lean and obese men and women yield conflicting results regarding the effects of gender and obesity.

Fatty acid and triglyceride metabolism in response to weight loss

Whole-body FFA Ra in plasma is reduced after weight loss, to an extent that is appropriate for the reduced body-fat mass.

Weight loss improves the sensitivity of adipose tissue lipolysis to the antilipolytic effect of insulin.

There are no studies evaluating gender differences in lipid metabolism in response to weight loss; such comparisons are likely complicated by differences in body composition as a result of weight loss between men and women.

Weight loss reduces plasma triglyceride and VLDL-triglyceride concentrations, predominantly by lowering hepatic VLDL-triglyceride secretion rates in both men and women.

Although a direct comparison of men and women is missing, weight loss apparently lowers hepatic VLDL-apoB-100 secretion in men but not in women.

Sex hormones, fatty acid and triglyceride metabolism

Variations in plasma female sex hormone concentrations, whether physiologic (ie, menstrual cycle) or exogenously induced, do not affect adipose tissue lipolysis and systemic plasma FFA availability.

Oral, but not transdermal, estrogens increase plasma triglyceride concentration because of increased hepatic VLDL-triglyceride secretion rate, whereas progestins oppose the effects of estrogens, most likely by stimulating VLDL-triglyceride clearance.

Normal cyclic variations in endogenous female sex hormone concentrations do not affect VLDL-triglyceride and VLDL-apoB-100 concentrations and kinetics.

The effect of menopause on VLDL metabolism in the postabsorptive state is not known. In the fed state, the removal rate of apoB-100 is lower in postmenopausal women than in young, premenopausal women, with no differences in the respective production rates, while there are no differences between postmenopausal women and age-matched men.

The effect of testosterone on lipid metabolism is not well understood.

effect on triglyceride secretion into plasma.[138,152] Although there is no evidence for progestins having an effect on hepatic triglyceride secretion, studies performed in vitro and in vivo in animals, and in postmenopausal women, indicate that progestins inhibit hepatic apoB-100 synthesis and secretion;[147,153–155] this suggests that progesterone increases the triglyceride content of VLDL secreted by the liver, which in turn may affect intravascular lipolysis of VLDL-triglyceride and VLDL-triglyceride plasma clearance, because larger, triglyceride-rich particles are more susceptible to lipolysis by lipoprotein lipase than smaller particles.[45,156]

The results from studies in which hormones were delivered orally, however, need to be interpreted with caution because of potential confounding by the "hepatic first-pass" effect. Unlike oral estrogen therapy, transdermal estrogen therapy (which more closely reflects the normal physiologic hormone delivery) is not associated with changes in plasma triglyceride concentration or may even reduce it,[148,157,158] most likely because it reduces the amount of estradiol delivered to the liver. In addition, the results from studies in which oral estrogen preparations were used are difficult to interpret because oral (but not transdermal) estradiol has been found to affect the plasma concentration of a variety of hormones that might confound the findings from studies in which oral estrogen preparations were given.[159–161] In contrast, progestins reduce plasma triglyceride concentration even if administered intramuscularly,[145] which supports their action in peripheral tissues and plasma triglyceride clearance rather than triglyceride secretion by the liver. Nonetheless, the authors recently demonstrated that normal physiologic variations in plasma progesterone concentrations in eumenorrheic women has no effect on VLDL-triglyceride metabolism.[136] This could be because of the relatively short progesterone withdrawal in normally menstruating women. It is also possible that normal cyclic variation in female sex steroid concentration is necessary for plasma triglyceride homeostasis and complete absence or disruption of this normal cycle affects plasma triglyceride metabolism and triglyceride concentration adversely. Support for this speculation comes from studies in which plasma triglyceride concentration was measured at regular intervals throughout several menstrual cycles in eumenorrheic women and was found to be remarkably stable,[162–164] whereas exercise-related secondary amenorrhea was found to significantly increase plasma triglyceride concentrations.[165]

The effects of menopause on the physiologic mechanisms that regulate plasma lipid concentrations are incompletely understood, and are often confounded by the concomitant differences in age as well as body composition. Indeed, in studies comparing premenopausal and postmenopausal women of similar age who were matched for BMI or abdominal fat distribution, menopause had little or no effect on fasting plasma and VLDL-triglyceride concentrations.[166–172] There are no studies evaluating VLDL-triglyceride kinetics in postmenopausal women in the basal, postabsorptive state, and only a few studies have evaluated apoB-100 kinetics in triglyceride-rich lipoproteins in the fed state. Results from these studies suggest that the removal rates of apoB-100 in the fed state are lower in postmenopausal women than in young, premenopausal women, with no differences in the respective production rates,[173] while there are no differences between postmenopausal women and age-matched men.[174] Impaired removal of triglyceride-rich lipoproteins may explain the exacerbated postprandial triglyceridemia associated with menopause in women (independently of any effects on fasting plasma triglyceride concentrations), which has been linked to delayed clearance of chylomicrons carrying dietary lipid.[175,176]

The effects of testosterone on plasma triglyceride concentration and metabolism are not entirely clear. Hypogonadal men have higher plasma triglyceride concentrations than eugonadal men,[177–179] and testosterone-replacement therapy normalizes plasma triglyceride concentrations.[177] This suggests that testosterone has hypotriglyceridemic properties. Although other investigators found no or only a marginally significant triglyceride-lowering effect of testosterone replacement,[179–183] some have even observed a further increase in plasma triglyceride concentration after testosterone therapy.[184] This discrepancy is probably because of differences in treatment regimens and study subjects. Also, female-to-male transsexuals experience a marked increase in plasma triglyceride concentration as a result of testosterone therapy.[185,186] However, addition of testosterone to hormone-replacement therapy in oophorectomized women apparently has no effect on plasma triglyceride concentration,[187,188] likely because of the lower dose of testosterone and the small rise in plasma free testosterone concentration, which actually failed to reach statistical significance in one[188] of the two studies.

Few studies have investigated the mechanisms responsible for the effects of testosterone on plasma triglyceride concentration and their results are inconclusive. Studies in vivo in rodents suggest that testosterone reduces plasma triglyceride concentration via increased VLDL-triglyceride clearance rather than reduced hepatic secretion;[189] although this study involved the use of fluoxymesterone, a low-potency synthetic testosterone analogue, which may have masked a potential effect of testosterone on the liver. Furthermore, it was found that VLDL-apoC-III concentration decreased after adding testosterone to oral estradiol-replacement therapy in surgically oophorectomized women,[190] which is in agreement with the increased plasma triglyceride clearance rate after testosterone administration in rodents (apoC-III inhibits VLDL-triglyceride lipolysis by lipoprotein lipase).[189] In vitro,[191] however, low doses of testosterone suppress hepatic triglyceride synthesis, whereas high doses of testosterone suppress it when fatty acid availability is low (<0.5 mM) and increase it when fatty acid availability is increased.

SUMMARY

A summary of the effects of gender and obesity on lipid metabolism is given in **Box 1**. Although differences in lipid metabolism between men and women and lean and obese subjects have been established, the underlying mechanisms are not clear and much remains to be learned.

REFERENCES

1. Magkos F, Mittendorfer B. Stable isotope-labeled tracers for the investigation of fatty acid and triglyceride metabolism in humans in vivo. Clin Lipidol 2009;4(2):215–30.
2. Coppack SW, Jensen MD, Miles JM. In vivo regulation of lipolysis in humans. J Lipid Res 1994;35(2):177–93.
3. Langin D. Control of fatty acid and glycerol release in adipose tissue lipolysis. C R Biol 2006;329(8):598–607.
4. Aguilera CM, Gil-Campos M, Canete R, et al. Alterations in plasma and tissue lipids associated with obesity and metabolic syndrome. Clin Sci (Lond) 2008; 114(3):183–93.
5. Boden G. Obesity and free fatty acids. Endocrinol Metab Clin North Am 2008; 37(3):635–46.
6. Jensen MD, Johnson CM. Contribution of leg and splanchnic free fatty acid (FFA) kinetics to postabsorptive FFA flux in men and women. Metabolism 1996;45(5):662–6.
7. Magkos F, Patterson BW, Mohammed BS, et al. Women produce fewer but triglyceride-richer very low-density lipoproteins than men. J Clin Endocrinol Metab 2007;92(4):1311–8.
8. Jensen MD, Cryer PE, Johnson CM, et al. Effects of epinephrine on regional free fatty acid and energy metabolism in men and women. Am J Physiol 1996;270 (2 Pt 1):E259–64.
9. Nielsen S, Guo Z, Albu JB, et al. Energy expenditure, sex, and endogenous fuel availability in humans. J Clin Invest 2003;111(7):981–8.
10. Nielsen S, Guo Z, Johnson CM, et al. Splanchnic lipolysis in human obesity. J Clin Invest 2004;113(11):1582–8.
11. Gormsen LC, Jensen MD, Schmitz O, et al. Energy expenditure, insulin, and VLDL-triglyceride production in humans. J Lipid Res 2006;47(10):2325–32.
12. Mittendorfer B, Magkos F, Fabbrini E, et al. Relationship between body fat mass and free fatty acid kinetics in men and women. Obesity (Silver Spring), in press.
13. Koutsari C, Jensen MD. Free fatty acid metabolism in human obesity. J Lipid Res 2006;47(8):1643–50.
14. Mittendorfer B, Patterson BW, Klein S. Effect of weight loss on VLDL-triglyceride and apoB-100 kinetics in women with abdominal obesity. Am J Physiol Endocrinol Metab 2003;284(3):E549–56.
15. Groop LC, Bonadonna RC, Simonson DC, et al. Effect of insulin on oxidative and nonoxidative pathways of free fatty acid metabolism in human obesity. Am J Physiol 1992;263(1 Pt 1):E79–84.
16. Shadid S, Kanaley JA, Sheehan MT, et al. Basal and insulin-regulated free fatty acid and glucose metabolism in humans. Am J Physiol Endocrinol Metab 2007; 292(6):E1770–4.
17. Owen OE. Resting metabolic requirements of men and women. Mayo Clin Proc 1988;63(5):503–10.
18. Jensen MD. Gender differences in regional fatty acid metabolism before and after meal ingestion. J Clin Invest 1995;96(5):2297–303.

19. Nguyen TT, Mijares AH, Johnson CM, et al. Postprandial leg and splanchnic fatty acid metabolism in nonobese men and women. Am J Physiol 1996;271(6 Pt 1): E965–72.
20. Carlson LA, Ericsson M. Quantitative and qualitative serum lipoprotein analysis. Part 1. Studies in healthy men and women. Atherosclerosis 1975;21(3):417–33.
21. Wahl PW, Warnick GR, Albers JJ, et al. Distribution of lipoproteins triglyceride and lipoprotein cholesterol in an adult population by age, sex, and hormone use—The Pacific Northwest Bell Telephone Company health survey. Atherosclerosis 1981;39(1):111–24.
22. Walden CE, Wahl PW, Knopp RH, et al. Hyperlipidemia in the Pacific Northwest Bell Telephone Company Health Survey. Part 1. Lipoprotein cholesterol and triglyceride concentrations. Arteriosclerosis 1983;3(2):117–24.
23. Gibbons GF, Wiggins D, Brown AM, et al. Synthesis and function of hepatic very-low-density lipoprotein. Biochem Soc Trans 2004;32(Pt 1):59–64.
24. Shelness GS, Sellers JA. Very-low-density lipoprotein assembly and secretion. Curr Opin Lipidol 2001;12(2):151–7.
25. Gibbons GF, Islam K, Pease RJ. Mobilisation of triacylglycerol stores. Biochim Biophys Acta 2000;1483(1):37–57.
26. Lewis GF. Fatty acid regulation of very low density lipoprotein production. Curr Opin Lipidol 1997;8(3):146–53.
27. Freedman DS, Otvos JD, Jeyarajah EJ, et al. Relation of lipoprotein subclasses as measured by proton nuclear magnetic resonance spectroscopy to coronary artery disease. Arterioscler Thromb Vasc Biol 1998;18(7):1046–53.
28. Hokanson JE, Austin MA. Plasma triglyceride level is a risk factor for cardiovascular disease independent of high-density lipoprotein cholesterol level: a meta-analysis of population-based prospective studies. J Cardiovasc Risk 1996;3(2):213–9.
29. Packard CJ. Understanding coronary heart disease as a consequence of defective regulation of apolipoprotein B metabolism. Curr Opin Lipidol 1999;10(3): 237–44.
30. Chan DC, Barrett HP, Watts GF. Dyslipidemia in visceral obesity: mechanisms, implications, and therapy. Am J Cardiovasc Drugs 2004;4(4):227–46.
31. Goff DC Jr, D'Agostino RB Jr, Haffner SM, et al. Insulin resistance and adiposity influence lipoprotein size and subclass concentrations. Results from the Insulin Resistance Atherosclerosis Study. Metabolism 2005;54(2):264–70.
32. Contois JH, McNamara JR, Lammi-Keefe CJ, et al. Reference intervals for plasma apolipoprotein B determined with a standardized commercial immunoturbidimetric assay: results from the Framingham Offspring Study. Clin Chem 1996;42(4):515–23.
33. Freedman DS, Otvos JD, Jeyarajah EJ, et al. Sex and age differences in lipoprotein subclasses measured by nuclear magnetic resonance spectroscopy: the Framingham Study. Clin Chem 2004;50(7):1189–200.
34. Johnson JL, Slentz CA, Duscha BD, et al. Gender and racial differences in lipoprotein subclass distributions: the STRRIDE study. Atherosclerosis 2004;176(2): 371–7.
35. Magkos F, Mohammed BS, Mittendorfer B. Effect of obesity on the plasma lipoprotein subclass profile in normoglycemic and normolipidemic men and women. Int J Obes (Lond) 2008;32(11):1655–64.
36. Magkos F, Mohammed BS, Mittendorfer B. Plasma lipid transfer enzymes in non-diabetic lean and obese men and women. Lipids, in press.
37. Nikkila EA, Kekki M. Polymorphism of plasma triglyceride kinetics in normal human adult subjects. Acta Med Scand 1971;190(1–2):49–59.

38. Olefsky J, Farquhar JW, Reaven GM. Sex difference in the kinetics of triglyceride metabolism in normal and hypertriglyceridaemic human subjects. Eur J Clin Invest 1974;4(2):121–7.
39. Schaefer JR, Rader DJ, Gregg RE, et al. VLDL apoB-100 and apoE metabolism in male and female subjects utilizing the stable isotope technique. In: Steinmetz A, Schneider J, Kaffarnik H, editors. Hormones in Lipoprotein Metabolism. Berlin: Springer-Verlag; 1993. p. 157–64.
40. Watts GF, Moroz P, Barrett PH. Kinetics of very-low-density lipoprotein apolipoprotein B-100 in normolipidemic subjects: pooled analysis of stable-isotope studies. Metabolism 2000;49(9):1204–10.
41. Mittendorfer B, Patterson BW, Klein S. Effect of sex and obesity on basal VLDL-triacylglycerol kinetics. Am J Clin Nutr 2003;77(3):573–9.
42. Streja D, Kallai MA, Steiner G. The metabolic heterogeneity of human very low density lipoprotein triglyceride. Metabolism 1977;26(12):1333–44.
43. Streja DA. Triglyceride removal from very low density lipoproteins in vivo as a function of their triglyceride content. Atherosclerosis 1979;32(1):57–67.
44. Verschoor L, Chen YD, Reaven EP, et al. Glucose and fructose feeding lead to alterations in structure and function of very low density lipoproteins. Horm Metab Res 1985;17(6):285–8.
45. Fisher RM, Coppack SW, Humphreys SM, et al. Human triacylglycerol-rich lipoprotein subfractions as substrates for lipoprotein lipase. Clin Chim Acta 1995; 236(1):7–17.
46. Karpe F, Bickerton AS, Hodson L, et al. Removal of triacylglycerols from chylomicrons and VLDL by capillary beds: the basis of lipoprotein remnant formation. Biochem Soc Trans 2007;35(Pt 3):472–6.
47. Egusa G, Beltz WF, Grundy SM, et al. Influence of obesity on the metabolism of apolipoprotein B in humans. J Clin Invest 1985;76(2):596–603.
48. Grundy SM, Mok HY, Zech L, et al. Transport of very low density lipoprotein triglycerides in varying degrees of obesity and hypertriglyceridemia. J Clin Invest 1979;63(6):1274–83.
49. Kesaniemi YA, Beltz WF, Grundy SM. Comparisons of metabolism of apolipoprotein B in normal subjects, obese patients, and patients with coronary heart disease. J Clin Invest 1985;76(2):586–95.
50. Kissebah AH, Alfarsi S, Adams PW. Integrated regulation of very low density lipoprotein triglyceride and apolipoprotein-B kinetics in man: normolipemic subjects, familial hypertriglyceridemia and familial combined hyperlipidemia. Metabolism 1981;30(9):856–68.
51. Howard BV, Zech L, Davis M, et al. Studies of very low density lipoprotein triglyceride metabolism in an obese population with low plasma lipids: lack of influence of body weight or plasma insulin. J Lipid Res 1980;21(8):1032–41.
52. Cummings MH, Watts GF, Pal C, et al. Increased hepatic secretion of very-low-density lipoprotein apolipoprotein B-100 in obesity: a stable isotope study. Clin Sci (Lond) 1995;88(2):225–33.
53. Riches FM, Watts GF, Naoumova RP, et al. Hepatic secretion of very-low-density lipoprotein apolipoprotein B-100 studied with a stable isotope technique in men with visceral obesity. Int J Obes Relat Metab Disord 1998;22(5):414–23.
54. Reaven GM, Bernstein RM. Effect of obesity on the relationship between very low density lipoprotein production rate and plasma triglyceride concentration in normal and hypertriglyceridemic subjects. Metabolism 1978;27(9):1047–54.
55. Barter PJ, Nestel PJ. Precursors of plasma triglyceride fatty acids in obesity. Metabolism 1973;22(6):779–83.

56. Gormsen LC, Nellemann B, Sorensen LP, et al. Impact of body composition on very-low-density lipoprotein-triglycerides kinetics. Am J Physiol Endocrinol Metab 2009;296(1):E165–73.
57. Bergman BC, Cornier MA, Horton TJ, et al. Effects of fasting on insulin action and glucose kinetics in lean and obese men and women. Am J Physiol Endocrinol Metab 2007;293(4):E1103–11.
58. Mittendorfer B, Horowitz JF, Klein S. Gender differences in lipid and glucose kinetics during short-term fasting. Am J Physiol Endocrinol Metab 2001; 281(6):E1333–9.
59. Horowitz JF, Coppack SW, Paramore D, et al. Effect of short-term fasting on lipid kinetics in lean and obese women. Am J Physiol 1999;276(2 Pt 1):E278–84.
60. Mittendorfer B, Horowitz JF, Klein S. Effect of gender on lipid kinetics during endurance exercise of moderate intensity in untrained subjects. Am J Physiol Endocrinol Metab 2002;283(1):E58–65.
61. Carter SL, Rennie C, Tarnopolsky MA. Substrate utilization during endurance exercise in men and women after endurance training. Am J Physiol Endocrinol Metab 2001;280(6):E898–907.
62. Moro C, Pillard F, de Glisezinski I, et al. Sex differences in lipolysis-regulating mechanisms in overweight subjects: effect of exercise intensity. Obesity (Silver Spring) 2007;15(9):2245–55.
63. Horowitz JF, Klein S. Oxidation of nonplasma fatty acids during exercise is increased in women with abdominal obesity. J Appl Physiol 2000;89(6):2276–82.
64. Mittendorfer B, Fields DA, Klein S. Excess body fat in men decreases plasma fatty acid availability and oxidation during endurance exercise. Am J Physiol Endocrinol Metab 2004;286(3):E354–62.
65. Magkos F, Patterson BW, Mohammed BS, et al. A single 1-h bout of evening exercise increases basal FFA flux without affecting VLDL-triglyceride and VLDL-apolipoprotein B-100 kinetics in untrained lean men. Am J Physiol Endocrinol Metab 2007;292(6):E1568–74.
66. Magkos F, Patterson BW, Mohammed BS, et al. Basal adipose tissue and hepatic lipid kinetics are not affected by a single exercise bout of moderate duration and intensity in sedentary women. Clin Sci (Lond) 2009;116(4): 327–34.
67. Henderson GC, Fattor JA, Horning MA, et al. Lipolysis and fatty acid metabolism in men and women during the postexercise recovery period. J Physiol 2007; 584(Pt 3):963–81.
68. Yale JF, Leiter LA, Marliss EB. Metabolic responses to intense exercise in lean and obese subjects. J Clin Endocrinol Metab 1989;68(2):438–45.
69. Vettor R, Macor C, Rossi E, et al. Impaired counterregulatory hormonal and metabolic response to exhaustive exercise in obese subjects. Acta Diabetol 1997;34(2):61–6.
70. Gustafson AB, Farrell PA, Kalkhoff RK. Impaired plasma catecholamine response to submaximal treadmill exercise in obese women. Metabolism 1990;39(4):410–7.
71. Abbasi F, McLaughlin T, Lamendola C, et al. The relationship between glucose disposal in response to physiological hyperinsulinemia and basal glucose and free fatty acid concentrations in healthy volunteers. J Clin Endocrinol Metab 2000;85(3):1251–4.
72. Campbell PJ, Carlson MG, Hill JO, et al. Regulation of free fatty acid metabolism by insulin in humans: role of lipolysis and reesterification. Am J Physiol 1992; 263(6 Pt 1):E1063–9.

73. Horowitz JF, Klein S. Whole body and abdominal lipolytic sensitivity to epinephrine is suppressed in upper body obese women. Am J Physiol Endocrinol Metab 2000;278(6):E1144–52.
74. McKeigue PM, Laws A, Chen YD, et al. Relation of plasma triglyceride and apoB levels to insulin-mediated suppression of nonesterified fatty acids. Possible explanation for sex differences in lipoprotein pattern. Arterioscler Thromb 1993;13(8):1187–92.
75. Sumner AE, Kushner H, Tulenko TN, et al. The relationship in African-Americans of sex differences in insulin-mediated suppression of nonesterified fatty acids to sex differences in fasting triglyceride levels. Metabolism 1997;46(4):400–5.
76. Sumner AE, Kushner H, Lakota CA, et al. Gender differences in insulin-induced free fatty acid suppression: studies in an African American population. Lipids 1996;31(Suppl):S275–8.
77. Sumner AE, Kushner H, Sherif KD, et al. Sex differences in African-Americans regarding sensitivity to insulin's glucoregulatory and antilipolytic actions. Diabetes Care 1999;22(1):71–7.
78. Horton TJ, Commerford SR, Pagliassotti MJ, et al. Postprandial leg uptake of triglyceride is greater in women than in men. Am J Physiol Endocrinol Metab 2002;283(6):E1192–202.
79. Burdge GC, Powell J, Calder PC. Lack of effect of meal fatty acid composition on postprandial lipid, glucose and insulin responses in men and women aged 50–65 years consuming their habitual diets. Br J Nutr 2006;96(3):489–500.
80. Koutsari C, Zagana A, Tzoras I, et al. Gender influence on plasma triacylglycerol response to meals with different monounsaturated and saturated fatty acid content. Eur J Clin Nutr 2004;58(3):495–502.
81. Perseghin G, Scifo P, Pagliato E, et al. Gender factors affect fatty acids-induced insulin resistance in nonobese humans: effects of oral steroidal contraception. J Clin Endocrinol Metab 2001;86(7):3188–96.
82. Frias JP, Macaraeg GB, Ofrecio J, et al. Decreased susceptibility to fatty acid-induced peripheral tissue insulin resistance in women. Diabetes 2001;50(6):1344–50.
83. Vistisen B, Hellgren LI, Vadset T, et al. Effect of gender on lipid-induced insulin resistance in obese subjects. Eur J Endocrinol 2008;158(1):61–8.
84. Mittendorfer B, Patterson BW, Klein S, et al. VLDL-triglyceride kinetics during hyperglycemia-hyperinsulinemia: effects of sex and obesity. Am J Physiol Endocrinol Metab 2003;284(4):E708–15.
85. Howard BV, Klimes I, Vasquez B, et al. The antilipolytic action of insulin in obese subjects with resistance to its glucoregulatory action. J Clin Endocrinol Metab 1984;58(3):544–8.
86. Lewis GF, Uffelman KD, Szeto LW, et al. Effects of acute hyperinsulinemia on VLDL triglyceride and VLDL apoB production in normal weight and obese individuals. Diabetes 1993;42(6):833–42.
87. Eckel RH, Sadur CN, Yost TJ. Deficiency of the insulin, glucose-mediated decrease in serum triglycerides in normolipidemic obese subjects. Int J Obes 1988;12(5):369–76.
88. Kelley DE, Goodpaster B, Wing RR, et al. Skeletal muscle fatty acid metabolism in association with insulin resistance, obesity, and weight loss. Am J Physiol 1999;277(6 Pt 1):E1130–41.
89. Magkos F, Wright DC, Patterson BW, et al. Lipid metabolism response to a single, prolonged bout of endurance exercise in healthy young men. Am J Physiol Endocrinol Metab 2006;290(2):E355–62.

90. Hartung GH, Lawrence SJ, Reeves RS, et al. Effect of alcohol and exercise on postprandial lipemia and triglyceride clearance in men. Atherosclerosis 1993; 100(1):33–40.
91. Sady SP, Thompson PD, Cullinane EM, et al. Prolonged exercise augments plasma triglyceride clearance. JAMA 1986;256(18):2552–5.
92. Cohen JC, Noakes TD, Benade AJ. Postprandial lipemia and chylomicron clearance in athletes and in sedentary men. Am J Clin Nutr 1989;49(3):443–7.
93. Simsolo RB, Ong JM, Kern PA. The regulation of adipose tissue and muscle lipoprotein lipase in runners by detraining. J Clin Invest 1993;92(5):2124–30.
94. Gill JM, Herd SL, Tsetsonis NV, et al. Are the reductions in triacylglycerol and insulin levels after exercise related? Clin Sci (Lond) 2002;102(2):223–31.
95. Gill JM, Al-Mamari A, Ferrell WR, et al. Effects of prior moderate exercise on postprandial metabolism and vascular function in lean and centrally obese men. J Am Coll Cardiol 2004;44(12):2375–82.
96. Cohn JS, Johnson EJ, Millar JS, et al. Contribution of apoB-48 and apoB-100 triglyceride-rich lipoproteins (TRL) to postprandial increases in the plasma concentration of TRL triglycerides and retinyl esters. J Lipid Res 1993;34(12): 2033–40.
97. Cohen JC, Noakes TD, Benade AJ. Serum triglyceride responses to fatty meals: effects of meal fat content. Am J Clin Nutr 1988;47(5):825–7.
98. Rivellese AA, Maffettone A, Vessby B, et al. Effects of dietary saturated, monounsaturated and n-3 fatty acids on fasting lipoproteins, LDL size and post-prandial lipid metabolism in healthy subjects. Atherosclerosis 2003;167(1):149–58.
99. Jackson KG, Wolstencroft EJ, Bateman PA, et al. Acute effects of meal fatty acids on postprandial NEFA, glucose and apo E response: implications for insulin sensitivity and lipoprotein regulation? Br J Nutr 2005;93(5):693–700.
100. Koutsari C, Malkova D, Hardman AE. Postprandial lipemia after short-term variation in dietary fat and carbohydrate. Metabolism 2000;49(9):1150–5.
101. Gill JM, Hardman AE. Exercise and postprandial lipid metabolism: an update on potential mechanisms and interactions with high-carbohydrate diets. J Nutr Biochem 2003;14(3):122–32.
102. Cohen JC, Berger GM. Effects of glucose ingestion on postprandial lipemia and triglyceride clearance in humans. J Lipid Res 1990;31(4):597–602.
103. Westphal S, Leodolter A, Kahl S, et al. Addition of glucose to a fatty meal delays chylomicrons and suppresses VLDL in healthy subjects. Eur J Clin Invest 2002; 32(5):322–7.
104. Malmstrom R, Packard CJ, Caslake M, et al. Effects of insulin and acipimox on VLDL1 and VLDL2 apolipoprotein B production in normal subjects. Diabetes 1998;47(5):779–87.
105. Lewis GF, Zinman B, Uffelman KD, et al. VLDL production is decreased to a similar extent by acute portal vs. peripheral venous insulin. Am J Physiol 1994;267(4 Pt 1):E566–72.
106. Lewis GF, Uffelman KD, Szeto LW, et al. Interaction between free fatty acids and insulin in the acute control of very low density lipoprotein production in humans. J Clin Invest 1995;95(1):158–66.
107. Cohn JS, McNamara JR, Cohn SD, et al. Postprandial plasma lipoprotein changes in human subjects of different ages. J Lipid Res 1988;29(4):469–79.
108. Couillard C, Bergeron N, Prud'homme D, et al. Gender difference in postprandial lipemia: importance of visceral adipose tissue accumulation. Arterioscler Thromb Vasc Biol 1999;19(10):2448–55.

109. Georgopoulos A, Rosengard AM. Abnormalities in the metabolism of postprandial and fasting triglyceride-rich lipoprotein subfractions in normal and insulin-dependent diabetic subjects: effects of sex. Metabolism 1989;38(8):781–9.
110. Matthan NR, Jalbert SM, Barrett PH, et al. Gender-specific differences in the kinetics of nonfasting TRL, IDL, and LDL apolipoprotein B-100 in men and premenopausal women. Arterioscler Thromb Vasc Biol 2008;28(10):1838–43.
111. Potts JL, Coppack SW, Fisher RM, et al. Impaired postprandial clearance of triacylglycerol-rich lipoproteins in adipose tissue in obese subjects. Am J Physiol 1995;268(4 Pt 1):E588–94.
112. Wideman L, Kaminsky LA, Whaley MH. Postprandial lipemia in obese men with abdominal fat patterning. J Sports Med Phys Fitness 1996;36(3):204–10.
113. Mekki N, Christofilis MA, Charbonnier M, et al. Influence of obesity and body fat distribution on postprandial lipemia and triglyceride-rich lipoproteins in adult women. J Clin Endocrinol Metab 1999;84(1):184–91.
114. Mamo JC, Watts GF, Barrett PH, et al. Postprandial dyslipidemia in men with visceral obesity: an effect of reduced LDL receptor expression? Am J Physiol Endocrinol Metab 2001;281(3):E626–32.
115. Lewis GF, O'Meara NM, Soltys PA, et al. Postprandial lipoprotein metabolism in normal and obese subjects: comparison after the vitamin A fat-loading test. J Clin Endocrinol Metab 1990;71(4):1041–50.
116. Vansant G, Mertens A, Muls E. Determinants of postprandial lipemia in obese women. Int J Obes Relat Metab Disord 1999;23(Suppl 1):14–21.
117. Taira K, Hikita M, Kobayashi J, et al. Delayed post-prandial lipid metabolism in subjects with intra-abdominal visceral fat accumulation. Eur J Clin Invest 1999; 29(4):301–8.
118. Couillard C, Bergeron N, Prud'homme D, et al. Postprandial triglyceride response in visceral obesity in men. Diabetes 1998;47(6):953–60.
119. Riemens SC, Ligtenberg JJ, Dullaart RP. Hyperglycemia-induced hyperinsulinemia acutely lowers plasma apolipoprotein B but not lipoprotein (a) in man. Clin Chim Acta 1997;261(2):149–58.
120. Bioletto S, Golay A, Munger R, et al. Acute hyperinsulinemia and very-low-density and low-density lipoprotein subfractions in obese subjects. Am J Clin Nutr 2000;71(2):443–9.
121. Klein S, Luu K, Gasic S, et al. Effect of weight loss on whole body and cellular lipid metabolism in severely obese humans. Am J Physiol 1996;270(5 Pt 1): E739–45.
122. Thyfault JP, Kraus RM, Hickner RC, et al. Impaired plasma fatty acid oxidation in extremely obese women. Am J Physiol Endocrinol Metab 2004;287(6): E1076–81.
123. Klein S, Mittendorfer B, Eagon JC, et al. Gastric bypass surgery improves metabolic and hepatic abnormalities associated with nonalcoholic fatty liver disease. Gastroenterology 2006;130(6):1564–72.
124. Jazet IM, Schaart G, Gastaldelli A, et al. Loss of 50% of excess weight using a very low energy diet improves insulin-stimulated glucose disposal and skeletal muscle insulin signalling in obese insulin-treated type 2 diabetic patients. Diabetologia 2008;51(2):309–19.
125. Goodpaster BH, Kelley DE, Wing RR, et al. Effects of weight loss on regional fat distribution and insulin sensitivity in obesity. Diabetes 1999;48(4):839–47.
126. Sartorio A, Maffiuletti NA, Agosti F, et al. Gender-related changes in body composition, muscle strength and power output after a short-term

multidisciplinary weight loss intervention in morbid obesity. J Endocrinol Invest 2005;28(6):494–501.
127. Tymitz K, Kerlakian G, Engel A, et al. Gender differences in early outcomes following hand-assisted laparoscopic Roux-en-Y gastric bypass surgery: gender differences in bariatric surgery. Obes Surg 2007;17(12):1588–91.
128. Wirth A, Steinmetz B. Gender differences in changes in subcutaneous and intra-abdominal fat during weight reduction: an ultrasound study. Obes Res 1998; 6(6):393–9.
129. Janssen I, Ross R. Effects of sex on the change in visceral, subcutaneous adipose tissue and skeletal muscle in response to weight loss. Int J Obes Relat Metab Disord 1999;23(10):1035–46.
130. Doucet E, St-Pierre S, Almeras N, et al. Reduction of visceral adipose tissue during weight loss. Eur J Clin Nutr 2002;56(4):297–304.
131. Ginsberg HN, Le NA, Gibson JC. Regulation of the production and catabolism of plasma low density lipoproteins in hypertriglyceridemic subjects. Effect of weight loss. J Clin Invest 1985;75(2):614–23.
132. Olefsky J, Reaven GM, Farquhar JW. Effects of weight reduction on obesity. Studies of lipid and carbohydrate metabolism in normal and hyperlipoproteinemic subjects. J Clin Invest 1974;53(1):64–76.
133. Viljanen AP, Iozzo P, Borra R, et al. Effect of weight loss on liver free fatty acid uptake and hepatic insulin resistance. J Clin Endocrinol Metab 2009;94(1):50–5.
134. Heiling VJ, Jensen MD. Free fatty acid metabolism in the follicular and luteal phases of the menstrual cycle. J Clin Endocrinol Metab 1992;74(4):806–10.
135. Horton TJ, Miller EK, Bourret K. No effect of menstrual cycle phase on glycerol or palmitate kinetics during 90 min of moderate exercise. J Appl Physiol 2006; 100(3):917–25.
136. Magkos F, Patterson BW, Mittendorfer B. No effect of menstrual cycle phase on basal very-low-density lipoprotein triglyceride and apolipoprotein B-100 kinetics. Am J Physiol Endocrinol Metab 2006;291(6):E1243–9.
137. Rebuffe-Scrive M, Enk L, Crona N, et al. Fat cell metabolism in different regions in women. Effect of menstrual cycle, pregnancy, and lactation. J Clin Invest 1985;75(6):1973–6.
138. Kissebah AH, Harrigan P, Wynn V. Mechanism of hypertriglyceridaemia associated with contraceptive steroids. Horm Metab Res 1973;5(3):184–90.
139. Jensen MD, Levine J. Effects of oral contraceptives on free fatty acid metabolism in women. Metabolism 1998;47(3):280–4.
140. Jensen MD, Martin ML, Cryer PE, et al. Effects of estrogen on free fatty acid metabolism in humans. Am J Physiol 1994;266(6 Pt 1):E914–20.
141. Jensen MD, Caruso M, Heiling V, et al. Insulin regulation of lipolysis in nondiabetic and IDDM subjects. Diabetes 1989;38(12):1595–601.
142. Magkos F, Patterson BW, Mittendorfer B. Reproducibility of stable isotope-labeled tracer measures of VLDL-triglyceride and VLDL-apolipoprotein B-100 kinetics. J Lipid Res 2007;48(5):1204–11.
143. Carr MC. The emergence of the metabolic syndrome with menopause. J Clin Endocrinol Metab 2003;88(6):2404–11.
144. Godsland IF. Effects of postmenopausal hormone replacement therapy on lipid, lipoprotein, and apolipoprotein (a) concentrations: analysis of studies published from 1974-2000. Fertil Steril 2001;75(5):898–915.
145. Kandeel KM, Nayel SA, Abaza MS. The effect of injectable contraceptive on lipid metabolism in women. Biomed Biochim Acta 1984;43(1):111–5.

146. Wolfe BM, Plunkett ER. Early effects of continuous low-dosage all-norgestrel administered alone or with estrogen. Maturitas 1994;18(3):207–19.
147. Wolfe BM, Huff MW. Effects of low dosage progestin-only administration upon plasma triglycerides and lipoprotein metabolism in postmenopausal women. J Clin Invest 1993;92(1):456–61.
148. Walsh BW, Li H, Sacks FM. Effects of postmenopausal hormone replacement with oral and transdermal estrogen on high density lipoprotein metabolism. J Lipid Res 1994;35(11):2083–93.
149. Fallat R, Glueck CJ. Effects of anabolic and progestational agents upon triglycerides and triglyceride kinetics in normals and hyperlipemic patients. Lipids 1974;9(2):117–20.
150. Glueck CJ, Fallat RW, Scheel D. Effects of estrogenic compounds on triglyceride kinetics. Metabolism 1975;24(4):537–45.
151. Tikkanen MJ, Kuusi T, Nikkila EA, et al. Very low density lipoprotein triglyceride kinetics during hepatic lipase suppression by estrogen. Studies on the physiological role of hepatic endothelial lipase. FEBS Lett 1985;181(1):160–4.
152. Kim HJ, Kalkhoff RK. Sex steroid influence on triglyceride metabolism. J Clin Invest 1975;56(4):888–96.
153. Cheng DC, Wolfe BM. Norethindrone acetate inhibition of triglyceride synthesis and release by rat hepatocytes. Atherosclerosis 1983;46(1):41–8.
154. Wolfe BM, Grace DM. Norethindrone acetate inhibition of splanchnic triglyceride secretion in conscious glucose-fed siwne. J Lipid Res 1979;20(2):175–82.
155. Khokha R, Wolfe BM. Hypotriglyceridemic effects of levonorgestrel in rats. Atherosclerosis 1984;52(3):329–38.
156. Breckenridge WC. The catabolism of very low density lipoproteins. Can J Biochem Cell Biol 1985;63(8):890–7.
157. Araujo DA, Farias ML, Andrade AT. Effects of transdermal and oral estrogen replacement on lipids and glucose metabolism in postmenopausal women with type 2 diabetes mellitus. Climacteric 2002;5(3):286–92.
158. Sanada M, Tsuda M, Kodama I, et al. Substitution of transdermal estradiol during oral estrogen-progestin therapy in postmenopausal women: effects on hypertriglyceridemia. Menopause 2004;11(3):331–6.
159. Sonnet E, Lacut K, Roudaut N, et al. Effects of the route of oestrogen administration on IGF-1 and IGFBP-3 in healthy postmenopausal women: results from a randomized placebo-controlled study. Clin Endocrinol (Oxf) 2007;66(5):626–31.
160. Shifren JL, Desindes S, McIlwain M, et al. A randomized, open-label, crossover study comparing the effects of oral versus transdermal estrogen therapy on serum androgens, thyroid hormones, and adrenal hormones in naturally menopausal women. Menopause 2007;14(6):985–94.
161. Qureshi AC, Bahri A, Breen LA, et al. The influence of the route of oestrogen administration on serum levels of cortisol-binding globulin and total cortisol. Clin Endocrinol (Oxf) 2007;66(5):632–5.
162. Basdevant A, De Lignieres B, Bigorie B, et al. Estradiol, progesterone and plasma lipids during the menstrual cycle. Diabete Metab 1981;7(1):1–4.
163. Demacker PN, Schade RW, Stalenhoef AF, et al. Influence of contraceptive pill and menstrual cycle on serum lipids and high-density lipoprotein cholesterol concentrations. Br Med J (Clin Res Ed) 1982;284(6324):1213–5.
164. Punnonen R. Total serum cholesterol, triglycerides and phospholipids during the normal menstrual cycle. Int J Gynaecol Obstet 1978;15(4):296–8.

165. Lamon-Fava S, Fisher EC, Nelson ME, et al. Effect of exercise and menstrual cycle status on plasma lipids, low density lipoprotein particle size, and apolipoproteins. J Clin Endocrinol Metab 1989;68(1):17–21.
166. Campos H, McNamara JR, Wilson PW, et al. Differences in low density lipoprotein subfractions and apolipoproteins in premenopausal and postmenopausal women. J Clin Endocrinol Metab 1988;67(1):30–5.
167. Mauriege P, Imbeault P, Prud'Homme D, et al. Subcutaneous adipose tissue metabolism at menopause: importance of body fatness and regional fat distribution. J Clin Endocrinol Metab 2000;85(7):2446–54.
168. Ozbey N, Sencer E, Molvalilar S, et al. Body fat distribution and cardiovascular disease risk factors in pre- and postmenopausal obese women with similar BMI. Endocr J 2002;49(4):503–9.
169. Peters HW, Westendorp IC, Hak AE, et al. Menopausal status and risk factors for cardiovascular disease. J Intern Med 1999;246(6):521–8.
170. Torng PL, Su TC, Sung FC, et al. Effects of menopause and obesity on lipid profiles in middle-aged Taiwanese women: the Chin-Shan Community Cardiovascular Cohort Study. Atherosclerosis 2000;153(2):413–21.
171. Tremollieres FA, Pouilles JM, Cauneille C, et al. Coronary heart disease risk factors and menopause: a study in 1684 French women. Atherosclerosis 1999;142(2):415–23.
172. Van Beek AP, de Ruijter-Heijstek FC, Jansen H, et al. Sex steroids and plasma lipoprotein levels in healthy women: The importance of androgens in the estrogen-deficient state. Metabolism 2004;53(2):187–92.
173. Matthan NR, Jalbert SM, Lamon-Fava S, et al. TRL, IDL, and LDL apolipoprotein B-100 and HDL apolipoprotein A-I kinetics as a function of age and menopausal status. Arterioscler Thromb Vasc Biol 2005;25(8):1691–6.
174. Welty FK, Lichtenstein AH, Barrett PH, et al. Human apolipoprotein (Apo) B-48 and ApoB-100 kinetics with stable isotopes. Arterioscler Thromb Vasc Biol 1999;19(12):2966–74.
175. Masding MG, Stears AJ, Burdge GC, et al. Premenopausal advantages in postprandial lipid metabolism are lost in women with type 2 diabetes. Diabetes Care 2003;26(12):3243–9.
176. Van Beek AP, de Ruijter-Heijstek FC, Erkelens DW, et al. Menopause is associated with reduced protection from postprandial lipemia. Arterioscler Thromb Vasc Biol 1999;19(11):2737–41.
177. Lanfranco F, Zitzmann M, Simoni M, et al. Serum adiponectin levels in hypogonadal males: influence of testosterone replacement therapy. Clin Endocrinol (Oxf) 2004;60(4):500–7.
178. Oppenheim DS, Greenspan SL, Zervas NT, et al. Elevated serum lipids in hypogonadal men with and without hyperprolactinemia. Ann Intern Med 1989;111(4): 288–92.
179. Zitzmann M, Brune M, Nieschlag E. Vascular reactivity in hypogonadal men is reduced by androgen substitution. J Clin Endocrinol Metab 2002;87(11): 5030–7.
180. Whitsel EA, Boyko EJ, Matsumoto AM, et al. Intramuscular testosterone esters and plasma lipids in hypogonadal men: a meta-analysis. Am J Med 2001; 111(4):261–9.
181. Berg G, Schreier L, Geloso G, et al. Impact on lipoprotein profile after long-term testosterone replacement in hypogonadal men. Horm Metab Res 2002;34(2): 87–92.

182. Snyder PJ, Peachey H, Berlin JA, et al. Effects of testosterone replacement in hypogonadal men. J Clin Endocrinol Metab 2000;85(8):2670–7.
183. Kapoor D, Goodwin E, Channer KS, et al. Testosterone replacement therapy improves insulin resistance, glycaemic control, visceral adiposity and hypercholesterolaemia in hypogonadal men with type 2 diabetes. Eur J Endocrinol 2006; 154(6):899–906.
184. Jockenhovel F, Bullmann C, Schubert M, et al. Influence of various modes of androgen substitution on serum lipids and lipoproteins in hypogonadal men. Metabolism 1999;48(5):590–6.
185. Meyer WJ 3rd, Webb A, Stuart CA, et al. Physical and hormonal evaluation of transsexual patients: a longitudinal study. Arch Sex Behav 1986;15(2):121–38.
186. Elbers JM, Giltay EJ, Teerlink T, et al. Effects of sex steroids on components of the insulin resistance syndrome in transsexual subjects. Clin Endocrinol (Oxf) 2003;58(5):562–71.
187. Floter A, Nathorst-Boos J, Carlstrom K, et al. Serum lipids in oophorectomized women during estrogen and testosterone replacement therapy. Maturitas 2004;47(2):123–9.
188. Leao LM, Duarte MP, Silva DM, et al. Influence of methyltestosterone postmenopausal therapy on plasma lipids, inflammatory factors, glucose metabolism and visceral fat: a randomized study. Eur J Endocrinol 2006;154(1):131–9.
189. Bagdade JD, Livingston R, Yee E. Effects of synthetic androgen fluoxymesterone on triglyceride secretion rates in the rat. Proc Soc Exp Biol Med 1975; 149(2):452–4.
190. Chiuve SE, Martin LA, Campos H, et al. Effect of the combination of methyltestosterone and esterified estrogens compared with esterified estrogens alone on apolipoprotein CIII and other apolipoproteins in very low density, low density, and high density lipoproteins in surgically postmenopausal women. J Clin Endocrinol Metab 2004;89(5):2207–13.
191. Elam MB, Umstot ES, Andersen RN, et al. Deprivation and repletion of androgen in vivo modifies triacylglycerol synthesis by rat hepatocytes. Biochim Biophys Acta 1987;921(3):531–40.

Cardiopulmonary Aspects of Obesity in Women

Gerald S. Zavorsky, PhD[a,b,*]

KEYWORDS

- Pulmonary • Cardiovascular • Exercise • Obesity
- Women • Gas exchange

Life expectancy has been increasing for women, from 75 years in 1970 to 80 years in 2005.[1] Despite this increased longevity, approximately half of all women of reproductive age in the United States today are overweight or obese.[2] Obesity causes or exacerbates many health problems, independently and in association with other diseases, and is among the most significant contributors to ill health.[3] Furthermore, obese women have a higher prevalence of depression compared with obese men (46% in women, 17% in men).[4] This issue of *Obstetrics and Gynecology Clinics of North America* is devoted specifically to the important and timely topic of women and obesity.

The National Institutes of Health classifies obesity in terms of body mass index (BMI) (weight in kilograms divided by height in meters squared [kg/m^2]). Overweight ranges from a BMI of 25.0 to 29.9 kg/m^2; obesity class I ranges from 30.0 to 34.9 kg/m^2; obesity class II ranges from 35.0 to 39.9 kg/m^2; and obesity class III (extreme obesity or morbid obesity) is a BMI greater than or equal to 40 kg/m^2. Because the prevalence of obesity class I and II in the United States has increased fourfold between 1986 and 2000[5] and because women in this class of obesity have a twofold higher risk for all-cause mortality compared with normal-weight women,[6] an immediate concern is reducing the prevalence of obesity in women, especially women who fall into the obese class III category.

This article discusses cardiopulmonary aspects of obesity as they pertain to women. This review article focuses specifically on cardiovascular and pulmonary complications of obesity in nonpregnant women and includes exercise-related topics.[7–18]

[a] Department of Obstetrics, Gynecology, and Women's Health, School of Medicine, Saint Louis University, Saint Mary's Health Center, 6420 Clayton Road, Suite 290, St. Louis, MO 63117, USA
[b] Department of Pharmacological and Physiological Science, School of Medicine, Saint Louis University, 402 South Grand Boulevard, St. Louis, MO 63104, USA
* Corresponding author. Department of Obstetrics, Gynecology, and Women's Health, School of Medicine, Saint Louis University, Saint Mary's Health Center, 6420 Clayton Road, Suite 290, St. Louis, MO 63117.
E-mail address: zavorsky@slu.edu

Obstet Gynecol Clin N Am 36 (2009) 267–284
doi:10.1016/j.ogc.2009.03.006 **obgyn.theclinics.com**

PULMONARY COMPLICATIONS

There are several parameters of pulmonary function that can be examined in women. Some of the most common tests of pulmonary function are spirometry; forced expiratory volume in 1 second; forced vital capacity; forced expiratory flow rate over the mid-expiratory phase; peak expiratory flow rate; DLCO and diffusing capacity of the lung for nitric oxide (DLNO), which is a reflection of alveolar-membrane conductance; and helium dilution or nitrogen washout tests that measure lung volumes, such as residual volume (RV), functional residual capacity, expiratory reserve volume, inspiratory reserve volume, and total lung capacity. Healthy women have reduced lung function compared with healthy men, because even when normalized for height and age, women have, on average, approximately a 660-mL lower alveolar volume and a 650-mL lower vital capacity than men.[7] Therefore, women have smaller lungs compared with men even when height and age are taken into account. In addition, DLCO and DLNO also are lower in women by approximately 3 mL/min/mm Hg and 18 mL/min/mm Hg, respectively, when normalized for lung volume and age.[7] This suggests that there may be a smaller number of alveoli per unit area in women compared with men. Therefore, obesity could be suspected of having a larger impact on the decrement of pulmonary function in women compared with men because women's lung diffusing abilities and lung volumes are reduced. That, however, is not the case. There are studies that suggest that obese women have relatively normal lung function in terms of pulmonary diffusing capacity and spirometry. Specifically, alveolar-membrane conductance, as reflected by DLNO, is reduced in morbidly obese men but not in morbidly obese women.[8] The DLCO, in terms of percent predicted, also is normal in morbidly obese women compared with morbidly obese men,[8] although this not always is the case.[19] For example, obese women who have a reduced DLCO have an increased prevalence of moderate or severe left ventricular diastolic dysfunction.[20] Weight loss from bariatric surgery can improve DLNO, as it reduces the waist-to-hip ratio (an indicator of abdominal obesity) such that alveolar volume increases, resulting in improved DLNO.[12] The waist-to-hip ratio plays a large role in lung function in the obese population. Obese women have a smaller waist circumference compared with obese men[8] and, therefore, a reduced waist-to-hip ratio compared with obese men.[8,14] As such, the effects of obesity on pulmonary diffusing capacity and pulmonary gas exchange are related to the waist-to-hip ratio.

Studies have demonstrated that pulmonary gas exchange expressed as the alveolar to arterial oxygen partial pressure difference ($AaDo_2$) or arterial partial pressure of oxygen (Pao_2) are significantly associated with the waist-to-hip ratio at rest.[8,14] Specifically, 21% to 32% of the variance in the $AaDo_2$ and 28% to 36% of the variance in Pao_2 are related to the waist-to-hip ratio,[8,14] signifying that as the waist-to-hip ratio increases, Pao_2 decreases and $AaDo_2$ increases. A decreasing Pao_2 and an increasing $AaDo_2$ indicate an increase in the impairment of pulmonary gas exchange. Furthermore, those studies show that morbidly obese women have better pulmonary gas exchange compared with morbidly obese men because women have a lower waist-to-hip ratio.[8,14] There are other variables that may be associated with pulmonary gas exchange, such as waist circumference and BMI. The waist circumference may be a better predictor of gas exchange impairment compared with the waist-to-hip ratio because the waist circumference gives a reflection of the amount of fat mass surrounding the abdomen. An abnormally high $AaDo_2$ and low Pao_2 may be attributed to ventilation-perfusion abnormalities, as the lower portions of the lung have been found to be underventilated and overperfused in obese individuals.[21] Because the expiratory reserve volume commonly is reduced in obesity, it follows that obese persons breathe closer to residual volume. Therefore, when seated upright, ventilation to lower lung zones is impaired, resulting in abnormally low ventilation-perfusion ratios.[21] Those individuals who have large waist circumferences could have a larger mismatching between ventilation and perfusion and increased atelectasis compared with those whose waist circumferences are smaller. Vaughan and colleagues[22] have demonstrated that as waist circumference decreases in morbidly obese patients, the $AaDo_2$ also decreases ($r^2 = 0.35$, $P<.05$), meaning that pulmonary gas exchange is related to abdominal obesity. They also showed a significant relationship between changes in expiratory reserve volume and Pao_2 ($r^2 = 0.35$) and $AaDo_2$ ($r^2 = 0.58$), demonstrating that as expiratory reserve volume increased from surgical weight loss due to the reduction in waist circumference, gas exchange improved.[22]

Although there are significant relationships between pulmonary gas exchange and waist circumference, they are not as strong as the relationship between pulmonary gas exchange and waist-to-hip ratio.[8,14] It has been speculated that a large fat mass surrounding the hips has protective effects against the abdominal fat mass such that the gas exchange impairment is reduced.[14] A large fat mass surrounding the hip may help keep the abdominal fat mass from sagging toward the ground. A sagging abdominal fat mass may result in more atelectasis and ventilation-perfusion mismatching compared with a nonsagging abdominal fat mass. Typically, women have more of a gynoid-shaped physique, where the fat mass is concentrated around the hip. Men tend to have a more android-shaped physique in which the fat mass is concentrated around the abdomen. Previous studies[8,14] show that if a large fat mass surrounds the abdomen and a large fat mass also surrounds the hip and thighs (as in women), the gas exchange impairment is not as severe. As to the reason why BMI is not associated with pulmonary gas exchange impairment, it could be that height also has particular protective effects. Approximately 65% of the variance in height in obese[14] and nonobese subjects[7] could be explained by vital capacity. A large vital capacity indicates that there should be a larger surface area for oxygen to diffuse through the alveolar-capillary membrane, especially in the upper part of the lung. This would compensate for the lower portions of the lung that are underventilated and overperfused in obese individuals.[21] There is no relationship, however, between height or vital capacity to pulmonary gas exchange in the morbidly obese.[14]

Although obese men have worse pulmonary gas exchange compared with obese women, there still is a larger than expected impairment of pulmonary gas exchange in obese women when compared with matched, nonobese women controls. **Fig. 1** illustrates the gender differences in pulmonary gas exchange at rest in morbidly obese men and women (nonpregnant). From **Fig. 1**, morbidly obese women who have an average BMI of 51 kg/m^2 have a gas exchange impairment ($AaDo_2$) that is threefold higher and a Pao_2 that is 7 mm Hg lower than matched, nonobese women controls. The predicted values are from Crapo and colleagues,[23] represented by the horizontal dashed line in **Fig. 1** for each arterial blood gas parameter. Nonetheless, percent arterial oxygen saturation (Sao_2), as measured by co-oximetry (multiwavelength oximetry), overall remains normal in those who are morbidly obese.

Exercise has the potential to alter pulmonary gas exchange in obese women, whose lung volumes are smaller than matched controls. For instance, even though spirometric function is normal or near normal in morbidly obese women,[8,13,24] functional residual capacity, expiratory reserve volume, and RV are approximately 80%, 50%, and 90%, respectively, of predicted in obese women (BMI of approximately 40 kg/m^2).[24] In **Fig. 2**, end-expiratory lung volume (EELV) is lower and inspiratory reserve volume higher in obese women than in normal-weight women at the start of exercise. The decrease in EELV is related to the cumulative effect of chest wall fat.[25] At peak exercise,

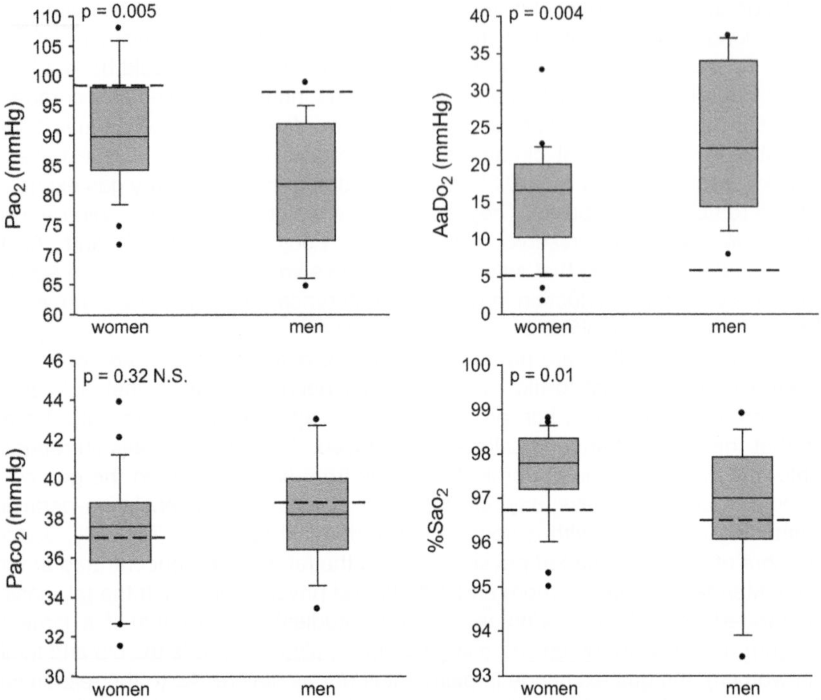

Fig. 1. Box plots showing gender differences in pulmonary gas exchange in the morbidly obese (n = 25 women, BMI 51 kg/m^2; n = 17 men, BMI 50 kg/m^2). At rest, there was a gender difference in Pao_2 (P = .005), $AaDo_2$ (P = .004), and percent Sao_2 (P = .01) but not $Paco_2$ (P = .32) at rest. Each box plot indicates 25th, 50th, and 75th percentile values. Bars indicate 5th and 95th percentile values. Outliers are indicated by the filled blacked circles. Horizontal, dashed lines indicate the predicted values for nonobese, healthy individuals. Morbidly obese men had lower Pao_2 (−9 mm Hg with standard error of ±3 mm Hg; 95% CI, −16 to −3 mm Hg), higher $AaDo_2$ (8 ± 3 mm Hg; 95% CI, 3 to 13 mm Hg), and lower percent Sao_2 (−1.0 ± 0.4%; 95% CI,−1.8 to −0.2%) compared with morbidly obese women. (*From* Zavorsky GS, Christou NV, Kim DJ, et al. Preoperative gender differences in pulmonary gas exchange in morbidly obese subjects. Obes Surg 2008;18:1587; with permission.)

obese women have an increase in EELV of approximately 400 mL compared with levels at the start of exercise, which is not observed in normal-weight women, suggesting that obese women experience dynamic hyperinflation throughout exercise, which is an attempt of the body to overcome the relatively shallow and rapid breathing pattern experienced by obese women at various levels of exercise (**Fig. 3**).

Expiratory flow limitation (EFL) also is increased in obese women. EFL is an assessment of breathing constraints at rest and during exercise. It is calculated as the percentage of tidal volume that encroaches on the maximal flow volume loop and the encroachment of flow at the midrange of tidal volume on the maximal flow volume loop at isovolume.[24] In approximately 50% of obese women, tidal volume is under some degree of EFL at rest (ie, 36% to 100% of the tidal volume overlaps the maximal flow-volume loop) (see **Fig. 3**). In contrast, normal-weight women are not flow limited at rest. During exercise, the flow limitation in obese women persists all the way up to peak exercise capacity whereas in normal-weight women no flow limitation is present except at peak exercise (see **Fig. 3**).

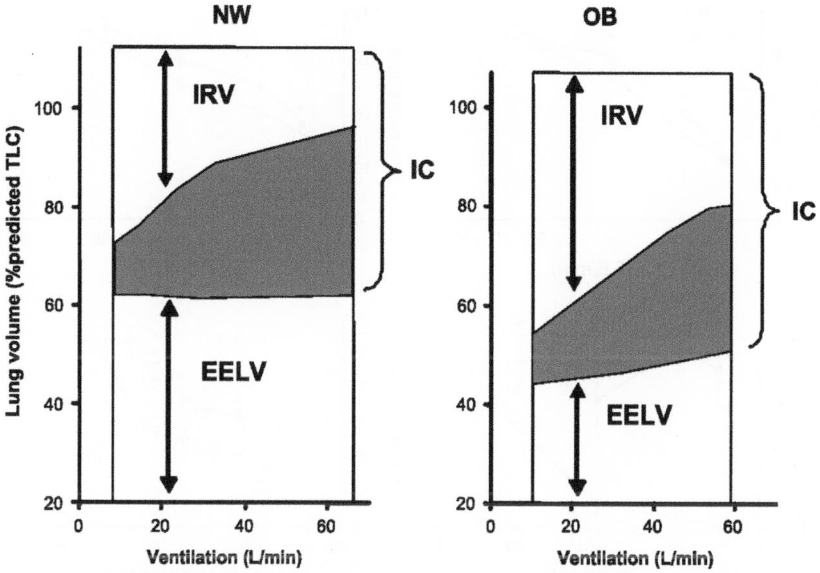

Fig. 2. Lung volumes from rest to peak exercise in obese (OB) (BMI = 40 ± 8 kg/m^2) and normal-weight (NW) (BMI 23 ± 1 kg/m^2) women. Significant increases in EELV by 0.38 ± 0.08 L (P<.05) were measured in OB, whereas no significant change in EELV was found in the NW subjects. Inspiratory reserve volume (IRV) was significantly (P<.05) higher at rest and throughout the exercise in OB women but did not reach a statistical significant difference at the peak of exercise. IC, inspiratory capacity; TLC, total lung capacity. (*From* Ofir D, Laveneziana P, Webb KA, et al. Ventilatory and perceptual responses to cycle exercise in obese females. J Appl Physiol 2007;102:2217; with permission.)

Therefore, because of reduced lung volume, dynamic hyperinflation, and increased EFL in obese women with exercise, it would be expected that they have worse gas exchange compared with normal-weight women. This, however, is not the case. Sa_{O_2} obtained from pulse oximetry is maintained above 96% from rest to peak exercise in obese women.[24] This is corroborated by another study in which percent Sa_{O_2} measured from the gold standard of multiwavelength oximetry was normal in morbidly obese women right up to peak exercise (**Fig. 4**).[8] Only 4% of arterial blood gas samples (8% of women) demonstrated hypoxemia with exercise.[8] Mild exercise-induced arterial hypoxemia (EIH) is defined as percent Sa_{O_2} as between 93% and 95%; moderate EIH as percent Sa_{O_2} of 88% to 93%; and severe EIH less than 88%.[26] Also, only 10% of the blood gas samples (13% of the women) had excessive gas exchange impairment during exercise (see **Fig. 4**). Excessive gas exchange impairment during exercise is defined as AaD_{O_2} greater than or equal to 25 mm Hg whereas an AaD_{O_2} greater than 35 mm Hg is severe.[26]

As such, the prevalence of EIH in morbidly obese women is approximately 8 times lower than the prevalence of EIH in healthy women reported elsewhere (67% to 76% have exercise-induced hypoxemia (EIH) when peak oxygen uptake ($\dot{V}_{O_{2peak}}$) = 2.8 to 3.5 L/min).[27,28] Only approximately 10% of women and 2% of men, however, have exercise-induced hypoxemia when $\dot{V}_{O_{2peak}}$ is less than 50 mL/kg per minute,[29] similar to the 8% prevalence found in morbidly obese women.[8] The highest $\dot{V}_{O_{2peak}}$ recorded in a morbidly obese woman was 18.5 mL/kg per minute (2.76 L/min).[8] Therefore, it seems that gas exchange limitations, which are more common in those who are capable of

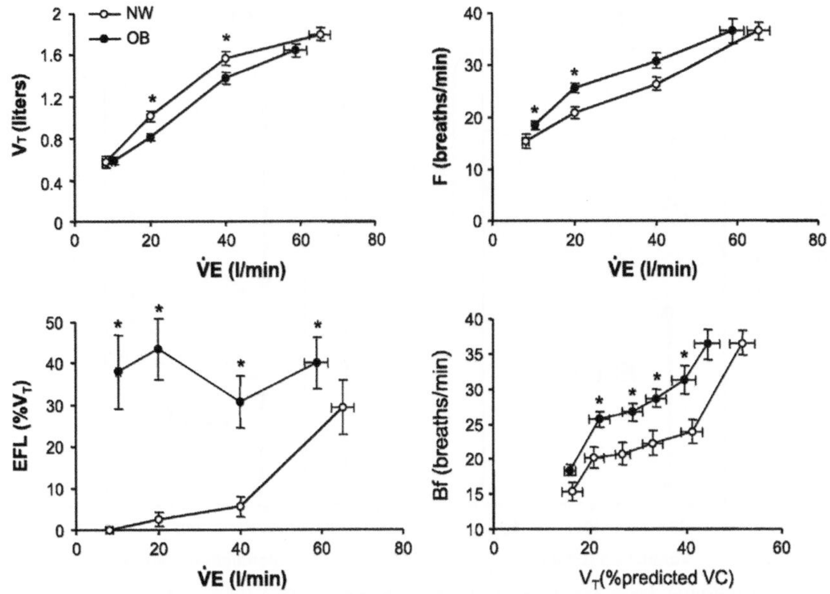

Fig. 3. Extent of EFL, tidal volume (V_T), and breathing frequency (F) are expired volume per unit time $\dot{V}E$ and breathing frequency (Bf) is expressed against V_T, during exercise in obese (OB) women (*filled circles*) and normal-weight (NW) women (*open circles*). Breathing pattern was relatively rapid and shallow in obese compared with normal-weight women. Values are means ± SE. VC, vital capacity. **P*<.05 OB versus NW. (*From* Ofir D, Laveneziana P, Webb KA, et al. Ventilatory and perceptual responses to cycle exercise in obese females. J Appl Physiol 2007;102:2217, 2007; with permission.)

a high level of work, are not found in morbidly obese women, as they have a very low peak $\dot{V}O_2$ (in mL/kg/min), and on average, are below the 10th percentile for $\dot{V}O_{2peak}$ for their age and gender.[30]

Correcting arterial blood gases for changes in body core temperature at rest may is usually not necessary, but it is necessary to do when blood gas sampling occurs throughout exercise, since increases in body core temperature affect blood gas readings.[13,26] A 1°C increase in core temperature caused by exercise underestimates PaO_2 and arterial partial pressure of carbon dioxide ($PaCO_2$) by approximately 5% and overestimates $AaDO_2$ by approximately 25% compared with the standard blood gas measurement at 37°C.[13,26]

Despite no appreciable impairment in pulmonary gas exchange occurring in obese women with exercise, they do not adequately hyperventilate during strenuous exercise despite high arterial plasma lactate concentrations.[8,13] This is evident from the data presented in **Fig. 3** and **Fig. 4**. Inadequate compensatory hyperventilation ($PaCO_2$ between 35.1 and 38.0 mm Hg)[26] or absence of a compensatory hyperventilatory response ($PaCO_2$ > 38.0 mm Hg) during intense exercise[26] is demonstrated in morbidly obese women.[8,13] Specifically, 75% of morbidly women demonstrate inadequate compensatory exercise hyperventilation at or near peak exercise.[8] In contrast, at the same level of oxygen uptake (ie, 1.8 to 2.1 L/min), non-obese women controls have a $PaCO_2$ of approximately 33 mm Hg.[31,32] The increased ventilatory constraints due to the large abdominal fat mass surrounding the chest that results from obesity[24,33] promotes ventilation-perfusion inequality (low ventilation-perfusion

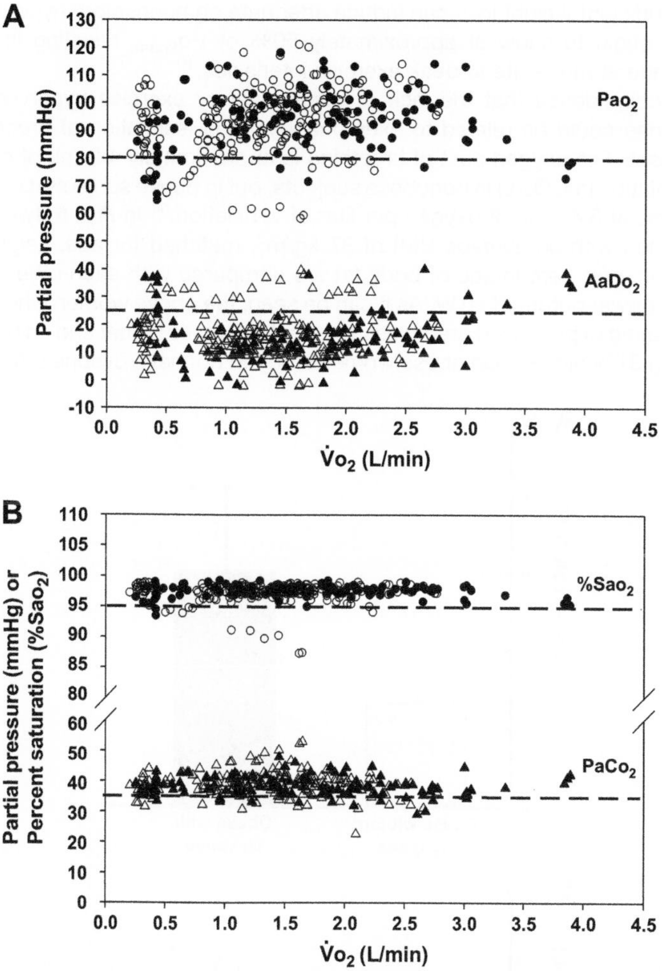

Fig. 4. Pulmonary gas exchange in morbidly obese men and women at various levels of physiologic stress. Approximately 340 temperature-corrected arterial blood gas samples were obtained from a total of 25 morbidly obese, nonpregnant women (BMI 51 ± 7 kg/m^2) and 17 morbidly obese men (BMI 50 ± 10 kg/m^2) in an upright position on a cycle-ergometer at sea level. (*A*) Pao_2 in men (*solid black circles*); Pao_2 in women (*open white circles*); $AaDo_2$ in men (*solid black triangles*); $AaDo_2$ in women (*open white triangles*). The horizontal dashed line for Pao_2 at 80 mm Hg indicates below which there is poor oxygenation. The horizontal dashed line for $AaDo_2$ at 25 mm Hg indicates above which there is a significant gas exchange impairment during exercise. (*B*) Percent Sao_2 in men (*solid black circles*); percent Sao_2 in women (*open white circles*); $Paco_2$ in men (*solid black triangles*); $Paco_2$ in women (*open white triangles*). The horizontal dashed line for percent Sao_2 at 95% indicates below which there is arterial hypoxemia. The horizontal dashed line for $Paco_2$ at 35 mm Hg indicates above which there is a lack of compensatory hyperventilation during intense exercise. (*Individual data obtained from* Zavorsky GS, Christou NV, Kim DJ, et al. Preoperative gender differences in pulmonary gas exchange in morbidly obese subjects. Obes Surg 2008;18:1587.)

ratios).[21] Sufficient weight loss can induce adequate compensatory hyperventilation, which can begin to show at approximately 50% of $\dot{V}o_{2peak}$ resulting in improved gas exchange at moderate to peak exercise intensities.[10]

It is no coincidence that the lack of compensatory exercise hyperventilation in obese women could be related to exertional dyspnea (sensation of breathlessness with exercise). The oxygen cost of breathing is approximately 1.2 mL of oxygen per liter of ventilation (mL O_2/L) in nonobese subjects, but in obese subjects it can be three times higher, at 3.45 mL of oxygen per liter of ventilation.[34] In **Fig. 5**, two groups of obese women with an average BMI of 37 kg/m^2, matched for age, height, weight, lung function, and percentage of body fat are compared with each other while they cycled at a power output of 60 W. As it can be seen, the obese women who had dyspnea had a rating of perceived breathlessness that is 3 times higher and an oxygen cost of breathing 37% higher than obese women who did not have dyspnea. Also, 72% of

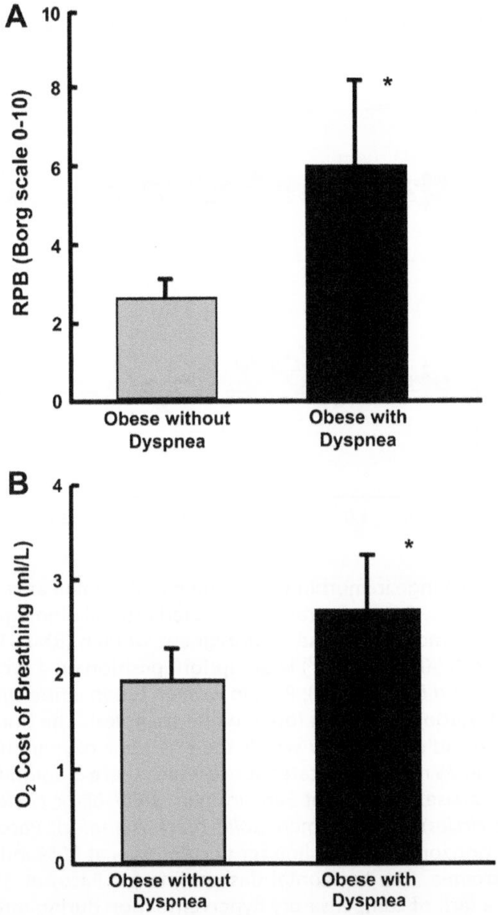

Fig. 5. (*A*) Rating of perceived breathlessness (RPB) and oxygen cost of breathing (*B*) during constant load cycling test at 60 W in obese women with (n = 8) and without exertional dyspnea (n = 8). Values are mean ± SD. *P<.01. (*From* Babb TG, Ranasinghe KG, Comeau LA, et al. Dyspnea on exertion in obese women: association with an increased oxygen cost of breathing. Am J Respir Crit Care Med 2008;178:116; with permission.) Copyright © 2008 American Thoracic Society.

the rating of perceived breathlessness can be explained by the increase in the oxygen cost of breathing.[19] Therefore, breathlessness during exercise in obese women is strongly associated with an increased oxygen cost of breathing not related to $\dot{V}O_{2peak}$.[19] Moreover, the hyperventilatory response to exercise (defined as the slope of the relationship between minute ventilation and carbon dioxide production) is not different between obese women who had dyspnea and obese women who did not have dyspnea[35] but is different compared with nonobese, physically active women.[13] For the same level of carbon dioxide production, minute ventilation is less in obese women compared with normal-weight women and, therefore, the slope is less in obese women (**Fig. 6**C).[13] This makes sense because $Paco_2$ remains unaltered between rest and peak exercise in obese women (see **Fig. 4**).[10,13] Weight loss increases the slope of the relationship between minute ventilation and carbon dioxide production in women during graded exercise.[10]

There are other respiratory complications that are a result of obesity. Some morbidly obese subjects have respiratory insufficiency (which is obesity hypoventilation syndrome [$Pao_2 \leq 55$ mm Hg or $Paco_2 \geq 47$ mm Hg on room air], obstructive sleep apnea, or both). The combination of obesity hypoventilation syndrome and obstructive sleep apnea is termed, *pickwickian syndrome*.[36] The literature has shown, however, that obesity hypoventilation syndrome occurs rarely, at most in approximately 10% of the morbidly obese population.[37–41] The prevalence of obstructive sleep apnea is more variable, in anywhere from 3% to 40% of the morbidly obese population.[37–41] The studies combined obese men and women so it is difficult to know whether or not there are gender differences in the prevalence of obesity hypoventilation syndrome or obstructive sleep apnea. In one study, however, 86% of the participants were women, and the prevalence rates were similar to the other studies, with 40% having obstructive sleep apnea and 8% with obesity hypoventilation syndrome.[38]

Weight loss surgery has been shown to virtually eliminate respiratory insufficiency in those who are morbidly obese.[37,39,41] Marti-Valeri and colleagues[39] noted that subjects who had obstructive sleep apnea and obesity hypoventilation syndrome presurgery were resolved within 1 year post surgery (61 kg of weight loss). Sugarman and colleagues[41] noted that 80% of the subjects had their respiratory insufficiency cured within 1 year post surgery (after 50 kg of weight loss).

CARDIOVASCULAR COMPLICATIONS

There are several parameters of cardiac function that can be examined in obesity with the worst-case end result becoming heart failure. Heart failure is a pathophysiologic condition that is associated with obesity. It has been well established that increased BMI is associated with increased risk for heart failure.[42] Compared with women who have a normal BMI, obese women have double the risk for heart failure.[42] **Fig. 7** shows the crude cumulative incidence of heart failure in women according to BMI category up to 18 years of follow-up. Obese women have the greatest incidence of heart failure compared with overweight and normal-weight women. Similarly, among the three obesity classes, the risk for heart failure increases in a graded fashion with increasing severity of obesity (**Fig. 8**).

One way to examine cardiac function in obese women is through ECG tracings. In a recent study that included mostly women, resting ECG tracings showed that 62% of subjects demonstrated conduction or ST-T wave abnormalities.[38] That same study demonstrated that none of the morbidly obese subjects who exercised to 85% of their theoretic maximal heart rate had a positive stress test. This demonstrates that, on average, obese women can have normal ECG tracings during exercise.

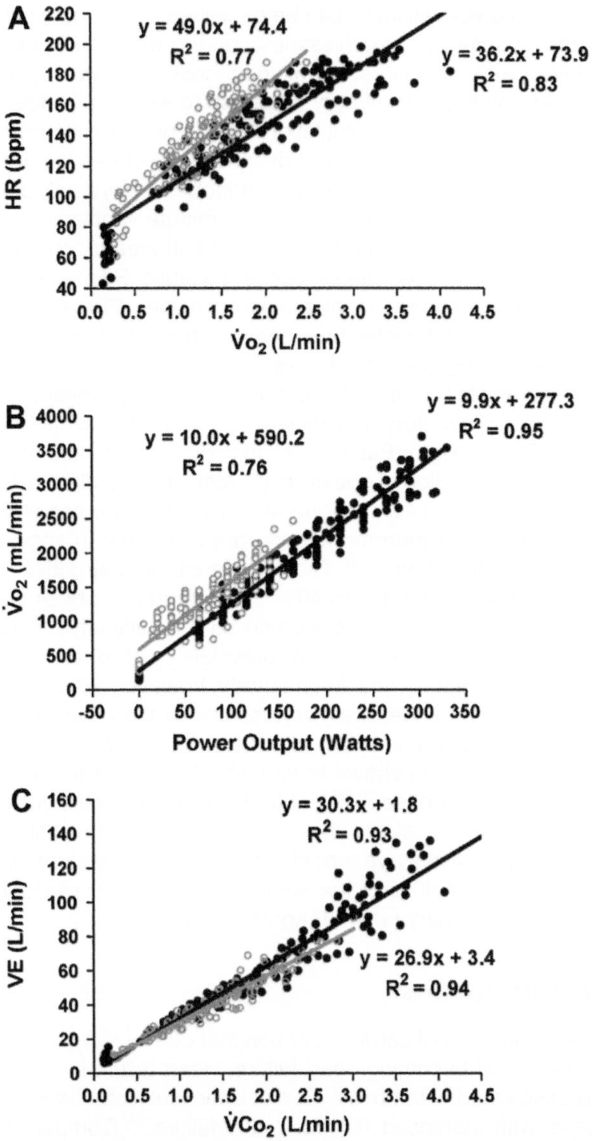

Fig. 6. Cardiopulmonary relationships during ramped cycling exercise. Pooled data. (*A*) Cardiac efficiency; (*B*) aerobic work efficiency; (*C*) ventilatory efficiency. A light gray regression line represents pooled data for morbidly obese women (*open gray circles*). The dark black line represents pooled data from fit nonobese women (*solid black circles*). Morbidly obese women have a poorer cardiac efficiency, a higher aerobic cost of exercise for the same power output, and a poorer ventilatory response to carbon dioxide production ($\dot{V}o_2$) compared with fit, nonobese women. (*From* Zavorsky GS, Murias JM, Kim DJ, et al. Poor compensatory hyperventilation in morbidly obese women at peak exercise. Respir Physiol Neurobiol 2007;159:187; with permission.)

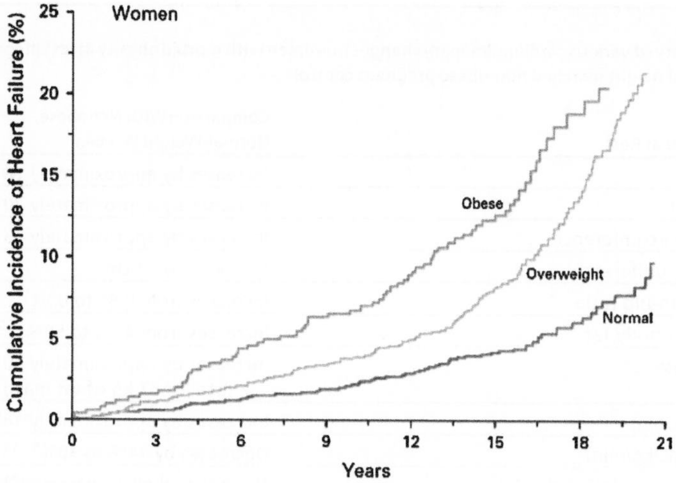

No. at Risk							
Normal	1729	1688	1634	1568	1477	1227	295
Overweight	955	929	880	815	757	634	248
Obese	493	477	448	409	372	296	104

Fig. 7. Cumulative incidence of heart failure according to category of BMI at base-line examination. BMI was 18.5 to 24.9 in normal subjects, 25.0 to 29.9 in overweight subjects, and 30.0 or more in obese subjects. (*From* Kenchaiah S, Evans JC, Levy D, et al. Obesity and the risk of heart failure. N Engl J Med 2002;347:305; with permission.)

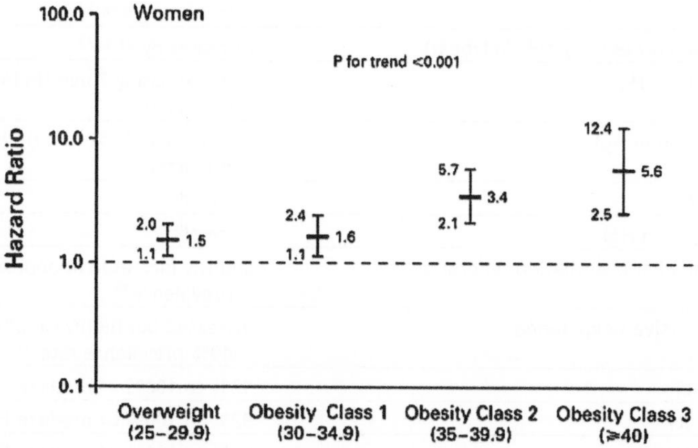

	Overweight (25–29.9)	Obesity Class 1 (30–34.9)	Obesity Class 2 (35–39.9)	Obesity Class 3 (≥40)
No. of events	108	40	21	7
No. at risk	955	339	111	43
Person-yr of follow-up	14,232	4909	1540	595

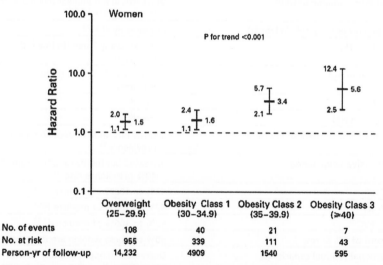

Fig. 8. Risk for heart failure in obese subjects, according to category of BMI at the base-line examination. I bars represent the 95% CI for the hazard ratios (HRs). HRs were adjusted for age, total serum cholesterol level, cigarette smoking, alcohol consumption, and presence or absence of valve disease, hypertension, diabetes mellitus, ECG evidence of left ventricular hypertrophy, and myocardial infarction at base line. Normal weight (BMI, 18.5 to 24.9) was the reference category. HRs on the Y axis are shown on a logarithmic scale. (*From* Kenchaiah S, Evans JC, Levy D, et al. Obesity and the risk of heart failure. N Engl J Med 2002;347:305; with permission.)

Table 1
Summary of various cardiopulmonary changes in women with morbid obesity at rest in comparison to age and height matched non-obese pregnant controls

Variable at Rest	Comparison With Nonobese, Normal-Weight Women
BMI	Increases by approximately twofold[11,24]
Weight	Increases by approximately 70 kg[11]
Waist circumference	Increases by approximately 53 cm[11]
Hip circumference	Increases by 51 cm[11]
Waist-to-hip ratio	Increases from 0.85 to 0.92[11]
Percent body fat	Increases from 45% to 50%[11,24]
Fat mass	Increases by approximately 50 kg (to a total of 67 kg of fat mass)[11]
$\dot{V}o_2$ (L/min)	Increases by approximately 14%[13]
$\dot{V}o_2$ (mL/kg/min)	Decreases by 14% to 30%[55,13]
Minute ventilation (L/min)	Normal or slightly increased[24,48]
HR (beats/min)	Increases by 15% to 30%[13,45]
Stroke volume (mL/beat)	Increases by approximately 20% (by 18 mL/beat)[44]
Ejection fraction	Decreases from 65% to 50% or 59%[44,45]
Cardiac output (L/min)	Increases by approximately 15% to 20% (by 0.8 to 1.4 L/min)[44,45]
Total blood volume (L)	Increases by approximately 14% (700 mL)[44]
Total blood volume (mL/kg)	Decreases in a nonlinear manner with increasing BMI[52]
Oxygen pulse ($\dot{V}o_2$/HR) (mL/beat)	Increases by 40%[13]
Pao_2 (mm Hg)	Approximately 7 mm Hg lower than predicted[8]
$AaDo_2$ (mm Hg)	Approximately 12 mm Hg higher than predicted[8]
Sao_2 (%)	Normal[8]
$Paco_2$ (mm Hg)	Normal[8]
Obesity hypoventilation syndrome	Slightly increased at approximately 10% prevalence[38]
Obstructive sleep apnea	Increased but highly variable, from 3% to 40% prevalence rate[37–41]
FVC (L)	92% to 100% of predicted[8,53]
FEV_1 (L)	92% to 100% of predicted[8,53]
FEV_1/FVC	92% to 100% of predicted[8,53]
Percent of EFL at rest	50% of obese women are flow limited[24]
Functional residual capacity (L)	Decreased to approximately 80% of predicted[24]
Expiratory reserve volume (L)	Decreased to 50% of predicted[24]
Residual volume (L)	Decreased to 90% of predicted[24]
Prevalence of dynamic hyperinflation	Increased[24]
EELV	Lower[24]

(*continued on next page*)

Table 1
(*continued*)

Variable at Rest	Comparison With Nonobese, Normal-Weight Women
Inspiratory reserve volume	Higher[24]
Pulmonary diffusing capacity for carbon monoxide (mL/min/mm Hg)	Approximately 100% of predicted[8]
Pulmonary diffusing capacity for nitric oxide (mL/min/mm Hg)	Approximately 100% of predicted[8]
Pulmonary Vc (mL)	Approximately 100% predicted[8,11]
Pulmonary Vc divided by VA (mL/L)	Increased to 120% or 130% of predicted[8]
Alveolar membrane diffusing capacity divided by VA (mL/min/mm Hg/min/L)	Increased to 120% or 130% of predicted[8]

Abbreviations: FEV_1, forced expiratory volume in 1 second; FVC, forced vital capacity; HR, heart rate; VA, alveolar volume; Vc, capillary blood volume; $\dot{V}O_2$, oxygen consumption.

Poor cardiac function in obesity includes lowered left ventricular ejection fraction,[43,44] decreased contractility,[45–47] and worsened cardiac efficiency reflected by the higher slope of the heart rate versus $\dot{V}O_2$ during graded exercise ($\Delta HR/\Delta\dot{V}O_2$)[13] compared with fit, nonobese women (see **Fig. 6**). The pooled data from **Fig. 6**A is comparable to other studies in which a similar cardiac efficiency index of 50 to 58 beats/L is reported in those who were morbidly obese.[48,49] The $\Delta HR/\Delta\dot{V}O_2$ that was higher and peak heart rate and O_2 pulse that were lower than predicted values in morbidly obese women[50,51] suggest poor cardiac accommodation in this population.

At rest, ejection fraction decreases with increasing BMI, whereas cardiac output, stroke volume, and total blood volume increase.[44] Blood volume expressed in mL/kg actually decreases, however, with increasing BMI in a nonlinear manner.[52] A substantial weight loss of 33 kg in obese women and men (from 117 to 84 kg) can decrease cardiac output, blood pressure, and heart rate by approximately 10% to 18% at rest whereas left ventricular ejection fraction can increase by 3%.[43] Cardiac output during exercise decreases in obese subjects at the same absolute workload.[45] With a reduction of weight by 55 kg (from 132 to 77 kg), cardiac output and stroke volume increased by 10% to 15% at a workload of 50 W in subjects who were previously morbidly obese.[45]

The change in oxygen uptake with changing workload ($\Delta\dot{V}O_2/\Delta W$) has been demonstrated to be a useful noninvasive index of aerobic work efficiency.[51] In several patient groups, this slope is lower, suggesting increased energetic contribution from anaerobic sources of ATP regeneration.[51] The aerobic work efficiency in morbidly obese women (see **Fig. 6**) is similar to the aerobic work efficiency reported elsewhere[53] and to predicted norms.[51] So, although the aerobic work efficiency was approximately the same in fit and obese groups, the relationship between oxygen consumption and power output shifted upward in obese women, demonstrating that a greater amount of oxygen must be consumed to accomplish the same power output as in nonobese individuals. Salvadori's group[54] also has shown that the relationship between oxygen consumption and power output shifted upward in the obese; however, in their study the aerobic work efficiency was approximately 20% lower (higher slope) in the obese compared with sedentary, fit individuals. More recent data suggest that obesity does not change the response slope ($\Delta\dot{V}O_2/\Delta W$), although it does displace the relationship upwards.[13,24,48,51] Weight loss does not change the slope, but it does displace the relationship downward.[10]

Table 2
Summary of various cardiopulmonary changes in women with morbid obesity during exercise in comparison to age and height matched non-obese pregnant controls

Variable During Submaximal Exercise or at Peak Exercise	Comparison With Nonobese, Normal-Weight Women
Power output at peak exercise (W)	Near normal to normal[8]
$\dot{V}O_2$ (L/min) at peak exercise	Near normal to normal[8,53]
$\dot{V}O_2$ (mL/kg/min) at peak exercise	Very much decreased. At or below 10th percentile of fitness when compared with American College of Sports Medicine normative data[8,53]
HR (beats/min) at peak exercise	Normal or slightly decreased[8,13]
Oxygen pulse ($\dot{V}O_2$/HR) at peak exercise	Normal[53] or decreased to 70% to 80% of predicted[8]
$\dot{V}E$ (L/min) at peak exercise	Normal or near normal[8,11]
Cardiac output (L/min)	Lower at the same submaximal power ouput[45]
Stroke volume (mL/beat)	Lower at the same submaximal power ouput[45]
Ejection fraction (%)	Lower at the same submaximal power ouput[45]
Cardiac efficiency (ΔHR/$\Delta\dot{V}O_2$)	Higher slope (indicating poor cardiac accommodation)[13]
Aerobic work efficiency ($\Delta\dot{V}O_2/\Delta$W)	Similar slope (10 to 11 mL/min/W) but higher Y intercept[13,24,48,51]
Ventilatory efficiency ($\Delta\dot{V}E/\Delta\dot{V}CO_2$)	Lower slope (worse)[13]
Breathing frequency (breaths/min) at the same $\dot{V}E$	Increased by approximately 3 to 5 breaths/min at same level of ventilation[24]
Tidal volume (L/breath)	Lower by approximately 200 mL/breath at the same level of ventilation[24]
Oxygen cost of breathing (mL of O_2 per L of ventilation)	3× higher (at 3.5 mL/L)[34]
Percent of EFL at exercise	50% of obese women are flow limited[24]
Prevalence of dynamic hyperinflation at exercise	Increased[24]
EELV at peak exercise	Approximately 400 mL higher[24]
PaO_2 at peak exercise (mm Hg)	Normal[8,53]
$AaDO_2$ (mm Hg)	Normal[8]
SaO_2 at peak exercise	Normal[8,53]
Prevalence of EIH	Approximately the same in morbidly obese women compared with nonobese women (at 10%) when $\dot{V}O_2$ at peak exercise is <50 kg/min[8,29]
$PaCO_2$ at peak exercise (mm Hg)	Inadequate compensatory exercise hyperventilation. Approximately 75% of morbidly obese women have a $PaCO_2$ > 35 mm Hg at peak exercise[8]
The slope of pulmonary diffusing capacity for carbon monoxide to $\dot{V}O_2$ (L/min)	Similar[11]
The slope of pulmonary diffusing capacity for nitric oxide to $\dot{V}O_2$ (L/min)	Similar[11]
The slope of pulmonary Vc to $\dot{V}O_2$ (L/min)	Similar[11]

Abbreviations: HR, heart rate; O_2, oxygen; Vc, capillary blood volume; $\dot{V}E$, expired volume per unit time; $\dot{V}O_2$ oxygen consumption, EIH, exercise-induced hypoexemia.

SUMMARY

Tables 1 and **2** summarize the mean differences in morbidly obese women compared with nonobese, normal-weight women. Morbid obesity was used as the comparison as it is this class of obesity that has the most profound changes in cardiopulmonary parameters compared with overweight or obese class I or II women. Some of the variables report only slight changes with morbid obesity, thus lower obesity classes would not likely perturb those same parameters. The predicted values from which morbid obesity in women is compared with are based on previously published reference equations for spirometry,[56] pulmonary diffusion,[7] arterial blood gases,[23] peak exercise variables,[51] and various slopes of dynamic responses to exercise.[51] Where reference equations are not available, a comparative nonobese group that is age and height matched are compared against the morbidly obese women.

This brief review of cardiopulmonary aspects of obesity in women shows that obese women—although not as affected as obese men—still have a worsened pulmonary gas exchange compared with predicted values at rest. Pulmonary function, such as spirometry and diffusing capacity, on the whole, remain relatively normal compared with predicted values. Few obese women have obesity hypoventilation syndrome. Despite EFL, dynamic hyperinflation, and inadequate compensatory exercise hyperventilation during exercise that occurs in obese women, few obese women develop hypoxemia and poor gas exchange even at peak exercise capacity. The low prevalence of hypoxemia during exercise, however, is due to the fact that peak exercise capacity in morbidly obese women is low, approximately at or below the 10th percentile of fitness, when aerobic capacity is expressed in mL/kg per minute. Obese women also have poor cardiac accommodation as reflected by a higher slope of the heart rate versus oxygen uptake during graded exercise and a lower oxygen pulse at peak exercise. Obesity increases the oxygen cost of exercise. Cardiac output, heart rate, and total blood volume is higher in obese women whereas the ejection fraction is lower compared with normal-weight women. Substantial weight loss in obese women lowers cardiac output and increases ejection fraction at rest. When these same women exercise at the same power output as before weight loss, they show an increase in cardiac output and stroke volume.

REFERENCES

1. Kung HC, Hoyert DL, Xu J, et al. Deaths: final data for 2005. Natl Vital Stat Rep 2008;56:1–120.
2. Ogden CL, Carroll MD, Curtin LR, et al. Prevalence of overweight and obesity in the United States, 1999–2004. JAMA 2006;295:1549–55.
3. Kopelman P. Health risks associated with overweight and obesity. Obes Rev 2007;8(Suppl 1):13–7.
4. Mahony D. Psychological gender differences in bariatric surgery candidates. Obes Surg 2008;18:607–10.
5. Sturm R. Increases in clinically severe obesity in the United States, 1986–2000. Arch Intern Med 2003;163:2146–8.
6. Calle EE, Thun MJ, Petrelli JM, et al. Body-mass index and mortality in a prospective cohort of U.S. adults. N Engl J Med 1999;341:1097–105.
7. Zavorsky GS, Cao J, Murias JM. Reference values of pulmonary diffusing capacity for nitric oxide in an adult population. Nitric Oxide 2008;18:70–9.
8. Zavorsky GS, Christou NV, Kim DJ, et al. Preoperative gender differences in pulmonary gas exchange in morbidly obese subjects. Obes Surg 2008;18:1587–98.

9. Zavorsky GS, Gow J, Murias JM. Potassium kinetics and its relationship with ventilation during repeated bouts of exercise in women. Eur J Appl Physiol 2007;99:173–81.
10. Zavorsky GS, Kim DJ, Christou NV. Compensatory exercise hyperventilation is restored in the morbidly obese after bariatric surgery. Obes Surg 2008;18: 549–59.
11. Zavorsky GS, Kim DJ, McGregor ER, et al. Pulmonary diffusing capacity for nitric oxide during exercise in morbid obesity. Obesity (Silver Spring) 2008;16:2431–8.
12. Zavorsky GS, Kim DJ, Sylvestre JL, et al. Alveolar-membrane diffusing capacity improves in the morbidly obese after bariatric surgery. Obes Surg 2008;18: 256–63.
13. Zavorsky GS, Murias JM, Kim DJ, et al. Poor compensatory hyperventilation in morbidly obese women at peak exercise. Respir Physiol Neurobiol 2007;159: 187–95.
14. Zavorsky GS, Murias JM, Kim do J, et al. Waist-to-hip ratio is associated with pulmonary gas exchange in the morbidly obese. Chest 2007;131:362–7.
15. Zavorsky GS, Saul L, Decker A, et al. Radiographic evidence of pulmonary edema during high-intensity interval training in women. Respir Physiol Neurobiol 2006;153:181–90.
16. Zavorsky GS, Saul L, Murias JM, et al. Pulmonary gas exchange does not worsen during repeat exercise in women. Respir Physiol Neurobiol 2006;153:226–36.
17. Zavorsky GS, Hoffman SL. Pulmonary gas exchange in the morbidly obese. Obes Rev 2008;9:326–39.
18. Zavorsky GS. Pulmonary gas exchange and diffusing capacity at rest and during exercise in those with morbid obesity: pre and post surgical intervention. In: Parsons WV, Taylor CM, editors. New research on morbid obesity. New York: Nova Science Publishers; 2008. p. 117–50.
19. Babb TG, Ranasinghe KG, Comeau LA, et al. Dyspnea on exertion in obese women: association with an increased oxygen cost of breathing. Am J Respir Crit Care Med 2008;178:116–23.
20. Ravipati G, Aronow WS, Sidana J, et al. Association of reduced carbon monoxide diffusing capacity with moderate or severe left ventricular diastolic dysfunction in obese persons. Chest 2005;128:1620–2.
21. Holley HS, Milic-Emili J, Becklake MR, et al. Regional distribution of pulmonary ventilation and perfusion in obesity. J Clin Invest 1967;46:475–81.
22. Vaughan RW, Cork RC, Hollander D. The effect of massive weight loss on arterial oxygenation and pulmonary function tests. Anesthesiology 1981;54:325–8.
23. Crapo RO, Jensen RL, Hegewald M, et al. Arterial blood gas reference values for sea level and an altitude of 1,400 meters. Am J Respir Crit Care Med 1999;160: 1525–31.
24. Ofir D, Laveneziana P, Webb KA, et al. Ventilatory and perceptual responses to cycle exercise in obese females. J Appl Physiol 2007;102:2217–26.
25. Babb TG, Wyrick BL, DeLorey DS, et al. Fat distribution and end-expiratory lung volume in lean and obese men and women. Chest 2008;134:704.
26. Dempsey JA, Wagner PD. Exercise-induced arterial hypoxemia. J Appl Physiol 1999;87:1997–06.
27. Richards JC, McKenzie DC, Warburton DE, et al. Prevalence of exercise-induced arterial hypoxemia in healthy women. Med Sci Sports Exerc 2004;36: 1514–21.
28. Harms CA, McClaran SR, Nickele GA, et al. Exercise-induced arterial hypoxaemia in healthy young women. J Physiol (Lond) 1998;507:619–28.

29. Harms CA. Does gender affect pulmonary function and exercise capacity? Respir Physiol Neurobiol 2006;151:124–31.
30. ACSM. ACSM's Guidelines for exercise testing and prescription. 8th edition. Baltimore (MD): Lippincott Williams & Wilkins; 2009.
31. Hopkins SR, Barker RC, Brutsaert TD, et al. Pulmonary gas exchange during exercise in women: effects of exercise type and work increment. J Appl Physiol 2000;89:721–30.
32. Olfert IM, Balouch J, Kleinsasser A, et al. Does gender affect human pulmonary gas exchange during exercise? J Physiol 2004;557:529–41.
33. Wang LY, Cerny FJ. Ventilatory response to exercise in simulated obesity by chest loading. Med Sci Sports Exerc 2004;36:780–6.
34. Babb TG. Mechanical ventilatory constraints in aging, lung disease, and obesity: perspectives and brief review. Med Sci Sports Exerc 1999;31:S12–22.
35. Wood HE, Semon TL, Comeau LA, et al. The ventilatory response to exercise does not differ between obese women with and without dyspnea on exertion. Adv Exp Med Biol 2008;605:514–8.
36. Burwell CS, Robin ED, Whaley RD, et al. Extreme obesity associated with alveolar hypoventilation; a Pickwickian syndrome. Am J Med 1956;21:811–8.
37. Catheline JM, Bihan H, Le Quang T, et al. Preoperative cardiac and pulmonary assessment in bariatric surgery. Obes Surg 2008;18:271–7.
38. Boone KA, Cullen JJ, Mason EE, et al. Impact of vertical banded gastroplasty on respiratory insufficiency of severe obesity. Obes Surg 1996;6:454–8.
39. Marti-Valeri C, Sabate A, Masdevall C, et al. Improvement of associated respiratory problems in morbidly obese patients after open Roux-en-Y gastric bypass. Obes Surg 2007;17:1102–10.
40. Reichel G. Lung volumes, mechanics of breathing and changes in arterial blood gases in obese patients and in Pickwickian syndrome. Bull Physiopathol Respir (Nancy) 1972;8:1011–20.
41. Sugerman HJ, Fairman RP, Baron PL, et al. Gastric surgery for respiratory insufficiency of obesity. Chest 1986;90:81–6.
42. Kenchaiah S, Evans JC, Levy D, et al. Obesity and the risk of heart failure. N Engl J Med 2002;347:305–13.
43. Karason K, Wallentin I, Larsson B, et al. Effects of obesity and weight loss on cardiac function and valvular performance. Obes Res 1998;6:422–49.
44. Licata G, Scaglione R, Barbagallo M, et al. Effect of obesity on left ventricular function studied by radionuclide angiocardiography. Int J Obes 1991;15: 295–02.
45. Alaud-din A, Meterissian S, Lisbona R, et al. Assessment of cardiac function in patients who were morbidly obese. Surgery 1990;108:809–18 [discussion: 1818–20].
46. de Divitiis O, Fazio S, Petitto M, et al. Obesity and cardiac function. Circulation 1981;64:477–82.
47. Garavaglia GE, Messerli FH, Nunez BD, et al. Myocardial contractility and left ventricular function in obese patients with essential hypertension. Am J Cardiol 1988;62:594–7.
48. Salvadori A, Fanari P, Fontana M, et al. Oxygen uptake and cardiac performance in obese and normal subjects during exercise. Respiration 1999;66:25–33.
49. Lafortuna CL, Proietti M, Agosti F, et al. The energy cost of cycling in young obese women. Eur J Appl Physiol 2006;97:16–25.
50. Jones NL, Makrides L, Hitchcock C, et al. Normal standards for an incremental progressive cycle ergometer test. Am Rev Respir Dis 1985;131:700–8.

51. Neder JA, Nery LE, Peres C, et al. Reference values for dynamic responses to incremental cycle ergometry in males and females aged 20 to 80. Am J Respir Crit Care Med 2001;164:1481–6.
52. Lemmens HJ, Bernstein DP, Brodsky JB. Estimating blood volume in obese and morbidly obese patients. Obes Surg 2006;16:773–6.
53. Dolfing JG, Dubois EF, Wolffenbuttel BH, et al. Different cycle ergometer outcomes in severely obese men and women without documented cardiopulmonary morbidities before bariatric surgery. Chest 2005;128:256–62.
54. Salvadori A, Fanari P, Mazza P, et al. Work capacity and cardiopulmonary adaptation of the obese subject during exercise testing. Chest 1992;101:674–9.
55. Byrne NM, Hills AP, Hunter GR, et al. The metabolic equivalent: one size does not fit all. J Appl Physiol 2005;99:1112–9.
56. Hankinson JL, Odencrantz JR, Fedan KB. Spirometric reference values from a sample of the general U.S. population. Am J Respir Crit Care Med 1999;159:179–87.

Pregnancy and Obesity

Yariv Yogev, MD[a,*], Patrick M. Catalano, MD[b]

KEYWORDS

- Obesity • Pregnancy • Gestational diabetes
- Metabolic syndrome

Obesity has become a worldwide epidemic.[1] The latest reports of the World Health Organization (WHO) indicate that in 2005, approximately 1.6 billion adults were overweight and at least 400 million adults were obese. Overweight and obesity are defined as abnormal or excessive percent-fat accumulation that may impair health. As a rule, women have more body fat than men, and it is widely agreed that men with more than 30% body fat and women with more than 25% body fat are obese. The WHO and the National Institutes of Health define underweight as a body mass index (BMI, wt/ht^2) 18.5 or less, normal weight as a BMI of 18.5 to 24.9, overweight as a BMI of 25 to 29.9, and obesity as a BMI of 30 or greater. Obesity is further characterized by BMI into class I (30–34.9), class II (35–39.9), and class III (greater than 40).[1] The WHO also projects that by 2015, approximately 2.3 billion adults will be overweight and more than 700 million will be obese. Results from the latest 2003–2004 United States National Health and Nutrition Examination Survey (NHANES) indicate that 66.3% of adults are either overweight (BMI $\geq$ 25) or obese, with 32.2% being obese (BMI $\geq$ 30). The prevalence of overweight and obesity among adults aged 20 to 74 years in the United States has increased from 47.0% (in the 1976–1980 survey) to 66.3% (in the 2003–2004 survey). Over the same period, the prevalence of obesity has doubled among women from 16.5% to 33.2%.[2,3]

As the prevalence of obesity is increasing, so is the number of women of reproductive age who are overweight and obese. In the United States, the incidence of obesity among pregnant women ranges from 18.5% to 38.3% according to different reports.[4–8] This article addresses issues concerning pregravid obesity and weight gain during pregnancy and their implication on gestational diabetes and pregnancy outcome.

THE INFLUENCE OF OBESITY ON PREGNANCY OUTCOME IN THE NONDIABETIC PATIENT

As the prevalence of obesity is increasing, so is the number of women in the reproductive age who are overweight and obese. The average BMI is increasing among all age

[a] Division of Perinatal, Helen Schneider Hospital for Women, Rabin Medical Center, Sackler Faculty of Medicine, Tel Aviv University, Petah-Tiqva 49100, Israel
[b] Department of Reproductive Biology, Case Western Reserve University at MetroHealth Medical Center, Cleveland, OH, USA
* Corresponding author.
E-mail address: yarivyogev@hotmail.com (Y. Yogev).

Obstet Gynecol Clin N Am 36 (2009) 285–300
doi:10.1016/j.ogc.2009.03.003

categories and women are entering pregnancy at higher weights. Women are also more likely to retain gestational weight with each successive pregnancy.

Human pregnancy is an insulin-resistant condition by itself, potentially compounded by increased pregravid insulin resistance in obese women. There is a 40% to 50% increase in insulin resistance during pregnancy (from pregravid condition).[9,10] It is now universally acknowledged that maternal overweight and obesity are linked with adverse pregnancy outcome. Maternal complications include hypertension, diabetes, respiratory complications (asthma and sleep apnea), thromboembolic disease, more frequent cesarean delivery with increased wound infection, endometritis, and anesthetic complications (mainly difficulties in intubation and placement of epidural). Newborn complications include congenital malformations, large-for-gestational-age (LGA) infants, stillbirths, shoulder dystocia, and long-term adolescent complications (obesity and diabetes). Severe class II and III obese women are prone to even more complications and adverse outcomes. A discussion of these complications should be the balance between the benefit/risk ratio of fetal and maternal perspectives.

Fertility

Several studies have shown an increased risk of anovulatory infertility in obese women (odds ration or OR 2–3) by mechanisms including hyperandrogenism and polycystic ovary syndrome, which share several pathophysiologic characteristics, namely insulin resistance.[11–15] Although some controversy still exists regarding the effect of obesity in patients who have in vitro fertilization, three large population-based retrospective studies have shown lower pregnancy rates in obese patients. Linsten and colleagues[16] reported the results of 8,457 in vitro fertilization patients showing significantly lower birth rate in women with a BMI greater than or equal to 27 (OR 0.67, 95% confidence interval or CI 0.48–0.94). Fedorcsak and colleagues[17] reviewed 5,019 in vitro fertilization cycles and found a lower cumulative live-birth rate in the obese group: 41.4% versus 50.3% in normal-weight women (95% CI 32.1–50.7; NS). Wang and colleagues[18] reported the results of 3,586 patients and established a significant linear reduction in fecundity from the moderately obese to the very obese group ($P<.001$). Body fat distribution in women of reproductive age seems to have more impact on fertility than age or obesity itself; a 0.1-unit increase in waist-hip ratio led to a 30% decrease in probability of conception per cycle (hazard ration or HR 0.7; 95% CI 0.5–0.8).[13]

Miscarriage

Although the relationship between obesity and first-trimester miscarriage has been investigated extensively, the results are far from conclusive and require further research. Whereas several studies suggest that obesity may increase the risk of miscarriage[19–23] because of adverse influences on the embryo, the endometrium, or both,[20] others found no association between miscarriage and obesity.[24–27] These studies lack consistency, however, mainly because of the use of different obesity classification systems that disregard the WHO criteria.

Thromboembolic Complications

Pregnancy itself is a prothrombotic state with increases in the plasma concentration of coagulation factors I, VII, VIII, and X, a decrease in protein S, and inhibition of fibrinolysis, resulting in a fivefold increased risk for venous thrombosis.[28,29] Other factors likely to be important in the etiology of pregnancy-associated vein thromboembolisem are advanced maternal age, high parity, operative delivery, preeclampsia, and obesity. Abdollahi and colleagues[30] evaluated in a case-controlled study, the risk of thrombosis because of overweight and obesity after a first episode of objectively diagnosed thrombosis. Obesity (BMI $\geq$ 30) increased the risk of thrombosis twofold. Obese individuals had higher levels of factor VIII and IX but not of fibrinogen. In addition, the combined effect of obesity and oral contraceptive pills among women aged 15 to 45 revealed that pill users had a 10-fold increased risk for thrombosis when BMI was greater than 25.

Hypertensive Disorders

Arterial blood pressure, hemoconcentration, and cardiac function are all altered by the hemodynamic changes brought about by obesity. Some investigators have suggested a 10-fold higher rate of chronic hypertension in obese compared with normal-weight women.[31–35] The risk of pregnancy-induced hypertension or preeclampsia are significantly greater if the mother is overweight as assessed by BMI in early pregnancy.[36,37] Studies suggest a two- to threefold increased risk for preeclampsia with a BMI of greater than 30. Sattar and colleagues[38] reported the results of the risk of hypertensive complications of pregnancy in association with a waist circumference of greater than 80 cm in data from 1,142 pregnant women. The risk of pregnancy-induced hypertension was twofold greater (OR 1; 89% CI 1.1–2.9) and preeclampsia threefold (OR 2.7; 95% CI 1.1–6.8) greater in association with visceral obesity. Waist circumference was demonstrated to be a more sensitive risk marker than BMI.[30] In a study of 287,213 pregnancies, Sebire and colleagues[35] included 176,923 (61.6%) normal weight (BMI 20–24.9), 79,014 (27.5%) overweight (BMI 25–29.9), and 31,276 (10.9%) obese (BMI $\geq$30) women. Obese women were two to three times more likely to develop proteinuric preeclampsia.

Birth weight above the nintieth percentile was also increased in obese women, as was intrauterine death. Intrapartum complications included an increased rate of induction of labor and delivery by cesarean section. In the postpartum period there was an increased rate of hemorrhage, genital tract infection, urinary tract infection, and wound infection. The investigators concluded that maternal obesity carries significant risk for both mother and fetus, with risk increasing with the degree of obesity. These risks persist after adjusting for confounding demographic factors. Bianco and colleagues[39,40] performed a retrospective cohort study of 613 obese (BMI > 35; class II and III) and 11,313 nonobese women. A fourfold increased risk for preeclampsia was reported in the obese women. There was a 50% increase in frequency of fetal distress and a twofold increase in cesarean delivery. Postpartum, obese women had a threefold increased incidence of endometritis. Kumari[31] evaluated 159 pregnant women with BMI greater than 40 and 300 women with normal BMI matched for age and parity. Women with pre-existing diabetes and hypertension were excluded. A BMI greater than 40 was associated with hypertensive disorder of pregnancy in 28.8%, compared with 2.9% in the nonobese group. Additionally, Stone and colleagues[41] reported that the only risk factors associated with the development of severe preeclampsia were severe obesity in all patients (OR 3.5, 95% CI 1.6–7.4) and a history of preeclampsia in multiparous patients (OR 7.2, 95% CI 2.7–18.7). Finally, a meta-analysis showed that the risk of preeclampsia doubled with each 5 kg/m^2 to 7 kg/m^2 increase in prepregnancy BMI. This relation persisted in studies that excluded women with chronic hypertension, diabetes mellitus or multiple gestations, and other confounders.[42]

Epidemiologic studies have reported a relationship between pregnancies complicated by preeclampsia and increased risk of maternal coronary heart disease in later life. The reported increase in the relative risk of death from ischemic heart disease in association with a history of preeclampsia/eclampsia is approximately twofold.[42]

Preeclampsia shares many common pathologic pathways with ischemic heart disease.

Stillbirth and Fetal Death

Stillbirth remains a serious reproductive failure, with a frequency of two to five per 1,000 births, and constitutes more than half of all perinatal deaths.[43,44] Prepregnancy BMI and fetal death were examined in the Danish National Birth Cohort among 54,505 pregnant women. They reported a fivefold increase in risk of stillbirth in obese women. Prepregnancy obesity correlated with an increased risk of both late spontaneous abortion and stillbirth expressed as follows: before week 14: HR 0.8 (CI 0.5–1.4); weeks 14 to 19: HR 1.6 (CI 1.0–2.5); weeks 20 to 27: HR 1.9 (CI 1.1–3.3); weeks 28 to 36: HR 2.1 (CI 1.0–4.4); weeks 37 to 39: HR 3.5 (CI 1.9–6.4); and weeks 40 to 40+: HR 4.6 (CI 1.6–13.4). Overweight women also experienced a higher risk after 28 weeks and especially after 40 weeks of gestation: HR 2.9 (CI 1.1–7.7).[45] In a large British register-based study, overweight and obesity were only modestly related to intrauterine death [OR 1.1 (CI 0.9–1.2) and OR 1.4 (C.I 1.1–1.7), respectively] after adjustment for obesity-related diseases in pregnancy.[35] In a large Swedish population-based cohort of 167,750 women, the odds ratios for late fetal death were increased among nulliparous women who were overweight and obese [OR 3.2 (CI 1.6–6.2) and OR 4.3 (CI 2.0–9.3), respectively]. Among parous women, only obese women had a significant increase in the risk of late fetal death OR 2.0 (CI 1.2–3.3).[46] Moreover, Salihu and colleagues[47] reported in a large cohort of 134,527 obese women that overall, obese mothers were approximately 40% more likely to experience stillbirth than nonobese women (adjusted HR 1.4; CI 1.3–1.5). The risk for stillbirth increased in a dose-dependent fashion with increasing BMI: class I, HR 1.3 (CI 1.2–1.4); class II HR 1.4 (CI 1.3–1.6); and class III HR 1.9 (CI 1.6–2.1) (*P* for trend <.01).

Preterm Delivery

Most investigators report both low prepregnancy weight and poor weight gain in low BMI women as risk factors for preterm birth.[48–50] Regarding obese women, reports are inconclusive. Current evidence suggests that obesity may be associated with induced preterm delivery but not spontaneous preterm birth. Smith and colleagues[51] reported that among nulliparous women, the risk of spontaneous preterm labor decreased with increasing BMI, whereas the risk of requiring an elective preterm delivery increased. Obese nulliparous women were at increased risk of all-cause preterm delivery. In contrast, obesity and elective preterm delivery were only weakly associated among multiparous women. Bhattacharya and colleagues[52] also reported that the frequency of induced labor increased with increasing BMI, the risk being lowest in underweight women (BMI ≤ 19.9) (OR 0.8; 95% CI 0.8–0.9) and highest in the class II obese (OR 1.8; 95% CI 1.3–2.5). In a large retrospective cohort study including 62,167 women within the Danish National Birth Cohort, the crude risks of preterm premature rupture of membranes and of induced preterm deliveries were higher in obese as compared with normal-weight women, especially before 34 completed weeks of gestation (HR 1.5; CI 1.2–1.9 and HR 1.2; CI 1.0–1.6, respectively).[53]

Cesarean Section

Studies report a nearly twofold increased risk of cesarean delivery in women who are obese even after controlling for other factors. Why obesity increases the risk for cesarean section with an even greater risk among very obese women needs further study. The increased risk of cesarean delivery in obese women is an issue of grave concern. Apart from the immediate operative risk, the increased cesarean rate in overweight and obese women is also associated with an increase in postoperative complications, such as wound infection/breakdown, excessive blood loss, deep venous thrombosis, and postpartum endometritis. In a large retrospective study of 26,682 nulliparous women with singleton term deliveries, the incidence of cesarean delivery increased with increased prepregnancy BMI from 14.3% for lean women (BMI < 19.8) to 42.6% for class II women. Among women without any complications, the estimated adjusted relative risk (RR) was 1.4 (95% CI 1.0–1.8) among overweight women, 1.5 (95% CI 1.1–2.1) among obese women, and 3.1 (95% CI 2.3–4.8) among very obese women.[54] Similar results were reported by Vahratian,[55] showing an unadjusted RR of 1.4 for cesarean delivery among overweight and obese women. After controlling for maternal height, education, weight gain during pregnancy, and labor induction, the adjusted RR for cesarean delivery among overweight women was 1.2 (95% CI 0.8–1.8) and for obese women 1.5 (95% CI 1.05–2.0). Weiss and colleagues[25] reported the rate of cesarean section among nulliparous women to be 20.7% for normal-weight women, 33.8% for class I obese, and 47.4% for class II obese patients. Similar results were reported by Holger and colleagues,[56] with the increased risk of cesarean section rising with increasing BMI: 25.1% class I, 30.2% class II, and 43.1% in class III obese women, mainly because of repeat cesarean deliveries. Another study conducted among 1,881 low-risk women reported an overall cesarean rate of 5.1%, but the rate rose to 7.7% for obese women (BMI > 29) compared with 4.1% for women with normal BMI. After adjustment for weight gain, short stature, advanced maternal age, parity, and intrapartum complications, the OR for cesarean delivery in obese patients was approximately 4 (95% CI 2.0–7.9, *P*<.001).[57] Interestingly, Brost and colleagues[58] found that for each one-unit increase in prepregnancy or 27- to 31-week BMI, there was a parallel increase in the odds of cesarean delivery of 7.0% and 7.8%, respectively. Obesity is also associated with increased risk of vaginal operative delivery: 33.8% in the obese and 47.4% in the very obese group versus 20.7% in controls.[59]

Birth Defects

Apart from the increase in failure to detect birth defects in obese women because of difficult interpretation of serum markers (changes in the volume of distribution) and suboptimal visualization of fetal anatomy by ultrasound examination, several studies report a significant increase in birth defects among obese women. In 1994, Waller and colleagues[60] first suggested that offspring of obese women were at increased risk of neural tube defects (OR 1.8; 95% CI 1.1–3.0), especially spina bifida (OR 2.6; 95% CI 1.5–4.5). These results have been confirmed in subsequent studies and have also shown increased risks of heart defects (OR 1.18; 95% CI 1.09–1.27)[61] and omphalocele (OR 3.3; 95% CI 1.0–10.3).[62] Because these types of congenital anomalies are often seen with pregestational diabetes, some investigators suggest that many of these obese women may have had undiagnosed type 2 diabetes.[62] Neural tube defects are associated with folic acid deficiencies, yet it is inconclusive if such a deficiency is a contributing factor to the increased risk of neural tube defect in obese women. Mojtabai[63] suggested that women with a BMI greater than 30 would need to increase their folate consumption by 350 mcg/day to achieve the same folate levels as women with BMI less than 20. In contrast, in a Canadian population Ray and colleagues[64] estimated whether the risk of neural tube defects was lower after flour was fortified with folic acid and surprisingly found the opposite result. Before fortification of flour, increased maternal weight was associated with a modest increased risk of neural tube defects (OR 1.4; 95% CI 1.0–1.8); after flour fortification, the risk actually increased (OR 2.8; 95% CI 1.2–6.6).

Fetal Overgrowth

Many variables have been associated with fetal overgrowth or macrosomia. Increasingly, maternal pregravid weight and decreased pregravid insulin sensitivity have been shown to strongly correlate with fetal growth, especially fat mass at birth.[65] Increased maternal insulin resistance may be associated with altered placental function in addition to increased feto-placental availability of nutrients in late gestation. These nutrients include glucose, but also free fatty acids and amino acids. As a result, women with gestational diabetes mellitus (GDM) are at increased risk of having a macrosomic infant; those who are obese with normal glucose tolerance are almost twice as likely to have a macrosomic infant.[66] Morbid obesity (BMI > 35) increases the risk of birth weights greater than 4,000 g (OR 2.1; 95% CI 1.3–3.2).[52] Ehrenberg and colleagues[67] reviewed the results of 12,950 pregnancies and found that obesity and pregestational diabetes both are independently associated an increased risk of macrosomia. After adjusting for confounding risk factors, these investigators found that compared with normal BMI subjects, obese women were at elevated risk for LGA newborn delivery (16.8% versus 10.5%; $P<.0001$), as were overweight women (12.3% versus 10.5%; $P = .01$). Baeten and colleagues[68] found that the risk of delivering a macrosomic infant was increased (albeit not in a dose-related fashion with each level of increasing BMI, independent of the diagnosis of diabetes; BMI >30: OR 2.1, 95% CI 1.9–2.4; BMI 25–29.9: OR 1.5, 95% CI 1.4–1.6; BMI 20–24.9: OR 1.2, 95% CI 1.2–1.3). Because the prevalence and frequency of overweight and obese women is nearly 10 times that of gestational diabetes (45% versus 4.5%), abnormal maternal body habitus is likely to have the strongest attributable risk on the prevalence of macrosomia.

The magnitude of effect of obesity on the risk of macrosomia in normal (nondiabetic) pregnancies varies considerably between different studies and has been reported to range from 1.4- to 18-fold.[8,69–74] Several studies have shown a continuous relationship between maternal obesity and risk for fetal macrosomia/LGA infants, so that the higher the BMI, the higher the risk.[8,25,71,75]

When studying effects of obesity on pregnancy outcome, it is often uncertain if adequate screening for GDM has been performed, and therefore it is often difficult to assess if effects are caused by obesity or by GDM. In a study by Jensen and colleagues,[76] all women with GDM were excluded. They evaluated pregnancy outcome and BMI in glucose-tolerant nondiabetic Danish women. They concluded that the risk of hypertensive complications, cesarean section, induction of labor, and macrosomia were all significantly increased in both overweight women (BMI 25.0–29.9) and obese women (BMI > 30) compared with women who were of normal weight (BMI 18.5–24.9). The frequencies of shoulder dystocia, preterm delivery, and infant morbidity other than macrosomia were not significantly associated with maternal BMI. This population-based study clearly demonstrates that prepregnancy overweight and obesity are associated with adverse pregnancy outcome in glucose-tolerant women. In a large multicenter study of more than 16,000 patients, class I and class II obesity were associated with an increased risk of fetal macrosomia (OR 1.7 and 1.9, respectively).[25] In another population-based study, the risk of delivering a macrosomic infant increased with each level of increasing BMI, using BMI less than 20 as the reference: BMI 20 to 24.9 (OR 1.2, 95% CI 1.2–1.3), BMI 25 to 29.9 (OR 1.5, 95% CI 1.4–1.6), BMI greater than 30 (OR 2.1, 95% CI 1.9–2.4).[68] Importantly, diabetes was excluded in these studies.

Thus, it appears that obesity, and probably overweight as well, has independent risk factors for macrosomia/LGA infants, and this risk is proportional to the level of obesity. The mechanism by which obesity affects neonatal birth weight is unclear. Possible explanations include obesity-related insulin resistance and genetic factors. The copresence of undetected type 2 or gestational diabetes, both of which have been shown to be associated with obesity, is another possible explanation.

Table 1 summarizes the approximate risk for the above-mentioned obstetric complications.

Weight Gain During Pregnancy and Fetal Overgrowth

Apart from pregravid maternal obesity, excessive weight gain during pregnancy has also been reported to be an independent risk factor for macrosomia.[69,77] In another study of women with varying levels of glucose intolerance, weight gain during pregnancy was found to be at least as important as glycemic control in affecting birth weight.[75] Furthermore, Ray and colleagues[69] calculated that for each 5-kg increase in weight during pregnancy, the risk for LGA infants is increased by 30%.

The time interval of weight gain during pregnancy is also of importance. In a prospective study of 389 uncomplicated pregnancies, weight gain during the first trimester was the best predictor of neonatal weight (31 g for each 1-kg maternal weight gain), followed by weight during the second trimester (26 g per 1 kg), while weight gain during the third trimester was not associated with newborn weight.[78]

THE ASSOCIATION BETWEEN MATERNAL OBESITY AND GDM

The association between obesity, hypertension, and insulin resistance in type 2 diabetes is well recognized. Approximately 3% to 15% of women develop GDM during pregnancy. Although many factors are related to this risk, including ethnicity, previous occurrence of GDM, age, parity, family history of diabetes, and degree of hyperglycemia in pregnancy, obesity is an independent risk for developing GDM, with a risk of about 20%.[26,27] It has been shown that even minor degrees of carbohydrate intolerance are related to obesity and pregnancy outcome.[75,78]

Sebire and colleagues[35] found a twofold increase in the rate of GDM (OR 1.68; 95% CI 1.53–1.84). Kumari,[31] comparing obese and nonobese patients, found a rate of GDM of 24.5% for the obese and 2.2% for the nonobese. Bianco and colleagues[39] reported a threefold increase in GDM for obese patients. A population-based cohort study of 96,801 singleton births found that not only obese women but also overweight women had a markedly increased risk for GDM (OR 5.0 and 2.4, respectively).[68]

Table 1
Average increased risk for obstetric complications associated with maternal obesity

Complication	Increased Odds Ratio
Infertility	2–3
Miscarriage	1.5–2
Thromboembolic complications	2–4
Hypertensive complications	2–3
Stillbirth	2–3
Preterm delivery	1.5–2
Cesarean section	2–3
Birth defects	1
Fetal overgrowth	1.5–2
Gestational diabetes	3–5

In a study of 6,857 women, Yogev and colleagues[79] found a direct association between glucose-screening categories, obesity, and rate of GDM. For patients with 50-g glucose challenge-test screening results from 130 mg/dL to 189 mg/dL, the rate of obesity was approximately 24% to 30%. Thereafter, at glucose challenge-test result greater than 190 mg, the rate of obesity increased twofold. In contrast, for nonobese women, the rate of GDM increased almost linearly for each 10-mg increment in glucose-screening value. These data demonstrate that the degree of obesity and glucose tolerance are both independently associated with the development of GDM. In another study, Yogev and colleagues[80] have shown that fetal size and cesarean section rate are associated with the degree of carbohydrate intolerance as represented by screening results. Furthermore, obesity was a significant and independent contributor impacting fetal growth.

Nondiabetic pregnant women have been the populations in the majority of studies in which the relationship between maternal prepregnancy weight and perinatal outcome have been addressed. However, there is scant data on obesity and overweight in GDM. The few studies reporting obesity in GDM lack information on the effect of achieving targeted levels of glycemic control and treatment modalities on pregnancy outcome.[81–83] Leiken and colleagues[81] demonstrated an independent risk for macrosomia among obese GDM women. They found that GDM had a frequency of macrosomia no different than that of nondiabetic subjects: nonobese GDM women with fasting hyperglycemia treated with diet and insulin therapy had a frequency of macrosomia no different than that of nondiabetic women. However, diet and insulin did not prevent excess macrosomia in women who were obese. These studies had small sample sizes, failed to provide information on glycemic control, and only evaluated single-outcome variables. Maternal age, parity, and obesity are all over-represented among GDM women. These variables need to be controlled to draw accurate conclusions that also control confounding effects. Therefore, it is not clear if obesity, level of glycemia, or treatment modalities is independently or cumulatively responsible for fetal-growth abnormalities.

In a previous study, Langer and colleagues[84] found that obese and overweight GDM patients achieving established levels of glucose control with insulin therapy showed no increased risk for composite outcome, macrosomia, and LGA in comparison to normal-weight GDM patients. In contrast, even when diet-treated obese patients achieved good glycemic control, there was no improvement in pregnancy outcome in comparison to normal-weight patients. Poorly controlled overweight and obese patients, regardless of treatment modality, had significantly higher rates of composite outcome, metabolic complications, macrosomia, and LGA. Although obesity in itself is related to adverse outcome in pregnancy, gestational diabetic women treated with insulin and possibly oral antidiabetic drugs, who achieve targeted levels of glycemic control, may have pregnancy outcomes comparable to those of normal-weight women. These findings are in contrast to the findings of Leiken and colleagues.[81] However, the improved outcome in the insulin-treated overweight and obese women may be because of an unidentified effect of insulin itself on the fetus or activation of other metabolic fuel pathways.

LONG-TERM IMPLICATIONS

The implications of maternal obesity far surpass intrauterine life, extending into infancy and even adulthood with severe health repercussions. Both the Barker[85,86] and fetal insulin hypotheses[87] have proposed that impaired adult cardiovascular health is programmed in utero by poor fetal nutrition, or by genetically-determined reduction of insulin-mediated fetal growth, that results in the birth of a small infant. Low birth weight may be a significant variable for the development of the metabolic syndrome in adulthood. Obesity was an independent risk factor in the diabetic populations studied. Therefore, the emphasis today may need to address sedentary lifestyle and issues related to obesity upon fetal programming, as under-nutrition is now infrequent in developed societies.

Maternal obesity long has been linked with the delivery of a macrosomic infant. Now there is abundant evidence linking macrosomia to increased overweight and obesity in adolescents as well as adults.[88–90] Perhaps more alarming is a recent retrospective cohort study by Whitaker[91] in over 8,400 children in the United States in the early 1990s, which reported that the prevalence of childhood obesity was between 2.4- and 2.7-times higher in offspring of obese women in the first trimester compared with children whose mothers' BMI was in the normal range at this early stage of pregnancy. These findings remained consistent even after controlling for additional risk factors, including birth weight, parity, weight gain, and smoking during pregnancy (RR 2.0; 95% CI 1.7–2.3).

The epidemic of obesity and subsequent risk of diabetes and components of the metabolic syndrome clearly may begin in utero with fetal overgrowth and adiposity. Fully 50% to 90% of adolescents with type 2 diabetes have a BMI greater than 27,[92] and 25% of obese children 4 to 10 years of age have impaired glucose tolerance.[93] Not surprisingly, an additional study reported evidence of a link between maternal obesity and cardiovascular disease in adult offspring, confirming Barker's hypothesis of higher adult death rates from coronary heart disease in men who were classified as low birth weight.[94] In addition, they observed a positive association between the mother's BMI upon admission and future death rate from coronary heart disease in male offspring. They concluded that the mother's obesity may be an independent yet additional contributing factor to infant low birth weight. Fall and colleagues[95] reported higher adult rates of type 2 diabetes in offspring of mothers who were above average weight in pregnancy. Therefore, there is an association between maternal obesity (but not paternal) and insulin resistance on the risk of offspring to develop cardiovascular disease in adulthood. In a further study, high maternal weight or BMI accounted for the association between birth weight and adult adiposity.[96]

Maternal Long-Term Implications

Some pregnancies are associated with excessive maternal weight gain. Mean weight retention after pregnancy ranges between 0.4 kg and 3.8 kg.[97–100] Weight retention after pregnancy has been attributed to various causative factors, including smoking cessation, changes in activity leading to a more sedentary life style, socioeconomic factors such as low income, and other such factors.

Additionally, increased weight gain during pregnancy remains the strongest factor for weight retention after pregnancy.[101] Linnè and colleagues[102] reported that women with a weight gain of 16 kg or more during pregnancy were 2.5 times more likely to be a high weight retainer 1-year postpartum.

Of equal importance, women diagnosed with GDM have a considerably higher risk of developing type 2 diabetes mellitus later in life. In a case-controlled study, including 28 women diagnosed with GDM in 1984 to 1985, and a control group of 53 women who gave birth at the same time period, Linné and colleagues performed a 2-hour oral glucose tolerance test 15 years later.[103] Ten women (35%) in the GDM group were diagnosed with type 2 diabetes mellitus versus none in the control group

($P<.001$). Mean BMI in the diabetic group was 27.4 and in the nondiabetic GDM group, 24.6 ($P<.05$).

OBESITY, GLUCOSE INTOLERANCE AND METABOLIC SYNDROME—A VICIOUS CYCLE

In 1988, Reaven proposed that resistance to insulin-stimulated glucose uptake (insulin resistance) and secondary hyperinsulinemia are involved in the etiology of three major related diseases: cardiovascular disease (CVD), type 2 diabetes, and hypertension. He coined the term "Syndrome X" that has been modified later to "Metabolic syndrome" to describe a group of abnormalities that increase the risk for CVD: resistance to insulin-stimulated glucose uptake, glucose intolerance, hyperinsulinemia, increased triglyceride, decreased high-density lipoprotein-cholesterol, and hypertension.[104] Obesity is the most important risk factor for the metabolic syndrome. In the NHANES study, metabolic syndrome was present in 4.6%, 22.4%, and 59.6% of normal weight, overweight, and obese men, respectively, and a similar distribution was observed in women.[105]

SUMMARY

Obesity has become an epidemic. It is associated with increased rate of infertility and with many pregnancy complications. Moreover, it is associated with GDM, which increases the risk of these complications. The primary objective in the management of obesity during pregnancy is prevention. Having obese women lose weight and achieve a normal BMI before conception would be the ideal goal, but realistically quite difficult to achieve. Infertility treatment should be preceded by weight reduction. The latter may result in spontaneous conception (and prevention of multiple gestations) and in a better outcome of pregnancy.

Treatment options during pregnancy using pharmacologic or surgical means are contraindicated. Studies are necessary to clarify the safety of a diet during pregnancy. However, increased physical activity in women who are sedentary and healthy food choices rather than fast foods may result in a better pregnancy outcome for both mother and child.

The worldwide epidemic of adolescent and adult obesity may not only be a result of our lifestyle of inadequate activity and poor diet; it may also be propagated and enhanced at a much earlier stage in life because of an abnormal metabolic milieu in utero during gestation. Because we know that lifestyle treatment of obesity is rarely successful in the long term, we need to give serious consideration to prevention. The potential of in utero therapy and prevention of fetal macrosomia, possibly through lifestyle measures before and during gestation, and achieving a desired level of glycemic control in pregnancies complicated with diabetes, should become a research focus of considerable interest relative to the short- and long-term prevention of obesity and progression into overt diabetes and metabolic syndrome. The same holds for prevention of obesity in early childhood, as it is known that type 2 diabetes is generally preceded by an excessive weight gain in early childhood. Therefore, prevention rather than treatment may offer the best hope of breaking the vicious cycle of obesity during pregnancy. Until we attain a better understanding of the underlying genetic predispositions, physiology, and mechanisms relating to maternal and feto-placental interactions relating to fetal growth and development, all treatments must by necessity be empiric.

REFERENCES

1. World Health Organization. Obesity: preventing and managing the global epidemic. Geneva (Switzerland): World Health Organization; 2000. WHO technical report series 894.
2. Flegal KM, Carroll MD, Kuczmarski RJ, et al. Overweight and obesity in the United States: prevalence and trends, 1960–1994. Int J Obes Relat Metab Disord 1998;22:39–47.
3. Hedley AA, Ogden CL, Johnson CL, et al. Prevalence of overweight and obesity among US children, adolescents, and adults, 1999–2002. JAMA 2004;291: 2847–50.
4. Abrams BF, Laros RK Jr. Prepregnancy weight, weight gain, and birth weight. Am J Obstet Gynecol 1986;154:503–9.
5. Naeye RL. Maternal body weight and pregnancy outcome. Am J Clin Nutr 1990; 52:273–9.
6. Taffel SM, Keppel KG, Jones GK. Medical advice on maternal weight gain and actual weight gain. Results from the 1988 National Maternal and Infant Health Survey. Ann N Y Acad Sci 1993;678:293–305.
7. Siega-Riz AM, Adair LS, Hobel CJ. Institute of Medicine maternal weight gain recommendations and pregnancy outcome in a predominantly Hispanic population. Obstet Gynecol 1994;84:565–73.
8. Cogswell ME, Serdula MK, Hungerford DW, et al. Gestational weight gain among average-weight and overweight women—what is excessive? Am J Obstet Gynecol 1995;172:705–12.
9. Catalano PM, Tyzbir ED, Roman NM, et al. Longitudinal changes in insulin release and insulin resistance in non-obese pregnant women. Am J Obstet Gynecol 1991;165:1667–72.
10. Catalano P. Editorial. Obesity and pregnancy—the propagation of a viscous cycle? J Clin Endocrinol Metab 2003;88(8):3505–6.
11. Green BB, Weiss NS, Daling JR. Risk of ovulatory infertility in relation to body weight. Fertil Steril 1988;50:721–6.
12. Grodstein F, Goldman MB, Cramer DW. Body mass index and ovulatory infertility. Epidemiology 1994;5:247–50.
13. Zaadstra BM, Seidell JC, Van Noord PA, et al. Fat and female fecundity: prospective study of effect of body fat distribution on conception rates. BMJ 1993;306:484–7.
14. Metwally M, Li TC, Ledger WL. The impact of obesity on female reproductive function. Obes Rev 2007;8(6):515–23.
15. Frisch RE. Body fat, menarche and ovulation. Baillieres Clin Obstet Gynaecol 1990;4:419–39.
16. Lintsen AM, Pasker-de Jong PC, de Boer EJ, et al. Effects of subfertility, cause, smoking and body weight on the success rate of IVF. Hum Reprod 2005;20: 1867–75.
17. Fedorcsák P, Dale PO, Storeng R, et al. Impact of overweight and underweight on assisted reproduction treatment. Hum Reprod 2004;19:2523–8.
18. Wang JX, Davies M, Norman RJ. Body mass and probability of pregnancy during assisted reproduction treatment: retrospective study. BMJ 2000;321: 1320–1.
19. Hamilton-Fairley D, Kiddy D, Watson H, et al. Association of moderate obesity with a poor pregnancy outcome in women with polycystic ovary syndrome treated with low dose gonadotrophin. Br J Obstet Gynaecol 1992;99:128–31.

20. WanG JX, Davies MJ, Norman RJ. Obesity increases the risk of spontaneous abortion during infertility treatment. Obes Res 2002;10:551–4.
21. Bussen S, Sutterlin M, Steck T. Endocrine abnormalities during the follicular phase in women with recurrent spontaneous abortion. Hum Reprod 1999;14: 18–20.
22. Lashen H, Fear K, Sturdee DW. Obesity is associated with increased risk of first trimester and recurrent miscarriage: matched case-control study. Hum Reprod 2004;19:1644–6.
23. Fedorcsak P, Dale PO, Storeng R, et al. The impact of obesity and insulin resistance on the outcome of IVF or ICSI in women with polycystic ovarian syndrome. Hum Reprod 2001;16:1086–91.
24. Douglas CC, Gower BA, Darnell BE, et al. Role of diet in the treatment of polycystic ovary syndrome. Fertil Steril 2006;85:679–88.
25. Weiss JL, Malone FD, Emig D, et al. FASTER Research Consortium. Obesity, obestetric complications and cesarean delivery rate: a population-based screening study. Am J Obstet Gynecol 2004;190:1091–7.
26. Gabbe S. Gestational diabetes mellitus. N Engl J Med 1986;315:1025–6.
27. Guttorm E. Practical screening for diabetes mellitus in pregnant women. Acta Endocrinol (Copenh) 1974;75:11–24.
28. Hellgren M, Blomback M. Studies on blood coagulation and fibrinolysis in pregnancy, during delivery and in the puerperium. I. Normal condition. Gynecol Obstet Invest 1981;12:141–54.
29. Greer IA. Haemostasis and thrombosis in pregnancy. In: Bloom AL, Forbes CD, Thomas DP, et al, editors. Haemostasis and Thrombosis in Pregnancy. Edinburgh (UK): Churchill Livingstone; 1994. p. 987–1015.
30. Abdollahi M, Cushman M, Rosendaal FR. Obesity: risk of venous thrombosis and the interaction with coagulation factor levels and oral contraceptive use. Thromb Haemost 2003;89:493–8.
31. Kumari A. Pregnancy outcome in women with morbid obesity. Int J Gynaecol Obstet 2001;73:101–7.
32. Martorell R, Kahn L, Hughes M. Obesity in Latin American women and children. J Nutr 1998;128:1464–73.
33. Lu GC, Rouse DJ, DuBard M, et al. The effect of the increasing prevalence of maternal obesity on perinatal morbidity. Am J Obstet Gynecol 2001;185:845–9.
34. Lederman S. Pregnancy weight gain and postpartum loss: avoiding obesity while optimizing the growth and development of the fetus. JAMA 2001;56:53–8.
35. Sebire NJ, Jolly M, Harris JP, et al. Maternal obesity and pregnancy outcome: a study of 287,213 pregnancies in London. Int J Obes 2001;25:1175–82.
36. Sibai BM, Gordon T, Thom E, et al. Risk factors for preeclampsia in healthy nulliparous women: a prospective multicenter study. The National Institute of Child Health and Human Development Network of Maternal-Fetal Medicine Units. Am J Obstet Gynecol 1995;172:642–8.
37. Sibai BM, Ewell M, Levine RJ, et al. Risk factors associated with preeclampsia in healthy nulliparous women. The Calcium for Preeclampsia Prevention (CPEP) Study Group. Am J Obstet Gynecol 1997;177:1003–10.
38. Sattar N, Clark P, Holmes A, et al. Antenatal waist circumference and hypertension risk. Obstet Gynecol 2001;97:268–71.
39. Bianco AT, Smilen SW, Davis Y, et al. Pregnancy outcome and weight gain recommendations for the morbidly obese woman. Obstet Gynecol 1998;91: 97–102.

40. Sattar N, Greer IA. Pregnancy complications and maternal cardiovascular risk: opportunities for intervention and screening? Br Med J 2002;325:157–60.
41. Stone JL, Lockwood CJ, Berkowitz GS, et al. Risk factors for severe preeclampsia. Obstet Gynecol 1994;83(3):357–61.
42. O'Brien TE, Ray JG, Chan WS. Maternal body mass index and the risk of preeclampsia: a systematic review. Epidemiology 2003;14:368–74.
43. Kalter H. Five-decade international trends in the relation of perinatal mortality and congenital malformations: stillbirth and neonatal death compared. Int J Epidemiol 1991;20:173–9.
44. Odlind V, Haglund B, Pakkanen M, et al. Deliveries, mothers and newborn infants in Sweden, 1973–2000. Trends in obstetrics as reported to the Swedish Medical Birth Register. Acta Obstet Gynecol Scand 2003;82:516–28.
45. Nohr EA, Bech BH, Davies MJ, et al. Prepregnancy obesity and fetal death. Obstet Gynecol 2005;106:250–9.
46. Cnattingius S, Bergström R, Lipworth L, et al. Prepregnancy weight and the risk of adverse pregnancy outcomes. N Engl J Med 1998;338(3):147–52.
47. Salihu HM, Dunlop A, Hedayatzadeh M, et al. Extreme obesity and risk of stillbirth among black and white gravidas. Obstet Gynecol 2007;110:552–7.
48. Schieve LA, Cogswell ME, Scanlon KS. Maternal weight gain and preterm delivery: Differential effects by body mass index. Epidemiology 1999;10:141–7.
49. Kramer MS, Coates AL, Michoud MC, et al. Maternal anthropometry and idiopathic preterm labor. Obstet Gynecol 1995;86:744–8.
50. Spinillo A, Capuzzo E, Piazzi G, et al. Risk for spontaneous preterm delivery by combined body mass index and gestational weight gain patterns. Acta Obstet Gynecol Scand 1998;77:32–6.
51. Smith GCS, Shah I, Pell JP, et al. Maternal obesity in early pregnancy and risk of spontaneous and elective preterm deliveries: a retrospective cohort study. Am J Public Health 2007;97(1):157–62.
52. Bhattacharya S, Campbell DM, Liston WA, et al. Effect of body mass index on pregnancy outcomes in nulliparous women delivering singleton babies. BMC Public Health 2007;24(7):168.
53. Nohr EA, Bech BH, Vaeth M, et al. Obesity, gestational weight gain and preterm birth: a study within the Danish National Birth Cohort. Paediatr Perinat Epidemiol 2007;21:5–14.
54. Dietz PM, Callaghan WM, Morrow B, et al. Population-based assessment of the risk of primary cesarean delivery due to excess prepregnancy weight among nulliparous women delivering term infants. Matern Child Health J 2005;9(3):237–44.
55. Vahratian A, Siega-Riz AM, Zhang J, et al. Maternal pre-pregnancy overweight and obesity and the risk of primary cesarean delivery in nulliparous women. Ann Epidemiol 2005;15:467–74.
56. Holger S, Scheithauer S, Dornhofer N, et al. Obesity as an obstetric risk factor: does it matter in a perinatal center? Obesity (Silver Spring) 2006;14:770–3.
57. Kaiser PS, Kirby RS. Obesity as a risk factor for cesarean in a low-risk population. Obstet Gynecol 2001;97:39–43.
58. Brost BC, Goldenberg RL, Mercer BM, et al. The Preterm Prediction Study: association of cesarean section with increases in maternal weight and body mass index. Am J Obstet Gynecol 1997;177:333–41.
59. Yu CK, Teoh TG, Robinson S. Obesity in pregnancy. BJOG 2006;113(10):1117–25.

60. Waller DK, Mills JL, Simpson JL, et al. Are obese women at higher risk for producing malformed offspring? Am J Obstet Gynecol 1994;170:541–8.
61. Cedergren MI, Kallen BA. Maternal obesity and infant heart defects. Obes Res 2003;11:1065–71.
62. Watkins ML, Rasmussen SA, Honeru MA, et al. Maternal obesity and risk for birth defects. Pediatrics 2003;111:1152–8.
63. Mojtabai R. Body mass index and serum folate in childbearing women. Eur J Epidemiol 2004;19:1029–36.
64. Ray JG, Wyatt PR, Vermeulen MJ, et al. Greater maternal weight and the ongoing risk of neural tube defects after folic acid flour fortification. Obstet Gynecol 2005;105:261–5.
65. Catalano P, Drago N, Amini S. Maternal carbohydrate metabolism and its relationship to fetal growth and body composition. Am J Obstet Gynecol 1995; 172:1464–70.
66. Kleigman R, Gross T. Prenatal problems of the obese mother and her infant. Obstet Gynecol 1985;66:299–306.
67. Ehrenberg HM, Mercer BM, Catalano PM. The influence of obesity and diabetes on the prevalence of macrosomia. Am J Obstet Gynecol 2004;191(3):964–8.
68. Baeten JM, Bukusi EA, Lambe M. Pregnancy complications and outcomes among overweight and obese nulliparous women. Am J Public Health 2001; 91:436–40.
69. Ray JG, Vermeulen MJ, Shapiro JL, et al. Maternal and neonatal outcomes in pregestational and gestational diabetes mellitus, and the influence of maternal obesity and weight gain: the DEPOSIT study. Diabetes Endocrine Pregnancy Outcome Study in Toronto. QJM 2001;94:347–56.
70. Perlow JH, Morgan MA, Montgomery D, et al. Perinatal outcome in pregnancy complicated by massive obesity. Am J Obstet Gynecol 1992;167:958–62.
71. Edwards LE, Dickes WF, Alton IR, et al. Pregnancy in the massively obese: course, outcome, and obesity prognosis of the infant. Am J Obstet Gynecol 1978;131:479–83.
72. Gross T, Sokol RJ, King KC. Obesity in pregnancy: risks and outcome. Obstet Gynecol 1980;56:446–50.
73. Galtier-Dereure F, Montpeyroux F, Boulot P, et al. Weight excess before pregnancy: complications and cost. Int J Obes Relat Metab Disord 1995;19: 443–8.
74. Galtier-Dereure F, Boegner C. Obesity and pregnancy: complications and cost. Am J Clin Nutr 2000;71:1242S–8S.
75. Jensen DM, Damm P, Sørensen B, et al. Pregnancy outcome and prepregnancy body mass index in 2459 glucose-tolerant Danish women. Am J Obstet Gynecol 2003;189:239–44.
76. Bo S, Menato G, Signorile A, et al. Obesity or diabetes: what is worse for the mother and for the baby? Diabetes Metab 2003;29:175–8.
77. Hutcheon JA, Platt RW, Meltzer SJ, et al. Is birth weight modified during pregnancy? Using sibling differences to understand the impact of blood glucose, obesity, and maternal weight gain in gestational diabetes. Am J Obstet Gynecol 2006;195:488–94.
78. Sermer M, Naylor CD, Gare DJ, et al. Impact of increasing carbohydrate intolerance on maternal-fetal outcomes in 3637 women without gestational diabetes: the Toronto Tri-Hospital Gestational diabetes Project. Am J Obstet Gynecol 1995;173:146–56.

79. Yogev Y, Langer O, Xenakis EM, et al. Glucose screening in Mexican-American women. Obstet Gynecol 2004;103(6):1241–5.
80. Yogev Y, Langer O, Xenakis EM, et al. The association between glucose challenge test, obesity and pregnancy outcome in 6390 non-diabetic women. J Matern Fetal Neonatal Med 2005;17(1):29–34.
81. Leiken EL, Jenkins JH, Graves WL. Prophylactic insulin in gestational diabetes. Obstet Gynecol 1987;70:587–92.
82. Lucas MJ, Lowe TW, Bowe L, et al. Class A1 gestational diabetes: a meaningful diagnosis? Obstet Gynecol 1993;82(2):260–5.
83. Casey BM, Lucas MJ, Mcintire DD, et al. Pregnancy outcomes in women with gestational diabetes compared with the general obstetric population. Obstet Gynecol 1997;90(6):869–73.
84. Langer O, Yogev Y, Xenakis EM, et al. Overweight and obese in gestational diabetes: the impact on pregnancy outcome. Am J Obstet Gynecol 2005;192(6):1768–76.
85. Barker DT, Gluckman PD, Godfrey KM, et al. Fetal nutrition and cardiovascular disease in adult life. Lancet 1993;341:938–41.
86. Barker DJ, Osmond C, Simmonds SJ, et al. The relation of small head circumference and thinness at birth to death from cardiovascular disease in adult life. Br Med J 1993;306:422–6.
87. Hattersley AT, Tooke JE. The fetal insulin hypothesis: an alternative explanation of the association of low birthweight with diabetes and vascular disease. Lancet 1999;353:1789–92.
88. Garn SM, Clark DC. Trends in fatness and the origins of obesity. Pediatrics 1976;57:443–56.
89. Garn SM, Cole PE, Bailey SM. Living together as a factor in family line resemblances. Hum Biol 1979;51:565–87.
90. Martorell R, Stein AD, Schroeder DG. Early nutrition and adiposity. J Nutr 2001;131:874S–80S.
91. Whitaker RC. Predicting preschooler obesity at birth: the role of maternal obesity in early pregnancy. Pediatrics 2004;114:e29–36.
92. Mokdad AH, Ford ES, Bowman BA, et al. Diabetes trends in the U.S. 1990–1998. Diabetes Care 2000;23:1278–83.
93. Sinha R, Fisch G, Teague B, et al. Prevalence of impaired glucose tolerance among children and adolescents with marked obesity. N Engl J Med 2002;346:802–10.
94. Forsén T, Eriksson JG, Tuomilehto J, et al. Mother's weight in pregnancy and coronary heart disease in a cohort of Finnish men: follow up study. Br Med J 1997;315:837–40.
95. Fall CH, Stein CE, Kumaran K, et al. Size at birth, maternal weight, and type 2 diabetes in South India. Diabet Med 1998;15:220–7.
96. Parsons TJ, Power C, Manor O. Fetal and early life growth and body mass index from birth to early adulthood in 1958 British cohort: longitudinal study. Br Med J 2001;323:1331–5.
97. Cederlof R, Kaij L. The effect of childbearing on body weight: a twin control study. Acta Psychiatr Scand Suppl 1970;219:47–9.
98. Forster J, Bloom E, Sorensen G, et al. Reproductive history and body mass index in black and white women. Prev Med 1986;15:685–91.
99. Smith DE, Lewis CE, Caveny JL, et al. Longitudinal changes in adiposity associated with pregnancy. The CARDIA Study. Coronary Artery Risk Development in Young Adults Study. JAMA 1994;271:1747–51.

100. Öhlin A, Rössner S. Maternal body weight development after pregnancy. Int J Obes Relat Metab Disord 1990;14:159–73.
101. Greene GW, Smiciklas-Wright H, Scholl TO, et al. Postpartum weight change: how much of the weight gained in pregnancy will be lost after delivery? Obstet Gynecol 1988;71:701–7.
102. Linne Y, Neovius M. Identification of women at risk of adverse weight development following pregnancy. Int J Obes 2006;30:1234–9.
103. Linnè Y, Barkeling B, Rössner S. Natural course of gestational diabetes mellitus: long term follow up of women in the SPAWN study. BJOG 2002;109(11):1127–31.
104. Reaven GM. Banting lecture 1988. Role of insulin resistance in human disease. Diabetes 1988;37(12):1595–607.
105. Ford ES, Giles WH, Dietz WH. Prevalence of the metabolic syndrome among US adults: findings from the third National Health and Nutrition Examination Survey. JAMA 2002;287(3):356–9.

Exercise Prescription for Overweight and Obese Women: Pregnancy and Postpartum

Michelle F. Mottola, PhD, FACSM[a,b,c,*]

KEYWORDS

- Maternal exercise • Overweight • Obese • Postpartum
- Weight management

Women of childbearing age are at an increased risk for obesity[1] and diabetes[2] because of excessive weight gain during pregnancy and weight retention after delivery.[3] Population estimates of maternal obesity and being overweight range from 34%[4] to 39%[5] worldwide, with an increasing prevalence of 69% over 10 years (1993 to 2003) in nine states in the United States.[6] A study of 18,633 patients collected from 1987 to 1997 showed a prevalence of 23% for overweight and obese pregnant women,[7] which may be an underestimation of the current situation.

Overweight women who have experienced previous weight retention start their next pregnancy with a higher early rate of weight gain.[8] This excessive weight gain during pregnancy has been strongly associated with maternal weight retention at 6 and 12 months postpartum, and each subsequent pregnancy is likely to result in more weight gain, with additional weight retention in the postpartum period.[9] This escalating problem may contribute to the obesity epidemic and other disease risks, as overweight women who gain 10% or more of their before-pregnancy mass are at higher risk for complications, such as gestational diabetes mellitus (GDM)[10] and pregnancy-induced hypertension.[9] Additionally, higher recurrence of GDM has been

This work is supported by the Canadian Institute of Health Research, The Lawson Foundation, and the Molly Towell Perinatal Research Foundation.
[a] Department of Anatomy and Cell Biology, Schulich School of Medicine and Dentistry, London, Ontario, Canada N6A 3K7
[b] Child Health Research Institute, Lawson Health Research Institute, London, Ontario, Canada N6A 3K7
[c] R. Samuel McLaughlin Foundation-Exercise and Pregnancy Laboratory, School of Kinesiology, Faculty of Health Science, The University of Western Ontario, London, Ontario, Canada N6A 3K7
* Corresponding author. R. Samuel McLaughlin Foundation-Exercise and Pregnancy Laboratory, The University of Western Ontario, London, Ontario, Canada N6A 3K7.
E-mail address: mmottola@uwo.ca

Obstet Gynecol Clin N Am 36 (2009) 301–316
doi:10.1016/j.ogc.2009.03.005
obgyn.theclinics.com

associated with greater before-pregnancy weight, body mass index (BMI), and pregnancy weight gain.[11]

Women who are overweight or obese have an increased risk of menstrual cycle irregularities, infertility,[12] and a diminished response to fertility treatments[13] that reduce the probability of conception. It has been shown that body fat distribution may influence fertility, as a 0.1 unit increase in the waist-to-hip ratio of women decreased the probability of conception by 30% per menstrual cycle.[14]

Overweight and obese women who do conceive have a higher risk of maternal and fetal complications, contributing to longer hospitalization[15] and increased instrumentation and delivery costs.[15] Infants of obese women are more likely to experience neonatal intensive care unit admission[16] and cesarean delivery.[15] The infants of Class III obese women (BMI $\geq$ 40 kg/m^2) are twice as likely to demonstrate fetal distress and low APGAR scores.[17] The high incidence of complications in overweight and obese women increases the cost of prenatal hospital care by fivefold.[15]

THE MATERNAL-FETAL-CHILD LINK TO OBESITY

Obesity begets obesity.[18,19] With childhood obesity on the rise worldwide, the recent release of the agenda for obesity research suggests that priority should be given to investigating critical periods throughout life. Three of these time points include early life: the fetal and neonatal periods, and pregnancy.[20]

Mothers of obese preschoolers have a higher prepregnancy BMI,[21] children of obese mothers are twice as likely to be large for gestational age (greater than the 95%ile) at birth, and large-for-gestational-age babies are more likely to be obese preschoolers.[21] Excess pregnancy weight gain and weight retention are precursors to obesity in midlife[2] and prepregnancy overweight and obesity may lead to a vicious cycle of excessive weight gain and adiposity passed on from the mother to her offspring.[22]

Although genetics are important, the robust link between the fetal environment and its profound influence on lifelong health and the future risk of chronic disease cannot be ignored.[18,22,23] The maternal metabolic state has a powerful influence on whether the offspring later develops obesity.[24] This altered metabolic state can be represented by an increasing hyperglycemia during pregnancy (GDM and impaired glucose tolerance), which is associated with increased risk of obesity in children 5 to 7 years of age.[25] This increased risk is modifiable if GDM is treated or prevented,[25] which strongly suggests that the influence of the intrauterine milieu can be passed on to the next generation nongenetically, and that by maintaining a healthy fetal environment, undesirable influences affecting the offspring can be reversed and prevented.[24,26–28]

The recent opinion statement from the American College of Obstetricians and Gynecologists (ACOG) on obesity during pregnancy strongly suggests aggressive preventative management in all overweight and obese pregnant women both before conception and after delivery.[29] This strong opinion and the overwhelming evidence linking maternal health to the fetal environment reinforce the idea that the best solution for obesity prevention may begin with promotion of a healthy maternal lifestyle. Furthermore, excessive weight gain and failure to lose pregnancy weight by 6 months after delivery is an important predictor of long-term obesity in the mother.[30]

Achievement and maintenance of a healthy weight needs to be encouraged and support provided to assist women in reaching and maintaining this goal during and after pregnancy.[31] Progressive weight loss between pregnancies with a multidisciplinary weight-management approach may help decrease the risk for GDM and hypertension in subsequent pregnancies.[9] One of the risk factors for developing GDM is a sedentary lifestyle and thus, a common link between obesity and GDM is physical inactivity, with both obesity and GDM as risk factors for type-2 diabetes.[32] Thus, prevention of excessive weight gain during pregnancy is highly recommended as an intervention to reduce the occurrence of GDM and prevent the development of true diabetes[11] and hypertension after pregnancy.

AEROBIC EXERCISE INTERVENTIONS FOR OVERWEIGHT OR OBESE PREGNANT WOMEN

Although the healthy lifestyle approach is intuitive,[33] to date only eight studies have examined the effectiveness of a combined nutrition and exercise intervention designed to prevent excessive weight gain during pregnancy, and not all exclusively examined overweight or obese women. As shown in **Table 1**, 63%[34–38] were not successful in preventing excessive pregnancy weight gain in overweight and obese women. Studies using education alone as an intervention[34–37] were not effective in preventing excess weight gain during pregnancy. Interventions for this population group need to be behavior-based because education programs increase knowledge but do not change behavior.[39] In addition, **Table 1** shows that behavior-based interventions without an individualized intervention of nutrition and exercise are not successful.[34]

The interventions that used dietary control in combination with exercise as part of a lifestyle change for overweight and obese pregnant individuals included a variety of activities. Although successful in preventing excessive weight gain, aqua-aerobic classes, designed for obese pregnant women and offered one or two times per week would not improve aerobic fitness.[40] Artal and colleagues[41] used a supervised moderate intensity (60% symptom-limited VO_{2max}) exercise session consisting of treadmill walking or cycling on a semirecumbent bike for obese GDM participants, once per week, followed by unsupervised exercise for the remaining 6 days at home. The exercise group had a mean exercise time of 153 plus or minus 91.4 minutes per week and 50% of them exercised more than 150 minutes per week.[41] Weekly weight gain was lower than in the diet-only group.

Although only partially successful (50%) in preventing excessive gestational weight gain, a pilot study using a mild walking program (30% of estimated heart-rate reserve) starting at 25 minutes per session three to four times per week, building slowly by adding 2 minutes per week until 40 minutes was reached, was successful in improving glucose regulation and reducing insulin requirements in overweight women with GDM.[38] Pedometers used to count steps accumulated during the walking sessions read approximately 2,600 steps at 25 minutes and increased to 4,200 steps at 40 minutes by the end of pregnancy. When these exercise step counts were added to the mean daily activity steps (6,500 steps), the women in the walking program were taking approximately 10,000 steps three to four times per week.[38] The low intensity of the walking program allows even previously sedentary overweight and obese women to follow this exercise prescription. Finally, excessive gestational weight gain was prevented with a nutrition and exercise intervention, which included a similar walking program (using a pedometer to count steps) for overweight and obese women.[42] By the end of the program, these women took over 10,000 steps three to four times per week, bringing them into the "active" category.[43] Because walking is the most popular activity for pregnant women,[44] the use of pedometers may aid in compliance for overweight and obese women.

Thus, it would appear that initiating a walking program during pregnancy,[38,42] or unstructured exercise at home,[41] may be better than structured aqua-aerobic classes,

Table 1
Summary of studies using an exercise intervention to prevent excessive gestational weight gain in overweight or obese women

Study	Population	Intervention	Results	Successful?
Gray-Donald et al[35]	Cree women of James Bay, 112 in intervention versus 107 historic controls; all BMI categories.	Goal to optimize gestational weight gain by use of exercise groups and dietary education via media campaign.	No difference between groups in weight gain or rate of weight gain.	Not successful. No exercise prescription given.
Polley et al[34]	Low income; 120 normal weight or overweight/obese in Pittsburgh.	Randomized into stepped behavior intervention or usual prenatal care; intervention received educational materials.	Among overweight/obese women, 59% had excessive weight gain in intervention group versus 32% in usual care group.	Not successful. Exercise intervention focused on increased walking and a more active lifestyle.
Olsen et al[36]	Low and middle/upper income in Upstate NY; 179 normal or overweight enrolled in intervention compared with 381 historic controls.	Goal to use 2 tiers: (a) health care provider information (b) materials mailed, including newsletter, postcards, and other reminders.	Among historic controls, 45% gained excessive versus 41% in intervention group, $P>.05$; found overweight low income women benefited most.	Not successful- except in low income women. No exercise prescription given.
Kinnunen et al[37]	Six maternity clinics from Finland; three clinics were intervention ($n = 49$); three were control ($n = 56$) and received standard care; all women were primiparous and from all BMI categories.	Individual counseling on diet and physical activity plus information on weight gain recommendations.	46% of women in intervention group versus 30% in control group exceeded weight gain, $P>.05$.	Not successful. Did not increase activity or prevent excessive weight gain. Supervised group-exercise sessions once per week, 45–60 min. Encouraged 800 MET minutes per week.

Claesson et al[40]	Prospective case-controlled intervention; used 155 for intervention versus 193 in control group, received standard care in Sweden; all women were obese.	To decrease total weight gain to < 7 kg using behavioral intervention by weekly motivational talk using trained midwife.	Intervention group had lower weight gain and lost more weight at postnatal check-up than control, but no difference in number of women who gained < 7 kg.	Successful in controlling weight gain for obese women, especially nulliparous. Offered aqua aerobic classes 1 to 2 times/week.
Artal et al[41]	Obese women with GDM; self-selected intervention.	Diet+exercise (n = 39) versus diet alone (n = 57); used standard GDM diet for both groups.	Weight gain/week lower in diet+exercise intervention group.	Successful in limiting weight gain. Encouraged 60% VO_{2peak} at least 5 days/week; 50% of exercise group = > 150 min/week.
Davenport et al[38]	GDM women; BMI ≥ 25kg/m^2; pilot study. Groups matched by age, BMI, and insulin usage.	Conventional management (CM) (n = 20) versus CM+walking (n = 10)	CM+walking group had improved glucose regulation and used fewer insulin units/kg/day in late pregnancy. 50% of women in both groups did not gain excessive weight.	Partially Successful in preventing excessive weight gain (50%); however GDM improved in CM+walking group. Walking = 25 min, added 2 min/week until 40 min, three to four times per week.
Mottola et al[42]	Single-arm intervention matched to historical controls for overweight and obese women starting at 16 weeks gestation.	Nutrition and exercise lifestyle intervention (NELIP) consisting of GDM dietary program with walking (n = 65), using pedometer to count steps.	Weight gained on NELIP was 6.8 kg ± 4.1 kg; 0.38 kg ± 0.2 kg/week; 80% did not gain excessively.	Successful in preventing excessive weight gain. Exercise prescription (30% heart rate reserve) started at 25 min, three to four times/week; adding 2 min per week; until 40 min reached.

as structured classes may be more difficult for time management and not all participants have access to a pool.

AEROBIC EXERCISE PRESCRIPTION FOR OVERWEIGHT AND OBESE PREGNANT WOMEN

A recent study in which 20 medically prescreened obese and 20 normal-weight pregnant women participated in a graded-treadmill exercise test to volitional fatigue, examined the impact of obesity on the ventilatory response to weight-bearing exercise during pregnancy.[45] The investigators concluded that exercise ventilatory response is increased during pregnancy but is not affected further by obesity during graded-treadmill exercise. This is important in that there is no apparent ventilatory limitation to submaximal weight-bearing exercise representing daily living activities, such as walking, in pregnant obese women, which lends support to the feasibility of exercise prescription in this population group.[45]

Evidence-based guidelines for exercise during pregnancy indicate that regular prenatal exercise is an important component of a healthy pregnancy.[46] In addition to maintaining physical fitness, exercise may be beneficial to prevent or treat maternal-fetal diseases.[32,47] Walking has been shown to be the most popular activity during pregnancy[44] and as three of the intervention studies have shown, walking in combination with nutritional control can be effective in preventing excessive weight gain in overweight and obese women.[38,41,42]

ACOG suggests that all pregnant women with low-risk pregnancies should exercise on most if not all days of the week.[48] The Physical Activity Guidelines for Americans (PAGA)[49] for healthy pregnant women recommends at least 150 minutes (2 hours and 30 minutes) of moderate-intensity aerobic activity per week, with this activity spread throughout the week. These guidelines also suggest that pregnant women who begin physical activity should increase the amount gradually over time.[49] Exercise prescription requires knowledge of the physical ability of the participant to engage in various activities.[50] With overweight or obese pregnant women, this information, included with a thorough clinical evaluation to ensure low obstetric risk, is extremely important before prescribing exercise. The PARmed-X for Pregnancy[46] is a tool that can be used by health care providers for medical prescreening in a simple checklist format. This document also provides more specific guidelines using the FITT principle for Frequency, Intensity, Time (duration) and Type of exercise after medical prescreening.[46]

Frequency of Exercise

ACOG[48] suggests exercise on most if not all days of the week for pregnant women, while the latest guidelines for Americans suggest that this activity be spread throughout the week.[49] A recent study would also suggest caution, as frequency of structured exercise, especially during late pregnancy, was a determinant of birth weight.[51] In a case-controlled study of 526 women, the odds of giving birth to a small-for-gestational-age baby was 4.61 times more likely for women who engaged in structured exercise more than five times per week and also 2.64 times more likely for those women who engaged in structured exercise two or less times per week.[51] Because small-for-gestational-age babies are at risk for obesity and cardiovascular disease later in life,[23] structured exercise performed three to four times per week would seem ideal. Starting an exercise program at three times per week with a day of rest between each exercise day may also help eliminate fatigue.[46]

Intensity of Exercise

Although it has been suggested that target heart-rate zones should not be used to monitor exercise intensity during pregnancy, recent evidence would suggest otherwise, especially for overweight and obese women. Using 106 medically prescreened overweight and obese women between 16 and 20 weeks of gestation, the relationship between aerobic capacity (VO_2) and heart rate (HR) was established over a full spectrum of exercise intensities.[52] Using regression analyses, it was found that $\%VO_{2reserve}$ ($VO_{2reserve} = VO_{2max} - VO_{2rest}$) is not equivalent to $\%HR_{reserve}$ ($HR_{reserve} = HR_{max} - HR_{rest}$) at intensities below 70% $VO_{2reserve}$. This indicates that if an exercise prescription is followed for moderate-intensity exercise, pregnant overweight and obese women may be exercising at a higher intensity ($\%VO_2$) than intended for a given heart rate, and that prescription describing $\%VO_{2reserve}$ as a proxy for $\%HR_{reserve}$ is appropriate for 70% and above, but not below.[52] Even though they are not equivalent below 70%, $\%HR_{reserve}$ is best described by $\%VO_{2\ reserve}$ and not VO_{2peak} in pregnant overweight and obese women.[52]

The American College of Sports Medicine[53] suggested that previously sedentary overweight and obese pregnant women should initiate an aerobic exercise program at an intensity equivalent to 20% to 39% $VO_{2reserve}$, which indicates the lowest level of physical activity that could provide health benefits.[53] However, values below 70% $VO_{2reserve}$ are not equal to $\%HR_{reserve}$ in pregnant overweight and obese women, and thus, the range of 20% to 39% $VO_{2reserve}$ was equivalent to 13% to 33% $HR_{reserve}$.[52] Target heart-rate zones based on age were developed and validated on the above population, equivalent to 13% to 33% $HR_{reserve}$. These target heart-rate zones are 110 to 131 beats per minute (bpm) for women 20 to 29 years of age and 108 to 127 bpm for women 30 to 39 years of age.[52] Low-risk pregnant overweight and obese women, who use these lower intensities, may be more compliant, especially when walking is used as the exercise modality. Even at these lower intensities, this population group will gain aerobic fitness. Alternate target heart-rate zones (validated on 156 pregnant women) have been suggested that also include the fitness level of the individual. Low-risk women who are not fit (in the bottom 25% of peak aerobic fitness), between the ages of 20 and 29 years (average BMI = 29.8 kg/m^2 $\pm$1.2 kg/m^2; $VO_{2peak} \leq$ 21mL/kg/min) and between 30 to 39 years (average BMI = 31.6 kg/m^2 $\pm$1.0 kg/m^2; $VO_{2peak} \leq$19.6mL/kg/min), can exercise safely between 128 and 144 bpm.[54] These target heart-rate zones were developed and validated, based on 60% to 80% of peak aerobic capacity and may not be appropriate for obese women, but may be offered as an alternative for overweight women who are not fit and wish to start an aerobic exercise program.

Rating of perceived exertion (RPE) is another indicator of appropriate intensity.[46,50] On the 6- to 20-point scale, an exertion rating of 12 to 14 (somewhat hard) indicates moderate activity.[46,50] Using the "talk test" will also confirm that the pregnant woman is not over exerting. The "talk test" indicates an appropriate intensity, as long as the woman can carry on a conversation while exercising.[46]

Time (Duration of Exercise Session)

Overweight and obese pregnant women should initially attempt 15 minutes, building slowly to a maximum of 30 minutes of aerobic activity at a specific target heart rate, even if it means reducing the intensity and using rest intervals.[46] All aerobic activity should be preceded by a brief 10- to 15-minute warm-up of low-intensity stretching or calesthenics and followed by a short 10- to 15-minute cool down.[46] A mild walking program starting at 25 minutes, adding 2 minutes per week until 40 minutes, and maintained until birth is also feasible for overweight and obese pregnant women.[42,52]

Structured exercise of a moderate intensity totaling 150 minutes per week, using a frequency of three sessions per week, would approximate 50 minutes of activity (30 minutes of which is at the appropriate target heart rate, with a 10-minute warm-up, followed by a 10-minute cool down), or 30 minutes per session, four times per week, with a 5-minute warm-up and a 5-minute cool down. These recommendations may provide a choice based on the initial fitness level and initial prepregnancy BMI of the participant. Individual prescription based on clinical evaluation is important in this population group.

Type of Exercise

Walking three to four times per week at the appropriate intensity is highly recommended to help prevent excessive gestational weight gain and other chronic disease risks for both the overweight and obese mother and the developing fetus.[42] Aerobic exercise in which large muscle groups are used, including walking, stationary cycling, aquatic exercise, or low-impact aerobics are appropriate for overweight and obese pregnant women. Active living should also be promoted in this group, in which women are encouraged to take the stairs, rather than the elevator, or park farther away from the door to increase daily step counts. Exercises that are contraindicated are those that increase the risk of falling, abdominal trauma, and collision, and contact sports, such as gymnastics, horseback riding, downhill skiing, soccer, and basketball.[49] Scuba diving should also be avoided and pregnant women are cautioned when they exercise at altitude.[50]

RATE OF PROGRESSION

The best time to progress is during the second trimester, when the risks and discomforts of pregnancy are lowest. Aerobic exercise should be increased gradually from a minimum of 15 minutes per session, three times per week at the appropriate target heart rate or RPE to a maximum of 30 minutes per session, four times per week (at the appropriate target heart rate or RPE), preceded by the warm-up and followed by the cool down.[46]

MUSCLE CONDITIONING AND STRENGTH TRAINING

Muscular strength and conditioning involves specific muscle groups that are stretched or moved through a specific range of motion, with or without added resistance to that muscle group.[46] The effects of muscle strength and conditioning exercise performed during pregnancy have rarely been examined, especially in the overweight or obese population. Muscle conditioning exercises in combination with aerobic activities provide a well-rounded fitness program for pregnant women who have no contraindications to exercise. Possible advantages to incorporating muscular strength and conditioning activities into an exercise program may be improvement in overall strength, posture, and core muscle strength that may help in labor and birth. By strengthening muscles of the body core, perhaps lower-back pain and pelvic-joint pain may be avoided as pregnancy progresses and the center of gravity shifts forward.[55] Strengthening the pelvic floor muscles during pregnancy have been shown to prevent urinary incontinence during gestation and 3 months after delivery.[56] Low back pain and pelvic pain are common complaints during pregnancy, which may interfere with activities of daily living.[57] The main factors associated with these complaints may be mechanical, because of an alteration in posture required to support the increase in body mass, the shift in the center of gravity, and hormonal changes (relaxin).[57] It was found that the higher the number of previous leisure-time physical activities, the lower the risk of low back and pelvic pain during pregnancy.[57]

Very little evidence-based literature reports guidelines on muscle conditioning for pregnant women, as most of the studies investigate the physiologic effects of aerobic exercise. Common sense and traditional medical advice have suggested that pregnant women avoid heavy lifting or straining, especially those activities that have a static or isometric exercise component.[58] Theoretical risks of resistance exercise during pregnancy have included changes in maternal blood pressure, especially if the Valsalva Maneuver (holding one's breath while working against a resistance) is initiated,[59] initiation of premature labor,[60] and transient fetal hypoxia (drop in oxygen levels).[61] High-resistance exercise may reduce blood flow and oxygen supply to the uterus, which may cause a mild transient decrease in fetal oxygen concentrations,[58] reflected by a drop in fetal heart rate (bradycardia).[62] A stable fetal heart-rate pattern during isotonic and isometric exercise has been reported in the literature,[55,58,62–64] while others revealed transient changes in fetal heart rate, especially during maternal exercise performed while lying on the back (supine position).[61,65] Thus, maternal strength conditioning exercises do not compromise maternal or fetal well-being in healthy pregnancies; however, exercises performed in the supine position should be avoided and this is reflected in several guidelines.[46,48,49]

One study examined the effects of circuit-type resistance training using rubber tubing on women with gestational diabetes. The exercise program consisted of eight exercises performed in a continuous circuit with short rests (< 1 minute) between stations, starting at two sets of 15 repetitions of each exercise and progressing to three sets of 20 repetitions. Intensity was monitored by instructing the participants to exercise at the level of "somewhat hard" on the RPE scale. Only those women who were overweight in the exercise intervention program had a reduced amount of insulin required to control their blood-glucose concentrations compared with a dietary intervention without exercise.[66] Because this was the only study investigating muscle strength and conditioning exercises during pregnancy, evidence-based research is lacking and this includes studies on yoga and Pilates.[67] Thus, muscle strength and conditioning activities should be conducted with caution and common sense.

POSTPARTUM

Maternal obesity has a negative association with the initiation of, and continuation of, breastfeeding, which may be attributed to excessive gestational weight gain, complications of pregnancy and delivery, or condition of the infant at birth.[68] Excessive fat may hinder mammary gland development and lactogenesis in obese women.[69] The greater the BMI of the mother before pregnancy, the less likely breastfeeding will be initiated[70] and the more likely she will terminate breastfeeding early.[71] Others have linked childhood obesity with parental control of feeding at 1 year of age[72] and rapid velocity of growth during infancy,[73] attributing this to formula-feeding.[39] In addition, it has been shown that the pattern of dietary intake of fats and energy among children resembles that of their parents, with the parental influence during early childhood as fundamental.[74]

POSTPARTUM EXERCISE INTERVENTIONS FOR OVERWEIGHT OR OBESE WOMEN

Two recent reviews suggest that dieting and exercise together is more effective than dieting alone in reducing weight retention after childbirth,[75] and that more interventions are necessary that focus primarily on weight management from a multi-level approach that includes the health care provider.[76] Problems exist in postpartum care, as education on the increased risk for development of type-2 diabetes mellitus and cardiovascular disease, the benefits of breastfeeding, and the importance of healthy lifestyle changes, such as increased physical activity and nutritional control, are not emphasized, especially for overweight and obese women.[30,77] Currently, only three studies exist in the literature in which an intervention program was specifically designed to reduce postpartum weight retention in overweight or obese women. Lovelady and colleagues[78] examined the effects of a 10-week calorie-reduced (by 500 kcal/day) and exercise program (4 days/week, 65%–80% of maximum HR) on infant growth in overweight, exclusively breastfeeding women. The exercise program, starting at 15 minutes per session, began at 4-weeks postpartum and was increased gradually until the women were walking, jogging, or aerobic dancing for 45 minutes per day. The women in the intervention group lost more weight and increased aerobic fitness compared with the control group. Infant growth patterns were not different between groups.[78] In a subsequent study, with the same protocol and the addition of supplementation of vitamin B_6, with a limitation of no less than 1,800 kcal/day for the dietary program, the results showed that a moderate weight loss of 0.5 kg per week did not affect B_6 status or infant growth in lactating overweight women.[79] More recently, overweight women in a structured diet (caloric deficit of 350 kcal/day) and exercise (increase energy expenditure by at least 150 kcal/day or > 1,050 kcal/week) program successfully lost weight and most maintained this weight loss by 1 year after delivery.[80] However, dropout rate was high and retention rate low (58%) in the follow-up period at 1 year after delivery.[80] This may be partially explained by the fact that women with children are 1.67 times more likely to quit an exercise program.[44] These findings may be important, in that in order for postpartum exercise programs to succeed, time management, social support, cultural sensitivity, and child care should be incorporated.[81] In addition, exercise sessions that include the infant, such as stroller walking, or muscle conditioning programs that include mother-child interaction may be more successful.

With obesity on the rise in reproductive age women, it is important that exercise and active living be introduced into the postpartum period to help diminish weight retention and promote safe weight loss. The literature suggests that lactation, reduction of daily energy intake (as long as at least 1,800 kcal/day are maintained), exercise, and weight loss (approximately 0.5 kg per week) are compatible, even in overweight or obese women.[78,79] More research is necessary to provide recommendations that are evidence-based.

EXERCISE GUIDELINES FOR OVERWEIGHT AND OBESE POSTPARTUM WOMEN

Exercise guidelines for postpartum women are virtually nonexistent[81] and certainly do not exist for overweight and obese women. Common sense, as indicated with recommendations for exercise during pregnancy, would suggest that postpartum women seek approval from their health care providers before beginning a moderate, structured exercise program. PAGA recommends at least 150 minutes (2 hours and 30 minutes) of moderate-intensity aerobic activity per week, with this activity spread throughout the week for postpartum women.[49] Although these guidelines are general, it is important that mode of delivery (vaginal, instrument-assisted, or caesarian) be considered and that the 6 to 8 week after-delivery assessment by the health care provider includes opportunity to discuss the issue of level of discomfort and other complicating factors, such as anemia or wound infection.[67] Care should be given to the c-section incision site, and stretching exercises should be avoided until the incision is healed.[81] Initiation of pelvic floor exercises is recommended in the immediate postpartum period to reduce the risk of future urinary incontinence.[67]

GENERAL GUIDELINES FOR BREASTFEEDING AND EXERCISE

Common-sense guidelines are available for postpartum women who wish to exercise. These include exercising after the baby has been fed or the breasts are empty to reduce discomfort. It is recommended that a good support bra be worn and that a sports bra be avoided because of breast compression.[81] Adequate nutrition and hydration should be maintained to support the energy demands of breastfeeding and exercise.[81] If there were no complications from delivery, a mild exercise program consisting of walking, pelvic floor exercises, relaxation, and light stretching of all muscle groups can begin in the immediate postpartum period.[81] Other activities, including walking up and down stairs and performing muscle-conditioning exercises can begin without delay after uncomplicated vaginal delivery.[82]

GUIDELINES FOR AEROBIC EXERCISE FOR OVERWEIGHT AND OBESE POSTPARTUM WOMEN

Every structured aerobic-exercise program should be based on the FITT principle. Once medical approval has been obtained, frequency of a moderate program should begin slowly at three times per week, and depending on the mother's fitness level, can be increased to four or five times per week.[81] Intensity can be monitored by the "talk test" and the RPE scale, where intensity should be of a moderate level (somewhat hard). If this is difficult for the overweight or obese woman, using an appropriate target heart rate estimating 20% to 39% of $VO_{2reserve}$ may be more appropriate.[53] This can be gradually increased as the participant's fitness level improves. Starting an exercise program at 15 minutes, with a 5- to 10-minute warm-up of lower intensity followed by a 5- to 10-minute cool down, including rest intervals to avoid fatigue may be recommended.[81] Exercise time at the target heart rate or RPE can progress from 15 minutes, adding 5 minutes per week, as long as the individual is not overly fatigued,[81] to at least 150 minutes (2 hours and 30 minutes) of moderate-intensity aerobic activity per week, with this activity spread throughout the week.[49] The type of activity recommended can include walking while pushing a stroller (also improves muscular strength), jogging, aerobic dancing,[78] or other activities that promote movement of major muscle groups.

Muscle-conditioning exercises for postpartum women may be more successful if the activity includes the infant and may help to overcome barriers to exercise.[44] The infant can be used as a resistance tool (the infant's head must be supported at all times before 6 months of age) for improving upper body strength.[81] Muscle-conditioning exercise can be resumed in the supine position and the infant can be placed on the abdominal muscles of the mother; while she is holding her thighs for support, the mother can perform abdominal exercise.[83] Muscle-conditioning activity that promotes maternal-infant interaction may also be successful in promoting active living.[81] More research is necessary to replace common-sense guidelines with evidence-based recommendations.

SUMMARY

To break the spiraling cycle of generations of unhealthy body weights and obesity-related health problems in adulthood, it is imperative to prevent excessive weight gain and to promote a healthy lifestyle during prenatal life and the postpartum period, especially for those women who are overweight and obese. The link between maternal lifestyle and the fetal environment reinforces the idea that the best solution for obesity prevention may begin with the promotion of a healthy lifestyle during pregnancy. Progressive weight loss between pregnancies with a multidisciplinary weight management approach may help decrease the risk for GDM and hypertension in subsequent pregnancies. Once a low-risk pregnancy has been established, walking, which is the most popular activity, combined with nutritional control may be the most effective in preventing excessive weight gain in overweight and obese women. Maternal exercise prescription should use the FITT principle, with a frequency of three to four times per week as ideal. Intensity based on a target heart-rate zone of 110 to 131 bpm for women 20 to 29 years of age and 108 to 127 bpm for women 30 to 39 years of age, coupled with use of the RPE scale and the "talk test" is suggested. A 5- to 10-minute warm-up preceding exercise starting at 15 minutes per session, building up to 30 minutes, should then be followed by a 5- to 10-minute cool down.

Dieting and exercise together are more effective than dieting alone in reducing weight retention after childbirth. Compliance may be improved by incorporating child care and children into the exercise routine. Exercise guidelines for postpartum women are virtually nonexistent and do not exist for overweight and obese women. Postpartum women should seek approval from their health care provider before beginning a moderate structured exercise program, which should begin slowly at three times per week, and increased to four or five times per week. Intensity, monitored by the "talk test" and the RPE scale, should be at a moderate level (somewhat hard), which can be adjusted as needed. Exercise can start from 15 minutes, adding 5 minutes per week, as long as the individual is not overly fatigued, to at least 150 minutes (2 hours and 30 minutes) of aerobic activity per week, with this activity spread throughout the week. The type of activity recommended includes walking while pushing a stroller, jogging, aerobic dancing, or other activities that promote movement of major muscle groups.

REFERENCES

1. Villamor E, Cnattingius S. Interpregnancy weight change and risk of adverse pregnancy outcomes: a population-based study. Lancet 2006;368:1164–70.
2. Lipscombe L, Hux J. Trends in diabetes prevalence, incidence, and mortality in Ontario, Canada 1995–2005: a population-based study. Lancet 2007;369:750–6.
3. Rooney B, Schauberger C, Mathiason M. Impact of perinatal weight change on long-term obesity and obesity-related illnesses. Obstet Gynecol 2005;106:1349–56.
4. Callaway L, Prins K, Johannes B, et al. The prevalence and impact of overweight and obesity in an Australian obstetric population. Med J Aust 2006;184(2):56–9.
5. LaCoursiere D, Bloebaum Y, Duncan L, et al. Population-based trends and correlates of maternal overweight and obesity, Utah 1991–2001. Am J Obstet Gynecol 2005;192(3):832–9.
6. Kim S, Dietz P, England L, et al. Trends in pre-pregnancy obesity in nine states, 1993–2003. Obes 2007;15:986–93.
7. Abenhaim H, Kinch R, Morin L, et al. Effect of prepregnancy body mass index categories on obstetrical and neonatal outcomes. Arch Gynecol Obstet 2007;275:39–43.
8. Muscati SK, Gray-Donald K, Koski KG. Timing of weight gain during pregnancy: promoting fetal growth and minimizing maternal weight retention. Int J Obes Relat Metab Disord 1996;20(6):526–32.
9. Pole JD, Dodds LA. Maternal outcomes associated with weight change between pregnancies. Can J Public Health 1999;90(4):233–6.

10. Artenisio A, Corrado F, Sobbrio G, et al. Glucose tolerance and insulin secretion in pregnancy. Diabetes Nutr Metab 1999;12:264–70.
11. Foster-Powell KA, Cheung NW. Recurrence of gestational diabetes. Aust NZ J Obst Gyn 1998;38:384–7.
12. Rich-Edwards JW, Goldman MB, Willett WC, et al. Adolescent body mass index and infertility caused by ovulatory disorder. Am J Obstet Gynecol 1994;171:171–7.
13. Dickey RP, Taylor SN, Curole DN, et al. Relationship of clomiphene dose and patient weight to successful treatment. Humanit Rep 1997;12:449–53.
14. Zaadstra BM, Seidell JC, Van Noord PA, et al. Fat and female fecundity: prospective study of effect of body fat distribution on conception rates. BMJ 1993;306:484–7.
15. Galtier-Dereure F, Montpeyroux F, Boulot P, et al. Weight excess before pregnancy: complications and cost. Int J Obes Relat Metab Disord 1995;19:443–8.
16. Rosenberg TJ, Garbers S, Chavkin W, et al. Prepregnancy weight and adverse perinatal outcomes in an ethnically diverse population. Obstet Gynecol 2003;102:1022–7.
17. Cedergren MI. Maternal morbid obesity and the risk of adverse pregnancy outcome. Obstet Gynecol 2004;103:219–24.
18. Catalano PM, Ehrenberg HM. The short- and long-term implications of maternal obesity on the mother and her offspring. BJOG 2006;113(10):1126–33.
19. Catalano PM. Editorial: obesity and pregnancy-the propagation of a viscous cycle? J Clin Endocrinol Metab 2003;88:3505–6.
20. Finegood DT. The agenda for obesity research in Canada. CMAJ 2007;176(8):111–4.
21. Veugelers P, Fitzgerald A. Prevalence of and risk factors for childhood overweight and obesity. CMAJ 2005;173:607–13.
22. Shankar K, Harrell A, Liu X, et al. Maternal obesity at conception programs obesity in the offspring. Am J Physiol Regul Integr Comp Physiol 2008;284:R528–38.
23. Oken E, Gillman MW. Fetal origins of obesity. Obes Res 2003;11(4):496–506.
24. Ismail-Beigi F, Catalano P, Hanson R. Metabolic programming: fetal origins of obesity and metabolic syndrome in the adult. Am J Physiol Endocrinol Metab 2006;291:E439–40.
25. Hillier T, Mullen J, Pedula K, et al. Childhood obesity and metabolic imprinting: the ongoing effects of maternal hyperglycemia. Diabetes Care 2007;30:2287–92.
26. Bayol S, Farrington S, Stickland N. A maternal "junk food" diet in pregnancy and lactation promotes an exacerbated taste for "junk food" and a greater propensity for obesity in rat offspring. Br J Nutr 2007;98:843–51.
27. Dunger D, Salgin B, Ong K. Early nutrition and later health. Early developmental pathways of obesity and diabetes risk. Proc Nutr Soc 2007;66:451–7.
28. Miles J, Huber K, Thompson N, et al. Moderate daily exercise activates metabolic flexibility to prevent prenatally induced obesity. Endocrin 2009;150(1):179–86.
29. American College of Obstetricians and Gynecologists (ACOG). Obesity in pregnancy. Obstet Gynecol 2005;106:671–4.
30. Rooney B, Schauberger C. Excess pregnancy weight gain and long-term obesity: one decade later. Obstet Gynecol 2002;100:245–52.
31. Neilsen R, Tapsell L. Gestational diabetes: weight control and dietary intake after pregnancy. Aust J Nutr Diet 1994;51(3):125–7.
32. Pivarnik JM, Chambliss H, Clapp JF, et al. Impact of physical activity during pregnancy and postpartum on chronic disease risk: An ACSM roundtable consensus statement. Med Sci Sports Exerc 2006;38(5):989–1005.

33. Althuizen E, van Poppel M, Seidell JC, et al. Design of the New Life(style) study: a randomized controlled trial to optimize maternal weight development during pregnancy. BMC Public Health 2006;6:168–75.
34. Polley BA, Wing RR, Sims CJ. Randomized controlled trial to prevent excessive weight gain in pregnant women. Int J Obes 2002;26:1494–502.
35. Gray-Donald K, Robinson E, Collier A, et al. Intervening to reduce weight gain in pregnancy and gestational diabetes mellitus in Cree communities: an evaluation. CMAJ 2000;163:1247–51.
36. Olsen CM, Strawderman MS, Reed RG. Efficacy of an intervention to prevent excessive gestational weight gain. Am J Obstet Gynecol 2004;191:530–6.
37. Kinnunen T, Pasanen M, Aittasalo M, et al. Preventing excessive weight gain during pregnancy-a controlled trial in primary health care. Eur J Clin Nutr 2007; 61:884–91.
38. Davenport MH, Mottola MF, McManus R, et al. A walking intervention improves capillary glucose control in women with GDM: a pilot study. Appl Physiol Nutr Metab 2008;33:511–7.
39. Berall G, Desantadina V. Prevention of childhood obesity through nutrition: review of effectiveness. CMAJ 2007;176:102–5.
40. Claesson IM, Sydsjo G, Brynhildsen J, et al. Weight gain restriction for obese pregnant women: a case-control intervention study. BJOG 2008;115:44–50.
41. Artal R, Catanzaro R, Gavard J, et al. A lifestyle intervention of weight-gain restriction: diet and exercise in obese women with gestational diabetes mellitus. Appl Physiol Nutr Metab 2007;32:596–601.
42. Mottola MF, Giroux I, Gratton R, et al. Nutrition and exercise prevents excess weight gain in pregnant overweight women. Med Sci Sports Exerc 2009 [Under 2nd revision].
43. Tudor-Locke C, Bassett D. How many steps/day are enough? Preliminary pedometer indices for public health. Sports Med 2004;43(1):1–8.
44. Mottola MF, Campbell MK. Activity patterns during pregnancy. Can J Appl Physiol 2003;28(4):642–53.
45. Davenport MH, Steinback CD, Mottola MF. Impact of pregnancy and obesity on cardiorespiratory responses during weight-bearing exercise. Respir Physiolo Neurobiol 2009 [Under second revision].
46. Wolfe LA, Mottola MF. PARmed-X for pregnancy: physical activity readiness medical examination. Ottawa (ON): Can Soc Exerc Physiol & Health Canada; 2002. p. 1–4.
47. Weissgerber T, Wolfe LA, Davies G, et al. Exercise in the prevention and treatment of maternal-fetal disease: a review of the literature. Appl Physiol Nutr Metab 2006;31:661–74.
48. American College of Obstetricians and Gynecologists. Exercise during pregnancy and the postpartum period. Obstet Gynecol 2002;99:171–3.
49. US Dept of Health & Human Services. Physical activity guidelines for Americans. Chapter 7. 2008. Available at: www.health.gov/paguidelines/guidleines/chapter7.aspx. Accessed January 22, 2009.
50. Artal R, O'Toole M, White S. Guidelines of the ACOG for exercise during pregnancy and the postpartum period. Br J Sports Med 2003;37:6–12.
51. Campbell MK, Mottola MF. Recreational exercise and occupational activity during pregnancy and birth weight: a case-control study. Am J Obstet Gynecol 2001; 184:403–8.
52. Davenport MH, Charlesworth S, Vanderspank D, et al. Development and validation of exercise target heart rate zones for overweight and obese pregnant women. Appl Physiol Nutr Metab 2008;33:984–9.

53. American College of Sports Medicine. Guidelines for exercise testing and exercise prescription. 7th edition. Philadelphia: Lippincott Williams & Wilkins; 2005.
54. Mottola MF, Davenport MH, Brun CR, et al. VO2peak prediction and exercise prescription for pregnant women. Med Sci Sports Exerc 2006;38:1389–95.
55. Hall DC, Kaufmann DA. Effects of aerobic and strength conditioning on pregnancy outcomes. Am J Obstet Gynecol 1987;157:1199–203.
56. Morkved S, Bo K, Schei B, et al. Pelvic floor muscle training during pregnancy to prevent urinary incontinence: a single blind randomized controlled trial. Obstet Gynecol 2003;101:313–9.
57. Mogren IM, Pohjanen A. Low back pain and pelvic pain during pregnancy. Spine 2005;30:983–91.
58. Avery ND, Stocking KD, Tranmer J, et al. Fetal responses to maternal strength conditioning exercises in late gestation. Can J Appl Physiol 1999;24:362–76.
59. Lotgering FK, van der Berg A, Struijk P, et al. Arterial pressure response to maximal isometric exercise in pregnant women. Obstet Gynecol 1992;166:538–42.
60. Durak E, Jovanovic-Peterson L, Peterson C. Comparative evaluation of uterine response to exercise on five aerobic machines. Am J Obstet Gynecol 1990; 162:754–6.
61. Green R, Schneider K, MacLennan AH. The fetal heart rate response to static antenatal exercises in the supine position. Aust J Physiother 1988;34:3–7.
62. Webb KA, Wolfe LA, Lowe-Wylde S, et al. A comparison of fetal heart rate (FHR) responses to maternal static and dynamic exercise [abstract]. Med Sci Sports Exerc 1991;23:S169.
63. Marsal K, Gennser G, Lofgren O. Effects on fetal breathing movements of maternal challenges. Acta Obstet Gynecol Scand 1979;58:335–42.
64. Ruissen C, Drongelen M, Hoogland H. The influence of maternal exercise on the pulsatility index of the umbilical artery blood velocity waveform. Eur J Obstet Gynecol Reprod Biol 1990;37:1–6.
65. Nelser CL, Hassett S, Cary S, et al. Effects of supine exercise on fetal heart rate in the second and third trimesters. Am J Perinatol 1988;5:159–63.
66. Brankston G, Mitchell B, Ryan E, et al. Resistance exercise decreases the need for insulin in overweight women with gestational diabetes mellitus. Am J Obstet Gynecol 2004;190:188–93.
67. Davies G, Wolfe LA, Mottola MF, et al. Joint SOGC/CSEP clinical practice guideline: exercise in pregnancy and the postpartum period. J Obstet Gynecol Can 2003;25(6):516–22.
68. Rasmussen KM. Association of maternal obesity before conception with poor lactation performance. Annu Rev Nutr 2007;27:103–21.
69. Oddy W, Li J, Landsborough L, et al. The association of maternal overweight and obesity with breastfeeding duration. J Pediatr 2006;149:185–91.
70. Manios Y, Grammatikaki E, Kondaki K, et al. The effect of maternal obesity on initiation and duration of breast-feeding in Greece: the GENESIS study. IP address: 129.100.136.178. Pub Health Nutr 2009;12:517–24.
71. Baker J, Michaelsen K, Sorensen T, et al. High prepregnant body mass index is associated with early termination of full and any breastfeeding in Danish women. Am J Clin Nutr 2007;86:404–11.
72. Farrow CV, Blissett J. Controlling feeding practices: cause or consequence of early child weight? Pediatrics 2008;121(1):e164–9.
73. McCarthy A, Hughes R, Tilling K, et al. Birth weight; postnatal, infant, and childhood growth; and obesity in young adulthood: evidence from the Barry Caerphilly Growth Study. Am J Clin Nutr 2007;86(4):907–13.

74. Oliveria S, Ellison R, Moore L, et al. Parent-child relationships in nutrient intake: the Framingham Children's Study. Am J Clin Nutr 1992;56(3):593–8.
75. Amorim A, Linne P, Lourenco P. Diet or exercise, or both, for weight reduction in women after childbirth. Cochrane Database Syst Rev;18(3):CD005627.
76. Keller C, Records K, Ainsworth B, et al. Interventions for weight management in postpartum women. J Obstet Gynecol Neonatal Nurs 2008:37:71–9.
77. Calfas K, Marcus B. 2007 Postpartum weight retention a mother's weight to bear? Am J Prev Med 2008;32(4):356–7.
78. Lovelady CA, Garner KE, Moreno K, et al. The effect of weight loss in overweight lactating women on the growth of their infants. N Engl J Med 2000;342:449–53.
79. Lovelady C, Williams J, Garner K, et al. Effect of energy restriction and exercise on vitamin B-6 status of women during lactation. Med Sci Sports Exerc 2001;33: 512–8.
80. O'Toole ML, Sawicki M, Artal R. Structured diet and physical activity prevent post-partum weight retention. J Women's Health (Larchmt) 2003;12:991–8.
81. Mottola MF. Exercise during the post partum period: practical applications. Curr Sports Med Rep 2002;1(12):362–8.
82. Bowes WA, Katz V. Postpartum care. In: Gabbe SC, Niebyl J, Simpson J, editors. Obstetrics: normal and problem pregnancies. New York: Churchill Livingstone; 2002. p. 701–26.
83. Kochan-Vintinner A. Active living during pregnancy: physical activity guidelines for mother and baby. In: Wolfe LA, Mottola MF, editors. Ottawa (ON): Canadian Society for Exercise Physiology and Health Canada; 1999. p. 27–32.

Childbearing and Obesity in Women: Weight Before, During, and After Pregnancy

Erica P. Gunderson, PhD

KEYWORDS

- Pregnancy • Postpartum period • Puerperium
- Gestational weight gain • Obesity • Parity
- Epidemiology • Women

The childbearing years are an important life stage for women that may result in substantial weight gain leading to the development of obesity. When compared with other age groups, US women aged 35 to 44 years have experienced the greatest increase in obesity prevalence in the past 45 years.[1] Furthermore, 45% of women begin pregnancy overweight or obese, up from 24% in 1983.[2] Gestational weight gain is also higher than ever before, with 43% of pregnant women gaining more than is recommended.[2]

Maternal overweight and obesity is the most common high-risk obstetric condition and is associated gestational diabetes mellitus, hypertensive disorders, and newborn macrosomia, among other perinatal complications.[3] Women who are already overweight or obese before a first pregnancy tend to retain or gain more weight after pregnancy than average weight women[4–7] despite larger newborns[8] and wider variability in gestational weight gain. Weight gain before, during, and after pregnancy not only affects the current pregnancy but may also be a primary contributor to the future development of obesity in women during midlife and beyond.[9–11]

Two types of prospective study designs have examined persistent weight changes related to pregnancy in women: (1) pregnancy cohort studies using self-reported pre-pregnancy weight, and (2) longitudinal cohorts of women of reproductive age that measured weights before and after pregnancies and controlled for secular trends by accounting for weight gain in non-parous women. The pregnancy cohort studies

This article was supported by a Career Development Award, grant K01 DK059944 from the National Institute of Diabetes, Digestive and Kidney Diseases, grant R01 HD050625 from the National Institute of Child Health and Human Development, and a Clinical Research Award from the American Diabetes Association.
Kaiser Foundation Research Institute, Kaiser Permanente Northern California, Division of Research, 2000 Broadway, Oakland, CA 94612, USA
E-mail address: epg@dor.kaiser.org

Obstet Gynecol Clin N Am 36 (2009) 317–332
doi:10.1016/j.ogc.2009.04.001
obgyn.theclinics.com
0889-8545/09/$ – see front matter

rely almost exclusively on self-report of pregravid weight, and estimates of postpartum weight retention may be inflated by weight gain from secular trends.[4,5,12] Moreover, pregnancy cohort studies have rarely obtained serial measurements of postpartum weight to differentiate net retention of gestational weight gain from subsequent postpartum weight gain or loss. By contrast, studies focusing on women of reproductive age more accurately estimate weight gain related to childbearing because body weight is measured before and after pregnancy. In addition, these studies remove weight gain due to secular trends and aging by estimating net weight gain for parous women relative to non-parous or nulliparous women during the same time interval.

Three outcome measures have been examined: (1) average weight change (retension), (2) substantial postpartum weight retention (ie, >=5 kg above pregravid weight), and (3) the incidence of overweight or obesity after pregnancy (body mass index [BMI] >26). Mean weight change or "retention" from preconception to postpartum is subject to high interindividual variability. Substantial weight retention (>=5 kg above pregravid weight) at 1 to 2 years postpartum may be a more useful clinical measure for identifying women who experience significant weight shifts after pregnancy.[4,13,14] The most clinically relevant health measure, the incidence of becoming overweight or obese after pregnancy, has rarely been assessed.[15,16]

The evidence[13,17–19] consistently shows that excessive gestational weight gain contributes to higher postpartum body weight; however, higher maternal body size before pregnancy and biologic factors are also important. For example, the age at menarche and a short interval from menarche to first birth may be as important as high gestational weight gain to the development of overweight after pregnancy.[16] Being heavy before a first pregnancy has important implications for long-term persistent weight changes. Most studies have examined the independent relationships of pregravid body size, gestational weight gain, and parity to postpartum weight retention with conflicting results. These traits were first proposed in the 1950s and again in the 1970s as important correlates of weight changes after pregnancy;[5,20] however, the joint influences of parity and pregravid body size on long-term weight changes have been examined in only a few large epidemiologic studies with sufficient numbers of primiparas across all BMI groups.[5–7] This article examines the evidence suggesting that gestational weight gain, primiparity, and maternal body size before pregnancy jointly influence long-term postpartum weight retention and the development of overweight and obesity among women of childbearing age.

GESTATIONAL WEIGHT GAIN AND LONG-TERM WEIGHT STATUS

Specifically, overweight and obese women are two to six times more likely to exceed the weight gain recommendations during pregnancy[21–23] than other BMI groups (**Table 1**). These women are also predisposed to higher postpartum weight gain (**Fig. 1**) and retention after pregnancy. Moreover, the incidence of high birth weight increases with higher gestational weight gain among average and high maternal BMI groups.[24] Obese women are also more likely to give birth to macrosomic infants, even with lower average pregnancy weight gain[8,21,25] and normal glucose tolerance.[26] Some evidence indicates that gestational weight gain below 15 lbs in obese women may lower the risk of large-for-gestational age infants.[27]

Gestational weight gain is strongly positively correlated with maternal weight change from preconception to beyond 6 months postpartum and exerts long-term effects on maternal body weight.[12,28–31] In multiple linear regression models, total gestational gain has accounted for 20% to 35% of the variability in the weight change.[4,12,28,31] Gunderson and colleagues[16] reported that gestational gain above

Table 1
Correlates of excessive gestational weight gain (GWG): pregravid BMI and race/ethnicity

Author, Year, Location, Study Period	Number of Subjects	Race (%)	Data Source	Excess GWG (%)	Adjusted OR (95% CI) of High GWG
Parker, 1993, USA, NMIHS, 1988	2119	Black, 47 White, 53	Survey	36 34	—
Keppel, 1993, USA, NMIHS, 1988	1592	Black, 17 White, 83	Survey	33 37	Mean GWG, 14.3 kg
Brawarsky, 2005, USA, Project WISH, San Francisco, 1980–1990	1100	Black, 16 White, 33 Latina, 36 Asian, 15	Telephone, chart review	61 57 51 47	NS for race Pregravid BMI (vs NW) OW: 2.3 (1.4–3.6)
Wells, 2006, USA, PRAMS, Denver, CO, 2000–2002	9115	Black, 4 White, 64 Hispanic, 28 Other, 3	Birth certificate	46 43 36 35	NS for race Pregravid BMI (vs NW) OW: 2.7 (2.0–3.4) OB: 6.6 (4.0–10.8)
Chasan-Taber, 2008, USA, West, MA	770	Hispanic (Puerto Rican), 100	—	45	Pregravid BMI (vs NW) OW: 2.2 (1.3–3.8)

Abbreviations: OR, odds ratio; NMIHS, National Maternal and Infant Health Survey; NW, normal weight; OB, obese; OW, overweight; WISH, Women and Infants Starting Healthy; PRAMS, pregnancy risk assessment and monitoring system.

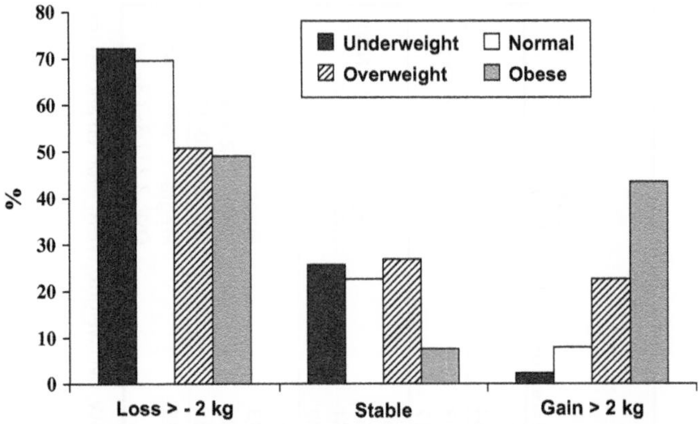

Fig. 1. Percentage of women within categories of late (6 weeks to 2 years) postpartum weight change (gain >2 kg, loss >2 kg, and stable ± 2 kg) according to pregravid BMI group. (*From* Gunderson EP, Abrams B, Selvin S. Does the pattern of postpartum weight change differ according to pregravid body size? Int J Obes Relat Metab Disord 2001;25:860; with permission.)

the recommended levels was associated with a threefold higher risk of becoming overweight after pregnancy (BMI ≥26) among women who were under or average weight before pregnancy in a large, multi-ethnic cohort.

Although gestational weight gain is linked to postpartum weight retention, primiparity and larger body size before pregnancy exert important influences. Findings on pregravid body size and primiparity have been inconsistent. Women who are overweight or obese before pregnancy are generally more likely to have excessive as well as inadequate gestational weight gains.[8,21] Their accelerated pregravid weight gain trajectories and other factors may make overweight women more susceptible to substantial weight gain related to pregnancy, as well as more severe levels of obesity in midlife.

Postpartum Weight Retention: Pregnancy Cohort Studies

In observational epidemiologic studies, the average weight change from preconception to the first year postpartum is referred to as "postpartum weight retention." Postpartum weight retention includes the weight gain during gestation (preconception through gestation), early postpartum weight loss (delivery to 6 weeks postpartum), and later postpartum weight changes (after 6 weeks postpartum). Few studies have obtained serial measurements during the 12 to 24 months postpartum to assess patterns of weight change (ie, weight loss versus gain).

Average postpartum weight retention (preconception to 6–18 months postpartum) is relatively small, ranging from 0.5 to 1.5 kg based on self-reported pregravid weights,[12,19,29,30,32,33] and has little impact on body weight for most women.[34] Nevertheless, the variability in postpartum weight change is large; 13% to 20% of women are 5 kg or more above their preconception weight by 1 year postpartum (**Table 2**).[12,29,30,32] Limitations of pregnancy cohort studies include the lack of control for secular trends in body weight changes, self-reported pre-pregnancy weight, and short-term postpartum weight retention (ie, 1 year or less).[4] The weight increases observed among black women versus white women in surveys may reflect differences in social, cultural, and behavioral factors rather than pregnancy itself. Long-term postpartum weight retension (beyond 1 to 2 years postpartum) has been examined in

Table 2
Percentage of women classified with substantial postpartum weight retention (weighing ≥5 kg above pre-pregnancy weight at postpartum measurement) in pregnancy cohort studies (n >500)

Author, Year, Country, Years Data Collected	Sample Size	Age Range (years)	Time of Postpartum Measurement	Overweight Before Pregnancy (%)	Substantial Weight Retention ≥5 kg (%)
Schauberger, 1995, USA, 1989–1990	790 463	Not stated	6 wks 6 mos	Not reported	>16
Ohlin, 1990, Sweden, 1971–1984	1423	17–49	12 mos	7[b]	14
Keppel, 1993,[a] USA, 1988	2944	>15	10–18 mos	10[b]	>20
Greene, 1988,[a] USA, 1959–1965	7116	23 ± 11	Variable (between 2 pregnancies)	24[d]	~20
Gunderson, 2001, USA, 1980–1990	1300	18–41 (mean, 27)	Variable (between 2 pregnancies)	13[b]	18
Olson, 2003, USA, not stated	540	18 to >40	12 mos	41[b]	~20
Huang, 2008, Taiwan, 2004	602	30 ± 4	6 mos	19[c]	25
Gunderson, 2008, USA, 1999–2003	940	33 ± 5	12 mos	25[b]	13

[a] Sample includes teenagers.
[b] Defined as BMI ≥ 26.
[c] Defined as BMI ≥ 24.
[d] Defined as >120% of ideal body weight for height.

relatively few studies.[5,25,35] Some evidence indicates that both gestational weight gain and weight retention at 1 year postpartum are directly associated with maternal body weight and overweight status decades after pregnancy.[9,36]

Both primiparity and maternal pregravid body size are directly associated with high gestational weight gain, which, in turn, is highly correlated with postpartum weight retention. Given this evidence, characterization of the interrelationships of these maternal attributes is essential to an understanding of postpartum weight changes and obesity.

HIGH PREGRAVID BODY SIZE

Pregravid body size exerts a strong influence on weight changes during and after pregnancy. As previously discussed, women who are overweight before pregnancy experience greater and more variable increases in body weight during and after pregnancy.[8] In 1957, McKeown and colleagues reported that weight change during the 12 months postpartum was largely influenced by the woman's weight before pregnancy; the heavier the woman, the larger amount of weight "retained."[20] Similarly, Aberdeen primiparas (1950s to 1960s) who were overweight in the first pregnancy were heavier by the middle of the subsequent pregnancy than other primiparas of average body size even after adjusting for weight increments related to age and secular trends.[5] The1988 National Maternal and Infant Health Survey (NMIHS) found that women who were overweight before pregnancy were more likely to experience substantial weight retention at 10 to 18 months postpartum than underweight and average weight groups.[32]

Several pregnancy cohort studies from developed countries have reported independent direct associations between pregravid weight or BMI and postpartum weight retention based on multivariable models,[18,28,29,34,37] although studies from a 1980s cohort reported no association.[12,38] A study of Brazilian women found an inverse association.[31] One explanation for the disparate findings is that studies with null findings included only white women, of whom only 7% were overweight before pregnancy (see **Table 2**), which limited the variation in gestational weight gain and pregravid BMI.

The bias in self-reported pregravid weight is greater for high pregravid body size groups and may inflate estimates of postpartum weight retention. In pregnancy cohort studies that utilized self-reported pregravid weight, substantial bias may be introduced because high BMI groups may underreport body weight by up to 5 kg versus 1 kg for other groups.[39,40] Gestational weight gain and postpartum weight retention are affected to a greater extent for high versus low BMI groups due to reporting bias. An underestimate of 5 kg may overestimate gestational weight gain by almost 50%, and an error of 1 kg may overestimate postpartum weight change by more than 100% to 200%. Measured weights at preconception, delivery, and postpartum provide more accurate estimates of average weight change as well as gestational weight gain, especially for overweight or obese women. Similarly, first trimester weight measurements may underestimate both gestational weight gain and postpartum weight retention because maternal fat deposition begins early in pregnancy, which has been estimated at 1.5 kg by 7 weeks' gestation.[41]

The pattern of postpartum weight changes has been assessed in relatively few studies and rarely according to pregravid body size groups. Gunderson and colleagues[25] examined the impact of pregravid body size on the pattern of weight changes during the early postpartum (delivery to 6 weeks' postpartum) and long-term postpartum (from 6 weeks' postpartum to a median 2 years) periods (see **Fig. 1**). Weight loss from delivery to 6 weeks' postpartum did not differ by pregravid

BMI group,[25] but high BMI groups were three to five times more likely to gain more than 2 kg in the long-term than the average BMI group (see **Fig. 1**). The group difference in long-term weight change was 4 kg on average (−0.3 kg for obese versus −4.3 kg for average weight women).[25] Early postpartum weight loss generally consists of the placenta and amniotic fluid and contraction of maternal blood volume and other body components, and largely represents the loss of nonadipose tissue accumulated during gestation; therefore, early postpartum weight loss is similar among BMI groups despite BMI group differences in gestational weight gain. Later postpartum weight changes may differ by BMI because they involve fat mass. Obese women may tend to gain rather than lose weight after 6 weeks postpartum.

Other studies report lower gestational fat mass gains among overweight and obese women when compared with underweight and average weight women (6.0 ± 2.6, 3.8 ± 3.4, 3.5 ± 4.1, and -0.6 ± 4.6 kg, respectively)[42] and much higher postpartum weight gains among heavier women.[37] The higher weight retention from preconception to postpartum observed among high BMI groups may be due to postnatal weight gain, particularly because these women have lower average gestational gains with greater variability when compared with women of average and low BMI.[23] These data suggest that retention of gestational gain is unlikely to explain the higher weight levels after pregnancy among obese women and to some extent among overweight women. Given that gestational gain is strongly correlated with higher postpartum weight, pregravid BMI is an important modifier of this relationship. For example, average size women may be more likely to retain gestational weight gain, and overweight or obese women may tend to lose less weight or to gain weight beyond the 6-week postpartum period.

Pregnancy Cohort Studies: Substantial Postpartum Weight Retention, Risk of Overweight

Substantial postpartum weight retention

Approximately 13% to 20% of pregnant women experience substantial weight retention by 1 year postpartum (see **Table 2**), defined as body weight at least 5 kg above preconception weight. Correlates of substantial postpartum weight retention based on epidemiologic studies include high gestational weight gain, pregravid overweight, primiparity, black race, low socioeconomic status, smoking cessation, and fewer than 5 hours of sleep per day.[4,13,19] The most important independent risk factors for not returning to within 5 kg of pre-pregnancy body weight are maternal overweight or obesity before pregnancy and excessive gestational weight gain.

Risk of becoming overweight after pregnancy: maternal characteristics

Approximately 6% to 14% of women are likely to become overweight within 1 year after delivery.[4,15] In the 1988 NMIHS, 8.2% of average weight white women were heavier by more than 9 kg at 10 to 18 months after delivery versus 22% of black women.[32]

Among pregnant women who were not overweight before pregnancy, Gunderson and colleagues[16] examined the racial and ethnic differences in becoming overweight after pregnancy. In this 1980 to 1990 multi-ethnic pregnancy cohort, overall, 6.4% became overweight by 1.5 years (median follow-up time) after the index pregnancy. Black women were about 40% more likely to become overweight within a median of 2 years after delivery when compared with white women (10% versus 7%). Although the adjusted risk estimate for black women was not statistically significant, it was comparable in magnitude to estimates from a population-based sample of women aged 30 to 55 years in which black women were 50% more likely than white women to gain 10 kg or more over 10 years.[43] Asian women had a greatly reduced risk of becoming overweight (2% versus 7%) when compared with white women, whereas Hispanic women had no increased risk when compared with white women.[8] Although these women did not become overweight, approximately 40% more Asians shifted from a BMI below 19.8 (underweight) to a BMI between 19.8 and 26.0 (normal weight), indicating that significant weight increments occurred among Asian women.

A higher prevalence of overweight and obesity for black women has been reported in population-based epidemiologic studies of US women.[43] In a 10-year prospective study of women aged 18 to 30 years at baseline, black women were three times more likely to become overweight than white women when controlling for age, parity, smoking, sociodemographics, and other risk factors.[16] The higher risk of becoming overweight among black women was not related to childbearing but to differences in secular trends in weight gain trajectories for black women versus white women.

Moreover, other studies found that maternal characteristics independently associated with a twofold to threefold higher risk of becoming overweight after pregnancy included gestational weight gain exceeding the Institute of Medicine (IOM) recommendations, age at menarche of less than 12 years, less than 8 years between menarche and first birth, first birth between age 24 to 30 years,[16] and short sleep duration (<5 hours per 24-hour period) at 6 months' postpartum.[13] These risk factors may indirectly represent genetic or biologic influences on adult body weight before pregnancy, socioeconomic differences in maternal age when childbearing begins, or postpartum changes. Although the strengths of associations were similar to total gestational weight gain, their lower prevalence in a population may result in relatively lower attributable risk from these factors for postpartum weight retention.

CHILDBEARING AND LONG-TERM WEIGHT GAIN: PRIMIPARITY AND PREGRAVID BODY SIZE

Among women of reproductive age, high pregravid body size and primiparity predispose women to substantial weight gain related to childbearing (paras versus nulliparas). Studies of weight gain related to childbearing (**Table 3**) are designed to estimate weight change due to pregnancy and its aftermath relative to weight changes that would normally occur among women of similar reproductive age who did not give birth during the same time interval (ie, removes weight gain due to secular trends and aging). Only four longitudinal studies have measured weight before and after pregnancy during fixed intervals and obtained estimates of weight gain attributed to childbearing by comparing changes among parous women with those among nulliparous or nonparous women.[6,44–46] A fifth study relied on survey methodology to estimate weight changes based on self-reported body weight associated with childbearing.[7] The evidence from these studies, as summarized herein, is consistent, except for one study[46] in which fewer than 27% of women were primiparas.

Specifically, population-based longitudinal studies, the NHANES I Epidemiologic Follow-up Study (NHEFS), the Coronary Artery Risk Development in Young Adults (CARDIA) Study, and the Black Women's Health Study (BWHS), prospectively estimated net weight changes from before to after pregnancy relative to the weight changes related to secular trends and aging in the population (see **Table 3**).[6,7,45,46] Two studies that measured body weight before and after pregnancy reported an average weight gain of 2 to 3 kg associated with a single birth versus no pregnancy in a biracial cohort (black and white women)[45] and a 1.7-kg weight increase per birth among white women.[46] These studies included fewer than 90 primiparas, limiting their ability to examine whether pregnancy-related weight gain varied by pregravid BMI.

Table 3
Longitudinal studies of women of reproductive age: weight gain associated with childbearing (nulliparous referent group and preconception and postpartum weight measurements, except self-reported weights by Rosenberg and colleagues)

Author, Year, Study	Number of Parous Subjects (primiparas)	Race, Age Range (yr) at Baseline	Study Period	Childbearing Weight Gain (kg) (Net Difference in Mean Gain for Paras versus Nulliparas)
Williamson, 1994, NHEFS, USA	308 (82)	White, 25–45	10 yrs (1971–1984)	Primiparas: 0 Multiparas: +1.7 kg per birth
Wolfe, 1997, NHEFS, USA	413 (not stated)	86% White, 25–45	10 yrs (1971–1984)	White race: Primiparas +0.5 kg Multiparas +3.2 kg Black race: Primi & Multiparas +2.3 kg
Smith, 1994, CARDIA study, USA	203 (89)	50% Black/white, 18–30	5 yrs (1985–1991)	Primiparas +2 – 3 kg
Gunderson, 2004, CARDIA study, USA	845 (557)	50% Black/white, 18–30	10 yrs (1985–1996)	Primiparas by Pregravid BMI: BMI < 25: +1 kg BMI >= 25: +3 –6 kg (3-way interaction: p<.001)[a]
Rosenberg, 2003, BWHS, USA	1230 (598)	Black, 21–39	4 yrs (1995–1999)	Primiparas by Pregravid BMI BMI < 25: +0.6 kg BMI>= 25: +3.0 kg or more

[a] Significant three-way interaction by parity, baseline BMI group (overweight and not overweight), and childbearing groups during follow-up. No significant interaction for race. Gunderson and colleagues (2004) and Rosenberg and colleagues (2003) had sufficient sample size to examine parity and pregravid BMI effect modification. NHEFS, NHANES I epidemiologic follow-up study; CARDIA, coronary artery risk development in young adults study; BWHS, black women's health study.

In the larger study cohorts, the CARDIA study and the BWHS, weight gain due to childbearing was greatest after the first birth (primiparas versus nulliparas), and this association depended on body size before pregnancy. The estimates from these two studies were remarkably similar; the average gain associated with having a first child was 3 to 6 kg among women who were overweight before pregnancy (BMI ≥25) and about 1 kg among women who were average weight (BMI <25) before pregnancy (**Fig. 2**), accounting for secular trends, aging, and changes in lifestyle versus nulliparas.[6,7]

The CARDIA data also provided evidence that weight gain attributed to childbearing did not differ between black women and white women[6] when weight changes were examined separately within pregravid body size categories and within parity groups (see **Fig. 2**). Among women nulliparous at baseline, black women gained more weight overall than white women during the 10-year follow-up period regardless of the number of births (0, 1, or 2+ birth groups); however, weight gain attributed to a first birth was similar by race (1 kg for normal BMI, and 3–6 kg for overweight BMI). Cultural as well as biologic and behavioral factors may influence the predisposition of overweight women to gain weight associated with childbearing. Similar gains in central adiposity (waist circumference) by race were linearly associated with the number of births during follow-up.[6]

In prospective longitudinal studies in women of reproductive age, the evidence indicates that persistent weight gain attributed to pregnancy occurs primarily after the first birth (ie, cumulative increases do not occur with subsequent births), and that weight gain is greater with increasing maternal body size. Steeper weight gain trajectories after pregnancy observed within certain race groups may be actually due to secular trends or differences in the prevalence of women who are overweight or obese before pregnancy.

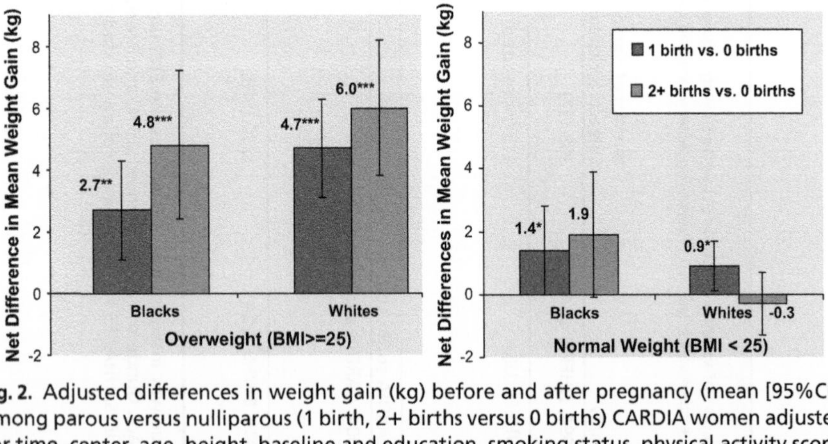

Fig. 2. Adjusted differences in weight gain (kg) before and after pregnancy (mean [95%CI]) among parous versus nulliparous (1 birth, 2+ births versus 0 births) CARDIA women adjusted for time, center, age, height, baseline and education, smoking status, physical activity score, and oral contraceptive use with race groups and pre-pregnancy BMI groups. Pairwise comparisons, *P < .05, **P < .01, ***P < .001. (*Data from* Gunderson EP, Murtaugh MA, Lewis CE, et al. Excess gains in weight and waist circumference associated with childbearing: the Coronary Artery Risk Development in Young Adults Study (CARDIA). Int J Obes Relat Metab Disord 2004;28:525–35.)

Childbearing and Risk of Becoming Overweight (Parous versus Nulliparous Women)

Childbearing is associated with the development of overweight in women of reproductive age.[11] A longitudinal study of US women aged 25 to 45 years at baseline found a 60% to 110% greater risk of becoming overweight among women with one birth when compared with women with no births during the 10-year follow-up period.[46] Limitations of this study included the relatively small number of parous women and the inclusion of peri- and postmenopausal women in the nongravid comparison group.

Another longitudinal study of women aged 18–30 years found that the risk of becoming overweight after pregnancy depended on smoking habits in women.[15] Among never smokers, those who bore children were twice as likely to become overweight as those who never gave birth (odds ratio [OR] = 2.66 [95%CI, 1.80–3.93] for one birth and 2.10 [95%CI, 1.24–3.56] for two or more births). Among current smokers, those who bore children were half as likely to become overweight as those who never gave birth (OR = 0.41 [95%CI, 0.17–0.96] for one birth and 0.36 [95%CI, 0.08–1.65] for two or more births).[15]

Other characteristics associated with becoming overweight among women of reproductive age (18–30 years at baseline) independent of parity included a higher risk for black versus white race (OR = 3.49 [95%CI, 2.59–4.69]), frequent weight cycling versus none (OR = 1.45 [95%CI, 1.03–2.04]), and a high school diploma or less versus 4 years of college (OR = 2.21 [95%CI, 1.50–3.26]). High versus low physical activity (OR = 0.62 [95%CI, 0.43–0.90]) was associated with a reduced risk of becoming overweight.[15] These findings are consistent with previous studies of postpartum weight changes.

Pregnancy and regional fat distribution and central adiposity

During pregnancy, fat is preferentially deposited in the femoral and abdominal regions. In a prospective study of 557 healthy women, subcutaneous body fat was measured via skinfold thicknesses before, during, and 6 weeks after pregnancy.[47] Central body fat gains in the subscapular area were relatively high during pregnancy but mobilized (or reduced) to a lesser extent than in triceps and thigh regions within the first 6 weeks' postpartum. Moreover, primiparas gained more at both thigh and subscapular locations than multiparas.[47] Another study using MRI tomographs found that 68% of gestational fat gain was deposited in the trunk, and that excess fat gain remaining at 1 year postpartum tended to be localized centrally.[48]

Regional fat distribution may differ for women already overweight or obese before pregnancy. Obese women experience more variable changes, including lower or higher gestational weight gains[23] and lower or similar gestational fat gains,[42] but have greater increases in central adiposity and fat deposition during the postpartum period when compared with lower BMI groups.[49] Body fat assessed via skinfold thicknesses and waist and hip circumferences in parous women (n = 47) showed that obese women developed more central obesity by 6 months' postpartum.[49] Women who are overweight before pregnancy accumulate excessive fat stores in response to pregnancy that continue into the postpartum period, or experience patterns of postpartum fat deposition that differ from those who are not overweight.

In population-based, cross-sectional studies, multiparity correlated positively with abdominal girth in women for whom childbearing ended many years earlier, and with larger waist-hip ratios (WHR) in both pre- and postmenopausal women.[50–52] Similarly, longitudinal studies of women of reproductive age reported greater increments in WHR[45] and waist circumference from preconception for up to several years postpartum associated with an increasing number of births independent of age, secular trends, preconception BMI, weight gain, education, and selected behavioral

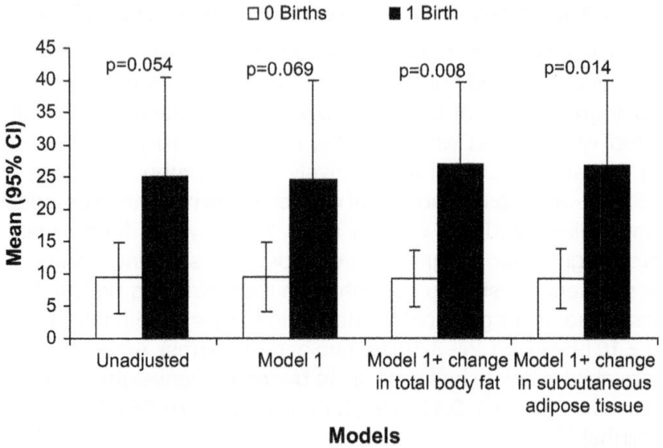

Fig. 3. Unadjusted and adjusted mean (95%CI) 5-year changes in visceral adipose tissue (cm^2) from before to after pregnancy for women with one birth and women with no births during the 5-year interval. (*From* Gunderson EP, Sternfeld B, Wellons MF, et al. Childbearing may increase visceral adipose tissue independent of overall increase in body fat. Obesity (Silver Spring) 2008;16(5):1078–84; with permission.)

attributes.[6] Parity-related increases in central adiposity were also similar for blacks and whites.

Longitudinal changes in visceral and overall adiposity from preconception to postpartum were examined in 122 premenopausal women (50 black, 72 white), of whom 14 gave birth and 108 did not give birth between 1995 and 2000.[53] Adipose tissue compartments were measured via CT and dual energy x-ray absorptiometry in 1995 to 1996 and again in 1999 to 2000. In multiple linear regression models adjusted for age, race, and changes in total and subcutaneous adiposity, visceral adipose tissue levels increased by 40% and 14% above initial levels for the 1 birth and 0 birth groups, respectively; the visceral fat level was 18.0 cm^2 (4.8–31.2) higher for 1 birth versus 0 births groups controlling for gain in total body fat and covariates ($P < .01$) (**Fig. 3**). There was a borderline greater increase in waist girth of 2.3 cm (0–4.5) ($P = .05$), a gain of 6.3 cm (4.1–8.5) versus 4.0 cm (3.2–4.8). This study provides evidence that pregnancy may be associated with preferential accumulation of adipose tissue in the visceral compartment for similar gains in total body fat.

SUMMARY

Epidemiologic studies that measure weight before and after pregnancy in primiparas and that control for secular trends and aging have consistently found that primiparity is associated with higher weight gain among women already overweight before pregnancy.[6,25] Furthermore, these findings consistently show that weight gain does not differ across racial and ethnic groups after controlling for pregravid body size groups.[6,25] Findings from pregnancy cohort studies in developed countries are somewhat mixed, but most report that higher postpartum weight retention is associated with high BMI before pregnancy. Bias in self-reported weight and a limited sample size (including a low percentage of overweight primiparas) may explain the conflicting findings. It is unclear whether becoming overweight after pregnancy is primarily due to high gestational gain, altered lifestyle habits during the postpartum period, or a combination of influences. Overall, the evidence supports the conclusion that substantial weight gain associated with childbearing is an important risk factor for the development of overweight and obesity in women during midlife.[11]

Further investigation is needed to confirm the links among primiparity, sleep duration, age at menarche, and young age at first birth in relation to becoming overweight after pregnancy, as well as the relative importance of these risk factors. More information regarding the influence of socioeconomic factors and culture practices, smoking cessation, lactation, and other behaviors on weight changes during or after pregnancy is also needed.

Within this context, future studies should identify women most likely to benefit from interventions that modify body size before conception, weight gain during pregnancy, or lifestyle during the postpartum period. Women who are most likely to benefit from interventions during one or more of these critical time periods are primiparas who are overweight or obese before pregnancy, and women who have excessive gestational weight gain regardless of parity or pregravid BMI. Morbidly obese women may be advised to gain very little during pregnancy and may benefit from intensive interventions postpartum to lose weight or slow their pre-pregnancy weight gain trajectory. Similarly, women who are moderately overweight before a first pregnancy may be advised to lose weight several months before pregnancy and to carefully control gestational weight gain from early gestation within IOM recommendations. Overweight and obese women who have modest gestational weight gain, as well as average weight women who have excessive gestational weight gain, may benefit primarily from interventions during the postpartum period to promote weight loss. Clinicians can identify women who are susceptible to substantial postpartum weight retention, to becoming obese, or to increased central adiposity after pregnancy. These women may require subsequent evaluation for primary prevention of midlife obesity and chronic diseases.

Weight gain and overweight during midlife are strong independent predictors of cardiovascular disease, particularly among women,[54] as well as the metabolic syndrome, type 2 diabetes, and early mortality.[55–57] Changes in body fat distribution and central obesity as a consequence of childbearing require further investigation. As a modifiable risk factor, weight gain during prenatal and postpartum periods may provide the critical window for conducting interventions to prevent substantial weight gain as well as the development of overweight and obesity in young women.

REFERENCES

1. Flegal KM, Carroll MD, Ogden CL, et al. Prevalence and trends in obesity among US adults, 1999–2000. JAMA 2002;288:1723–7.
2. Centers for Disease Control & Prevention. Pediatric & pregnancy nutrition surveillance system. 2009. Available at: http://www.cdc.gov/pednss/pnss_tables/tables_health_indicators.htm. Accessed April 27, 2009.
3. Catalano PM. Increasing maternal obesity and weight gain during pregnancy: the obstetric problems of plentitude. Obstet Gynecol 2007;110:743–4.
4. Gunderson EP, Abrams B. Epidemiology of gestational weight gain and body weight changes after pregnancy. Epidemiol Rev 1999;21:261–75.
5. Billewicz WZ. Body weight in parous women. Br J Prev Soc Med 1970;24:97–104.
6. Gunderson EP, Murtaugh MA, Lewis CE, et al. Excess gains in weight and waist circumference associated with childbearing: the Coronary Artery Risk Development in Young Adults Study (CARDIA). Int J Obes Relat Metab Disord 2004;28:525–35.

7. Rosenberg L, Palmer JR, Wise LA, et al. A prospective study of the effect of childbearing on weight gain in African-American women. Obes Res 2003;11:1526–35.
8. Institute of Medicine. Nutrition during pregnancy. Washington, DC: National Academy of Sciences; 1990.
9. Rooney BL, Schauberger CW, Mathiason MA. Impact of perinatal weight change on long-term obesity and obesity-related illnesses. Obstet Gynecol 2005;106:1349–56.
10. Linne Y, Dye L, Barkeling B, et al. Weight development over time in parous women: the SPAWN study–15 years follow-up. Int J Obes Relat Metab Disord 2003;27:1516–22.
11. Gunderson EP, Sternfeld B, Wellons MF, et al. Childbearing may increase visceral adipose tissue independent of overall increase in body fat. Obesity 2008;16(5): 1078–84.
12. Ohlin A, Rossner S. Maternal body weight development after pregnancy. Int J Obes 1990;14:159–73.
13. Gunderson EP, Rifas-Shiman SL, Oken E, et al. Association of fewer hours of sleep at 6 months postpartum with substantial weight retention at 1 year postpartum. Am J Epidemiol 2008;167:178–87.
14. Schmitt NM, Nicholson WK, Schmitt J. The association of pregnancy and the development of obesity: results of a systematic review and meta-analysis on the natural history of postpartum weight retention. Int J Obes 2007;31: 1642–51.
15. Gunderson EP, Quesenberry CP Jr, Lewis CE, et al. Development of overweight associated with childbearing depends on smoking habit: the Coronary Artery Risk Development in Young Adults (CARDIA) Study. Obes Res 2004;12: 2041–53.
16. Gunderson EP, Abrams B, Selvin S. The relative importance of gestational gain and maternal characteristics associated with the risk of becoming overweight after pregnancy. Int J Obes Relat Metab Disord 2000;24:1660–8.
17. Oken E, Taveras EM, Popoola FA, et al. Television, walking, and diet: associations with postpartum weight retention. Am J Prev Med 2007;32:305–11.
18. Parker JD, Abrams B. Differences in postpartum weight retention between black and white mothers. Obstet Gynecol 1993;81:768–74.
19. Olson CM, Strawderman MS, Hinton PS, et al. Gestational weight gain and postpartum behaviors associated with weight change from early pregnancy to 1 y postpartum. Int J Obes Relat Metab Disord 2003;27:117–27.
20. McKeown T, Record RG. The influence of weight and height on weight changes associated with pregnancy in women. J Endocrinol 1957;15:423–9.
21. Brawarsky P, Stotland NE, Jackson RA, et al. Pre-pregnancy and pregnancy-related factors and the risk of excessive or inadequate gestational weight gain. Int J Gynaecol Obstet 2005;91:125–31.
22. Chasan-Taber L, Schmidt MD, Pekow P, et al. Predictors of excessive and inadequate gestational weight gain in Hispanic women. Obesity 2008;16(7):1657–66.
23. Wells CS, Schwalberg R, Noonan G, et al. Factors influencing inadequate and excessive weight gain in pregnancy: Colorado, 2000–2002. Matern Child Health J 2006;10(1):55–62.
24. Cogswell ME, Serdula MK, Hungerford DW, et al. Gestational weight gain among average-weight and overweight women: what is excessive? Am J Obstet Gynecol 1995;172:705–12.
25. Gunderson EP, Abrams B, Selvin S. Does the pattern of postpartum weight change differ according to pregravid body size? Int J Obes Relat Metab Disord 2001;25:853–62.

26. Jensen DM, Damm P, Sorensen B, et al. Pregnancy outcome and prepregnancy body mass index in 2459 glucose-tolerant Danish women. Am J Obstet Gynecol 2003;189:239–44.
27. Kiel DW, Dodson EA, Artal R, et al. Gestational weight gain and pregnancy outcomes in obese women: how much is enough? Obstet Gynecol 2007;110:752–8.
28. Boardley DJ, Sargent RG, Coker AL, et al. The relationship between diet, activity, and other factors, and postpartum weight change by race. Obstet Gynecol 1995; 86:834–8.
29. Greene GW, Smiciklas-Wright H, Scholl TO, et al. Postpartum weight change: how much of the weight gained in pregnancy will be lost after delivery? Obstet Gynecol 1988;71:701–7.
30. Schauberger CW, Rooney BL, Brimer LM. Factors that influence weight loss in the puerperium. Obstet Gynecol 1992;79:424–9.
31. Kac G, Benicio MH, Velasquez-Melendez G, et al. Gestational weight gain and prepregnancy weight influence postpartum weight retention in a cohort of Brazilian women. J Nutr 2004;134:661–6.
32. Keppel KG, Taffel SM. Pregnancy-related weight gain and retention: implications of the 1990 Institute of Medicine guidelines. Am J Public Health 1993; 83:1100–3.
33. Kac G, D'Aquino Benicio MH, Valente JG, et al. Postpartum weight retention among women in Rio de Janeiro: a follow-up study. Cad Saude Publica 2003; 19(Suppl 1):S149–61.
34. Harris HE, Ellison GT, Holliday M, et al. The impact of pregnancy on the long-term weight gain of primiparous women in England. Int J Obes Relat Metab Disord 1997;21:747–55.
35. Maddah M, Nikooyeh B. Weight retention from early pregnancy to three years postpartum: a study in Iranian women. Midwifery 2008, Mar 27 [Epub ahead of print].
36. Linne Y, Dye L, Barkeling B, et al. Long-term weight development in women: a 15-year follow-up of the effects of pregnancy. Obes Res 2004;12:1166–78.
37. Butte NF, Ellis KJ, Wong WW, et al. Composition of gestational weight gain impacts maternal fat retention and infant birth weight. Am J Obstet Gynecol 2003;189:1423–32.
38. Muscati SK, Gray-Donald K, Koski KG. Timing of weight gain during pregnancy: promoting fetal growth and minimizing maternal weight retention. Int J Obes Relat Metab Disord 1996;20:526–32.
39. Stevens-Simon C, Roghmann KJ, McAnarney ER. Relationship of self-reported prepregnant weight and weight gain during pregnancy to maternal body habitus and age. J Am Diet Assoc 1992;92:85–7.
40. Rowland ML. Self-reported weight and height. Am J Clin Nutr 1990;52:1125–33.
41. Clapp JF III, Seaward BL, Sleamaker RH, et al. Maternal physiologic adaptations to early human pregnancy. Am J Obstet Gynecol 1988;159:1456–60.
42. Lederman SA, Paxton A, Heymsfield SB, et al. Body fat and water changes during pregnancy in women with different body weight and weight gain. Obstet Gynecol 1997;90:483–8.
43. Williamson DF, Kahn HS, Byers T. The 10-y incidence of obesity and major weight gain in black and white US women aged 30-55 y. Am J Clin Nutr 1991;53: 1515S–8S.
44. Rookus MA, Rokebrand P, Burema J, et al. The effect of pregnancy on the body mass index 9 months postpartum in 49 women. Int J Obes 1987;11: 609–18.

45. Smith DE, Lewis CE, Caveny JL, et al. Longitudinal changes in adiposity associated with pregnancy: the CARDIA Study. Coronary Artery Risk Development in Young Adults Study. JAMA 1994;271:1747–51.
46. Williamson DF, Madans J, Pamuk E, et al. A prospective study of childbearing and 10-year weight gain in US white women 25 to 45 years of age. Int J Obes Relat Metab Disord 1994;18:561–9.
47. Sidebottom AC, Brown JE, Jacobs DR Jr. Pregnancy-related changes in body fat. Eur J Obstet Gynecol Reprod Biol 2001;94:216–23.
48. Sohlstrom A, Forsum E. Changes in adipose tissue volume and distribution during reproduction in Swedish women as assessed by magnetic resonance imaging. Am J Clin Nutr 1995;61:287–95.
49. Soltani H, Fraser RB. A longitudinal study of maternal anthropometric changes in normal weight, overweight, and obese women during pregnancy and postpartum. Br J Nutr 2000;84:95–101.
50. Troisi RJ, Wolf AM, Mason JE, et al. Relation of body fat distribution to reproductive factors in pre- and postmenopausal women. Obes Rev 1995;3:143–51.
51. denTonkelaar I, Seidell JC, van Noord PA, et al. Fat distribution in relation to age, degree of obesity, smoking habits, parity and estrogen use: a cross-sectional study in 11,825 Dutch women participating in the DOM-project. Int J Obes 1990;14:753–61.
52. Kaye SA, Folsom AR, Prineas RJ, et al. The association of body fat distribution with lifestyle and reproductive factors in a population study of postmenopausal women. Int J Obes 1990;14:583–91.
53. Gunderson EP, Murtaugh MA, Lewis CE, et al. Excess gains in weight and waist circumference associated with childbearing: The coronary artery risk development in young adults study (CARDIA). Int J Obes Relat Metab Disord 2004;28(4):525–35.
54. Hubert HB, Feinleib M, McNamara PM, et al. Obesity as an independent risk factor for cardiovascular disease: a 26-year follow-up of participants in the Framingham Heart Study. Circulation 1983;67:968–77.
55. Willett WC, Manson JE, Stampfer MJ, et al. Weight, weight change, and coronary heart disease in women: risk within the 'normal' weight range. JAMA 1995;273:461–5.
56. Ford ES, Williamson DF, Liu S. Weight change and diabetes incidence: findings from a national cohort of US adults. Am J Epidemiol 1997;146:214–22.
57. Colditz GA, Willett WC, Rotnitzky A, et al. Weight gain as a risk factor for clinical diabetes mellitus in women. Ann Intern Med 1995;122:481–6.

Obesity and Its Relationship to Infertility in Men and Women

J. Ricardo Loret de Mola, MD, FACOG, FACS[a,b,*]

KEYWORDS

• Obesity • PCOS • Infertility female • Infertility male
• Reproduction • Metabolic syndrome

Obesity has become a new worldwide health problem and epidemic with significant impact on morbidity and mortality from cardiovascular disease, diabetes, hypertension, and related disorders. Obesity is defined as a body mass index (BMI) of 30 kg/m^2 or more, whereas overweight is defined as a BMI of 25 to 29.9 kg/m^2. The rate of obesity among young men and women is constantly increasing and how these weight changes will affect new generations and their future fertility is at this point unknown. In addition, similar rises have been observed in the pregnant population, with one in five women making an appointment for antenatal care being clinically obese. The rate of obesity has more than doubled over the past decade[1]; therefore, it is of vital importance that physicians involved in the care of women be familiar with how obesity affects the reproductive system in men and women, its endocrinology, obstetrics, and related health issues.

A condition frequently associated with obesity and reproductive disorders is the polycystic ovary syndrome (PCOS), which is observed in 4% to 7% of all women.[2] Obese patients who have PCOS frequently suffer from infertility as a result of anovulation; however, they also may have an increased risk for recurrent miscarriages and complications during pregnancy. Although the pathophysiology of PCOS may have a genetic component, its escalating rates in the general population also may be associated with environmental factors, such as changes in dietary habits and lack of regular exercise. Obesity increases the risk for the metabolic syndrome, which is associated with several cardiovascular risk parameters, such as insulin resistance, central obesity, glucose intolerance, and hypertension. The metabolic syndrome also is associated with PCOS.[3]

[a] Department of Obstetrics and Gynecology, Southern Illinois University School of Medicine, 751 N Rutledge Street, Room 0100, PO BOX 19637, Springfield, IL 62794-9637, USA
[b] Carol Jo Vecchie Women's Health, Springfield, IL, USA
* Corresponding author. Department of Obstetrics and Gynecology, Southern Illinois University School of Medicine, Springfield, IL.
E-mail address: rloretdemola@siumed.edu

Obstet Gynecol Clin N Am 36 (2009) 333–346
doi:10.1016/j.ogc.2009.03.002
0889-8545/08/$ – see front matter. Published by Elsevier Inc.

The relationship between obesity and male infertility has been largely ignored until recently. The increasing rates of obesity in both genders also are expected to affect the reproductive status of many men. Recent reports have described the relationships between obesity and semen characteristics, reproductive endocrine function, sexual function, and male infertility.

This review focuses on the negative impact of obesity in reproduction by considering (1) the pathophysiology of obesity and infertility in men and women, (2) the influence of obesity on the prevalence of PCOS, and (3) the benefits of weight loss on reproduction and on menstruation, ovulation, semen parameters, and reproductive outcomes.

THE PREVALENCE OF OBESITY AND INFERTILITY AMONG MEN AND WOMEN

We are facing a worldwide epidemic of obesity, which is particularly troublesome as these rates are highest among the American population. Obesity has long been associated with several medical conditions and social and psychologic disorders. There is a significant increase in the risk for type 2 diabetes mellitus and cardiovascular disease among obese individuals and, more recently, a relationship between obesity and fertility-related disorders and cancers has been recognized.[4–7] Among men, BMI is associated with infertility with an odds ratio (OR) of 1.12 (95% CI, 1.01–1.25, after correlation for female BMI, male and female age, smoking status, alcohol use, and exposure to solvents and pesticides). BMI seems to have its maximum negative effect on fertility at the range of 32 to 43 kg/m^2 and the effect plateaus beyond that point.[7] Although there have been several criticisms as to selection bias in the reports associating BMI to infertility in men, they have brought attention to the association between BMI and infertility among men.[8,9] A more recent male infertility study derived from a Norwegian database also demonstrated an association with being overweight (BMI 25–29.9 kg/m^2), with an OR for infertility of 1.19 (95% CI, 1.03–1.62); obese men had an OR for infertility of 1.36 (95% CI, 1.12–1.62). BMI affected male fertility in a relationship directly related to weight, reaching a plateau at a high BMI of greater than 35 kg/m^2.[10] Although several of these studies had selection biases and there are concerns with the study populations, they bring into the forefront the possibility that obesity affects fertility not only in women but also in men. There seems to be an increased incidence of obesity among men attending fertility clinics; abnormal semen analysis parameters among obese men have been reported by several groups.[11–13] There seems to be good evidence that obesity can be associated with reduced sperm concentration, and this observation exhibits a clear dose-response relationship.[14–16] Furthermore, when infertile couples were divided into patients who had male factor infertility (abnormal sperm concentration and motility), unexplained infertility, and female factor infertility, the incidence of obesity was three times higher in men who had male factor infertility than in any of the other groups.[11]

The rate of female obesity, alternatively, is associated in at least 30% of cases with PCOS; in some regions of the world, it is as high as 75% of cases.[2] Azziz and colleagues[17] reported that in 400 unselected consecutive premenopausal women who attended a clinic, the prevalence of PCOS was 6.6% and overweight and obesity in that patient population were 24% and 32%, respectively. **Table 1** shows a report of a large cohort of 320 women who had PCOS over the past 10 years and their different BMI categories.

EFFECTS OF MALE OBESITY ON THE SEMEN ANALYSIS

Studies of the relationship between obesity and sperm quality in infertile populations are based on the changes in semen parameters. A decrease in sperm concentration

Table 1
Prevalence of obesity in a large cohort of 320 women who had PCOS attending the Division of Endocrinology, S. Orsola-Malpighi Hospital, Bologna, in the past 10 years

BMI Categories	Number	Age (years)	Waist Circumference (cm)	Waist-To-Hip Ratio
≤19	14	22.7 ± 6.0	75.5 ± 2.8	0.81 ± 0.09
19.1–25	110	25.2 ± 6.2	70.6 ± 5.2	0.76 ± 0.06
25.1–30	58	23.9 ± 5.5	83.6 ± 6.6	0.81 ± 0.07
30.1–35	65	24.9 ± 5.9	95.7 ± 6.9	0.85 ± 0.07
35.1–40	42	26.9 ± 7.5	102.2 ± 7.6	0.87 ± 0.07
>40	31	27.2 ± 8.3	113.7 ± 9.1	0.92 ± 0.11
P values	—	<0.05	<0.001	<0.001

BMI categories are defined according to the World Health Organization document.
Data from Pasquali R, Gambineri A, Pagotto. The impact of obesity on reproduction in women with polycystic ovary syndrome. BJOG 2006;113:1148–59.

and motility is associated with decreased fertility.[18,19] Sperm morphology also is an independent feature closely correlated with male infertility.[20] A study of military personnel in Denmark showed that overweight and obese men had mean sperm concentrations that were lower than those of men with normal weight. The prevalence of oligospermia (sperm concentration <20 million sperm/mL) was higher in overweight and obese men than in normal weight controls (24.4% versus 21.7%). Moreover, overweight and obese men were found to have a 21.6% (95% CI, 4%–39.4%) reduction in their sperm concentration after correction for other conditions.[21]

Other investigators have made similar negative correlations between BMI and sperm concentration and total sperm count.[11] Specific physical features associated with obesity also have been correlated with abnormal sperm counts among infertile couples, whereas hip circumference correlated negatively with sperm concentration and weight and waist and hip circumferences correlated negatively to total sperm count.[22] Studies that have focused on the relationship between male obesity and sperm motility and morphology have been more conflicting. In the Danish study (previously described),[21] there was no relation between male BMI and percent of total motile sperm or morphology; however, other studies have shown a clear negative correlation between BMI and sperm motility.[23]

Increased DNA fragmentation has been associated with male infertility; there was a direct correlation between infertility and a high percentage of sperm DNA fragmentation. When sperm chromatin integrity was evaluated using the flow cytometry method (sperm chromatin structure assay) in different BMI groups, increasing BMI was directly correlated with the DNA fragmentation index, which was higher in obese and overweight men (27% and 25.8%, respectively) compared with normal-weight men (19.9%).[23]

In summary, there is good evidence that obesity can be associated with reduced sperm concentrations and DNA fragmentation but inconclusive evidence regarding motility and morphology.

EFFECTS OF MALE OBESITY ON THE ENDOCRINOLOGY AND FUNCTION OF THE HYPOTHALAMIC-PITUITARY-TESTICULAR AXIS

Although male infertility likely is multifactorial, with lifestyle being the most important, the hormonal alterations associated with obesity and its associated disorders are likely pivotal to the reproductive changes responsible for sperm production. In addition, obese men have erectile dysfunction and reduced coital frequency.[24] The relationship between obesity and erectile dysfunction can be explained by decreased testosterone levels and elevated pro-inflammatory cytokines, which induce endothelial dysfunction through the nitric oxide pathway.[25] Increased testicular temperature also affects spermatogenesis.[26] Obesity often is associated with decreased physical activity and increased fat deposition in the abdomen and scrotum,[27] which may increase local testicular temperature.

Obese men have hypogonadotropic hyperestrogenic hypoandrogenemia, characterized by decreased total and free testosterone, decreased gonadotropins, and increased circulating estrogen levels. The hypoandrogenemia is directly proportional to the degree of obesity,[28,29] with estrone and estradiol levels increased from increased peripheral aromatization of androgens.[30] Estrogen itself has a direct negative effect on spermatogenesis, as demonstrated in men taking high doses of diethylstilbestrol.[31] Estrogen acts on the hypothalamus, modifying GnRH pulsatility and reducing gonadotropins (luteinizing hormone [LH] and follicle-stimulating hormone [FSH]) in the pituitary.[32] The subsequent relative hypogonadotropic environment reduces testicular function and testosterone production, with lowered intratesticular and circulating testosterone serum levels. Studies in obese men in which aromatase inhibitors were used to reduce the aromatization of estrogens from androgens caused elevations of LH and testosterone,[33] and similar effects are expected from the use of the antiestrogen, clomiphene citrate. A decrease in the testosterone/estrogen ratio has been shown associated with infertility.[34] Inhibin B is a marker of Sertoli's cell function and its associated spermatogenic activity,[35] and inhibin B levels are altered in obese men, which may be directly causative of decreased spermatogenesis. The low inhibin B levels would predict elevations in FSH; however, relative hyperestrogenemia is believed possibly causative of this inappropriate low FSH response.[36] A similar negative relationship between inhibin B levels and BMI also was found in women who had PCOS and in fertile control patients.[37,38] Sex hormone–binding globulin (SHBG) and albumin levels also are reduced as a result of hyperinsulinemia and insulin resistance of obesity,[39] increasing circulating testosterone, which magnifies the negative feedback effect of the elevated total estradiol levels. Sleep apnea also may worsen the low serum testosterone levels in obese men.[40,41] Endorphins also are elevated in obesity, which in return further suppress GnRH pulsatility as evidenced by studies in which naloxone suppression of opiates increases LH secretion.[42] Leptin also is affected in obesity, and leptin deficiency or mutations in the leptin receptor are associated with severe early-onset obesity, delayed puberty, and hypogonadism.[43]

EFFECTS OF FEMALE OBESITY ON THE ENDOCRINOLOGY AND FUNCTION OF THE HYPOTHALAMIC-PITUITARY-OVARIAN AXIS

The association between obesity and infertility is partially related to oligo-ovulation or anovulation. PCOS is commonly associated with ovulatory dysfunction, hyperandrogenemia, and PCOS-appearing ovaries on ultrasound and frequently is associated with BMI values greater than 25 kg/m^2. In addition, obese PCOS women have higher rates of anovulation than leaner patients who have the same diagnosis,[3] and the response and doses used for induction of ovulation also are higher with suboptimal ovulatory responses.[44,45] An additional barrier to adequate response to ovulation induction medications is the hyperinsulinemia and insulin resistance associated with the increase in fat, in particular the abdominal phenotype of obesity, which defines it as a condition of relative functional hyperandrogenism. Adipose tissue also is able to store lipid soluble steroids, including androgens, which seem preferentially concentrated within the adipose tissue rather than in the blood. Therefore, because there is more abundant fat tissue than blood in obese patients, steroid concentrations are greater than in normal-weight individuals.[46] Furthermore, fat represents a site of intense sex hormone metabolism resulting from steroidogenic enzymes, such as 3β-dehydrogenase, 17β-hydroxydehydrogenase, and aromatase.[3,6,46] Estradiol levels from increased peripheral aromatization of androgens also have a direct negative effect on the hypothalamus, modifying GnRH pulsatility and reducing gonadotropins (LH and FSH) at the pituitary. The subsequent relative hypogonadotropic environment results in anovulation.

Insulin has a negative effect on the synthesis of SHBG by the liver; truncal obesity is associated with insulin resistance[47] and increases in free testosterone and dihydrotestosterone.[48] Levels of SHBG are regulated by other complex factors, including estrogens, iodothyronines, and growth hormone as stimulating agents and androgens and insulin as inhibiting factors.[49] Insulin binds with low affinity to the LH receptor in the theca cell, and hyperinsulinemia may stimulate compensatory ovarian theca cell steroidogenesis and androgen production via the saturation of the receptor, which may inhibit normal ovulation via premature follicular atresia and premature luteinization.[50] Part of the new Rotterdam criteria for the diagnosis of PCOS includes the ultrasound appearance of PCOS-appearing ovaries, where abundant follicles at the antral stage in the ovarian cortex are responsible for this endocrine milieu. Follicular development may be affected by increased reactive oxygen species.[51] In addition, leptin, a surrogate marker for fat mass, can directly modulate granulosa, theca, and interstitial cells,[52] with inhibition of steroidogenesis[52] and oocyte maturation,[53] thereby providing an additional potential mechanism for anovulation.

The endocannaboid system also plays a pivotal role in the anovulation of obesity. Its primary negative effect is in the hypothalamus, although some down-regulating influences may be mediated directly at the level of the pituitary and ovary. By suppressing the secretory pulsatility of LH,[54] endocannabinoids can down-regulate serum LH levels,[55] but administration of gonadotropins or pulsatile GnRH can restore ovulation and LH release. These effects are mediated by neurotransmitters known to facilitate GnRH secretion, such as norepinephrine and glutamate, and by stimulating those modulators known to down-regulate GnRH secretion, such as dopamine, γ-aminobutyric acid, opioids, and corticotropin releasing hormone.[56]

THE EFFECTS OF OBESITY ON PREGNANCY

Obesity significantly increases the risk for maternal complications during pregnancy, with strong associations with hypertensive disorders, diabetes, infection, thromboembolism, altered mood, and complications during labor and delivery, such as fetal distress, arrest of active phase of labor and dystocia (including shoulder), abnormal presentation, and an increased rate of instrumental delivery and cesarean section.[57–59] Even if pregnancy is achieved spontaneously[60] or after assisted reproductive techniques,[61,62] obesity is associated with increased risk for early and recurrent miscarriage. A recent meta-analysis suggested that PCOS is not associated with an increased risk for miscarriage after in vitro fertilization.[63] In women who have recurrent miscarriage, hyperinsulinemia seems to have an important etiologic role.[64,65] The risk for fetal death is not restricted to early pregnancy, however, as the risk for second- and third-trimester fetal loss increases consistently with increasing BMI. The risk for fetal death after 28 weeks compared with lean women triples among those who are overweight and quadruples among those who are obese,[66,67] with 1 in 121 women who have a BMI greater than 40 kg/m^2 experiencing a stillbirth.[67] Maternal obesity also has a significant detrimental impact on fetal development, probably secondary to glucose intolerance and gestational diabetes mellitus, with an increased risk for isolated and multiple fetal anomalies,[68–71] with folic acid supplementation reducing this risk. It is unclear if obesity alone is a risk factor for fetal anomalies; however, there seems to be a 7% increase in risk for fetal anomalies for each 1-unit increment in BMI above 25 kg/m^2.[68] Another significant problem in obese women who are pregnant is the equipment limitations to identify anomalies given the poor penetration of ultrasound waves through the abdominal fat tissue,[72] with 10% of obese women having suboptimal four-chamber views of the heart between 22 and 24 weeks' gestation.[73] The risk for death of the child is not, however, restricted to the antenatal period, with obesity having a significant impact on neonatal and infant mortality.[67,74] Prematurity is strongly associated with obese mothers, mostly related to induction of labor and cesarean section from preeclampsia.[74] The risk not only is limited to the fetus but also affects the mother because obesity increases the risk for operative delivery and its associated complications, including injuries, delayed healing, and wound infections. Therefore, given these maternal and fetal risks, it is important to emphasize the importance of weight loss before spontaneous or assisted conception for optimal pregnancy outcomes.[75]

TREATMENTS OF OBESITY AND INFERTILITY

Weight loss is the cornerstone of the treatment of obesity-associated infertility. There are limited data on the effect of weight loss in obese men on sperm production and fertility. Most studies have focused on the effects of weight loss on the hormonal profile of obese men. SHBG and testosterone levels improve after a very-low-energy diet[76] and gastroplasty.[77] In addition, physical activity and leanness are associated with a reduced risk for erectile dysfunction.[24]

Obesity independent of PCOS is associated with anovulation, and weight loss is an effective therapy for ovulation, alone or associated with medical induction of ovulation in obese women and obese PCOS women. Consequently, lifestyle changes that encourage weight loss, including diet, exercise, and folic acid supplementation, all should be instituted in advance of ovulation induction therapy. Women who have a BMI above 35 kg/m^2 should lose weight before conception, and this should be an integral part of any fertility program's management of all overweight and obese patients. Most of the evidence for lifestyle modification as an intervention comes from studies of obese PCOS women. Weight loss of 5% to 10% of total body weight can achieve a 30% reduction of visceral adiposity,[78] an improvement in insulin sensitivity, and restoration of ovulation.[79,80] Lifestyle modification is not enough to achieve a pregnancy[80]; therefore, weight loss should be part of all fertility treatments to improve the likelihood of ovulation. Weight loss is feasible with a 6-month program of exercise and calorie restriction and with the addition of pharmacologic therapies, such as sibutramine.[81,82] Although metformin also may induce weight loss and a reduction in visceral adiposity, the effect is modest[83] but enhanced in combination with lifestyle modification.[84,85] Bariatric surgery also is increasingly common for morbidly obese patients and is associated with significant weight loss, improvement in menstrual pattern,[86] and a reduction in obstetric complications.[87,88] The severe ketosis associated with the initial weight loss may induce fetal anomalies, and it is recommended that patients wait for a period of 1 year before attempting pregnancy. Collectively these techniques in conjunction with appropriate psychologic support should help obtain an optimal maternal metabolic profile before fertility treatments or pregnancy. Many obese women presenting at infertility clinics are diagnosed with PCOS and a reduced frequency of ovulation but may have concomitant oligospermia or tubal causes and, therefore, should be evaluated for these conditions concomitantly; infertility should not be assumed related purely to ovulatory dysfunction.[89] Normal first-line practice is to treat women who have ovulation induction using the antiestrogen, clomiphene citrate,[90] with perhaps lower success expected in obese couples but pregnancies do occur: there is a conception rate of up to 50% after three to six cycles and 75% within nine cycles.[91,92] A significant proportion, 5% to 10%, however, is multiple gestations.[93,94] The main factors that predict a favorable treatment outcome are the degree of obesity, hyperandrogenemia, and age (**Fig. 1**). The starting dosage of clomiphene is 50 mg per day (for 5 days, starting any day from cycle day 2 through 5 after a spontaneous or progestin-induced menstruation). The maximum dosage should be limited to 150 mg per day, because efficacy at higher doses is limited, and consistent with Food and Drug Administration recommendations of 750 mg per treatment cycle.

Suggestions that metformin, alone or as a cotreatment with clomiphen, may increase pregnancy rates in women who have PCOS and in obese women who have PCOS[95] have been disproved by recent large prospective trials (**Table 2**).[94] Treatment with metformin alone has a modest impact on ovulation rates, equating to one ovulation per five woman months,[96] and is most effective among women of normal weight and reduced central adiposity.[97] It is unclear why metformin has such a poor impact on success if the hyperinsulinemia is believed to be the key pathologic mechanism in anovulation, which suggests that alternative metabolic signaling pathways also may be disrupted. In patients who are obese, have PCOS, and have glucose intolerance, there still may be value in the use of metformin in association with clomiphene citrate, because this patient population has not been addressed properly in such studies.[94] The response to gonadotropins for ovulation induction in

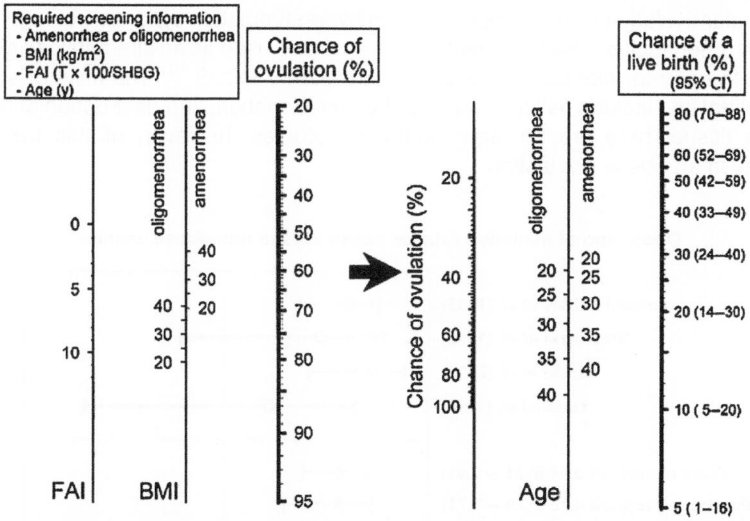

Fig. 1. Nomogram designed to predict chances for live birth in clomiphene citrate induction of ovulation. Note the two different steps. FAI, free androgen index; T, testosterone. (*From* Imani B, Eijkemans MJ, te Velde ER, et al. A nomogram to predict the probability of live birth after clomiphene citrate induction of ovulation in normogonadotropic oligoamenorrheic infertility. Fertil Steril 2002;77:91–7; with permission.)

Table 2
Randomized trial from the National Institutes of Health Reproductive Medicine Network

	Clomiphene Citrate	Metformin	Combination
N	209	208	209
Ovulation	49[a]	29	60[b]
Conception	20[a]	12	38[a]
Pregnancy	24[a]	9	31[a]
Live birth	23[a]	7	27[a]
Multiple	6	0	3

[a] $P<.001$.
[b] $P<.001$ (combination versus clomiphene citrate).
Data from Legro RS, Barnhart HX, Schlaff WD, et al. Clomiphene, metformin, or both for infertility in the polycystic ovary syndrome. N Engl J Med 2007;356:551–66.

obese women who have World Health Organization group II anovulatory infertility also is attenuated, with a higher threshold for ovarian hyperstimulation (**Fig. 2**). Despite requiring longer periods of stimulation and greater total dose of gonadotropins,[98] however, equivalent ovulation and pregnancy rates to those in controls[99,100] usually are observed. Similarly, the controlled ovarian stimulation of obese women requires higher doses of gonadotrophins[101,102]; however, a detrimental impact on live birth has been observed only in some studies[61,103] but not all.[101,104] Overall, patients undergoing assisted reproductive techniques require higher follicle-stimulating hormone dosing and a modestly increased incidence of cycle cancellation due to failure to produce enough follicles (5% of cycles compared with 2% for those of normal weight), with a cumulative conception rate over three cycles of 41% compared with 50% for those with normal weight.[103] Laparoscopic ovarian drilling also has been advocated recently for the treatment of anovulation in patients who have PCOS and can achieve unifollicular ovulation with no risk for ovarian hyperstimulation syndrome or high-order multiple pregnancies. This treatment modality can be used as an alternative to gonadotropin therapy for clomiphene-resistant anovulatory PCOS.[104] The risks of surgery are minimal and include risk for ovarian adhesion formation, and destruction of normal ovarian tissue.There are no large controlled studies, however, of this treatment modality in an obese population.

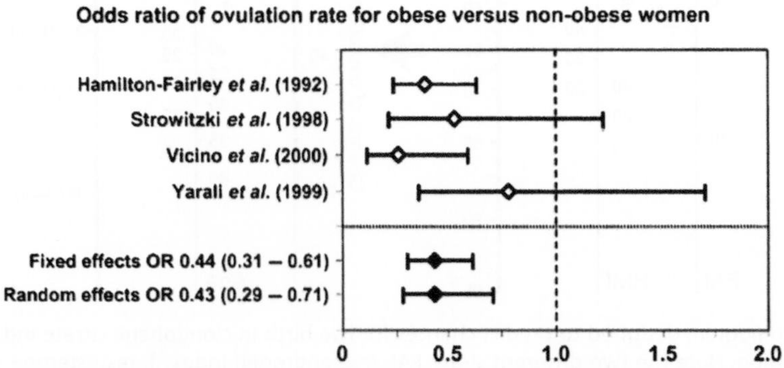

Fig. 2. Association between obesity and ovulation rate in gonadotrophin ovulation induction, with a pooled OR and 95% CI. (*From* Consensus on infertility treatment related to polycystic ovary syndrome. Hum Reprod 2008;23:462–77; with permission.)

SUMMARY

Obesity is a major health problem throughout the world. It seems that obesity is associated with reduced male and female fertility. Although the effects in men are modest, the increasing rates of obesity in the general population may cause more dramatic increases in infertility rates among men in the years to come. Obesity independent of PCOS is associated with anovulation and infertility in women, and weight loss is an effective therapy for improving ovulation, alone or associated with medical induction of ovulation in obese women and in obese women who have PCOS. Consequently, lifestyle changes that encourage weight loss, including diet and exercise, and folic acid supplementation, should be instituted in advance of ovulation induction therapy in women and to improve semen parameters among men.

REFERENCES

1. James PT. Obesity: the worldwide epidemic. Clin Dermatol 2004;22:276–80.
2. Ehrmann DA. Polycystic ovary syndrome. N Engl J Med 2005;352:1223–36.
3. Gambineri A, Pelusi C, Vicennati V, et al. Obesity and the polycystic ovary syndrome. Int J Obes Relat Metab Disord 2002;26:883–96.
4. Ford ES. Prevalence of the metabolic syndrome in US population. Endocrinol Metab Clin North Am 2004;33:333–50.
5. Linné Y. Effects of obesity on women's reproduction and complications during pregnancy. Obes Rev 2004;5:137–43.
6. Pasquali R, Pelusi C, Genghini S, et al. Obesity and reproductive disorders in women. Hum Reprod Update 2003;9:359–72.
7. Reddy UM, Wapner RJ, Rebar RW, et al. Infertility, assisted reproductive technology, and adverse pregnancy outcomes: executive summary of a National Institute of Child Health and Human Development workshop. Obstet Gynecol 2007;109:967–77.
8. Jimenez Torres M, Campoy Folgoso C, Canabate Reche F, et al. Organochlorine pesticides in serum and adipose tissue of pregnant women in southern Spain giving birth by cesarean section. Sci Total Environ 2006;372:32–8.
9. Munoz-de-Toro M, Beldomenico HR, Garcia SR, et al. Organochlorine levels in adipose tissue of women from a littoral region of Argentina. Environ Res 2006; 102:107–12.
10. Nguyen R, Wilcox A, Skjaerven R, et al. Men's body mass index and infertility. Hum Reprod 2007;17:2488–93.
11. Magnusdottir EV, Thorsteinsson T, Thorsteinsdottir S, et al. Persistent organochlorines, sedentary occupation, obesity and human male subfertility. Hum Reprod 2005;20:208–15.
12. Hanafy S, Halawa FA, Mostafa T, et al. Serum leptin correlates in infertile oligozoospermic males. Andrologia 2007;39:177–80.
13. Zorn B, Osredkar J, Meden-Vrtovec H, et al. Leptin levels in infertile male patients is correlated with inhibin B, testosterone and SHBG but not with sperm characteristics. Int J Androl 2007;30:439–44.
14. Castilla JA, Alvarez C, Aguilar J, et al. Influence of analytical and biological variation on the clinical interpretation of seminal parameters. Hum Reprod 2006;21: 847–51.
15. Hammoud AO, Gibson M, Peterson CM, et al. Effect of sperm preparation techniques by density gradient on intra-individual variation of sperm motility. Arch Androl 2007;53:349–51.

16. Keel BA. Within- and between-subject variation in semen parameters in infertile men and normal semen donors. Fertil Steril 2006;85:128–34.
17. Azziz JR, Sanchez LA, Knochenhauer ES, et al. Androgen excess in women: experience with over 1000 consecutive patients. J Clin Endocrinol Metab 2004;89:453–62.
18. Bonde JP, Ernst E, Jensen TK, et al. Relation between semen quality and fertility: a population-based study of 430 first-pregnancy planners. Lancet 1998;352: 1172–7.
19. Slama R, Eustache F, Ducot B, et al. Time to pregnancy and semen parameters: a cross-sectional study among fertile couples from four European cities. Hum Reprod 2002;17:503–15.
20. Guzick DS, Overstreet JW, Factor-Litvak P, et al. Sperm morphology, motility, and concentration in fertile and infertile men. N Engl J Med 2001;345:1388–93.
21. Jensen TK, Andersson AM, Jorgensen N, et al. Body mass index in relation to semen quality and reproductive hormones among 1,558 Danish men. Fertil Steril 2004;82:863–70.
22. Fejes I, Koloszar S, Szollosi J, et al. Is semen quality affected by male body fat distribution? Andrologia 2005;37:155–9.
23. Kort HI, Massey JB, Elsner CW, et al. Impact of body mass index values on sperm quantity and quality. J Androl 2006;27:450–2.
24. Bacon CG, Mittleman MA, Kawachi I, et al. Sexual function in men older than 50 years of age: results from the health professionals follow-up study. Ann Intern Med 2003;139:161–8.
25. Sullivan ME, Thompson CS, Dashwood MR, et al. Nitric oxide and penile erection: is erectile dysfunction another manifestation of vascular disease? Cardiovasc Res 1999;43:658–65.
26. Mieusset R, Bujan LE, Massat G, et al. Inconstant ascending testis as a potential risk factor for spermatogenesis in infertile men with no history of cryptorchism. Hum Reprod 1997;12:974–9.
27. Shafik A, Olfat S. Lipectomy in the treatment of scrotal lipomatosis. Br J Urol 1981;53:55–61.
28. Giagulli VA, Kaufman JM, Vermeulen A. Pathogenesis of the decreased androgen levels in obese men. J Clin Endocrinol Metab 1994;79:997–1000.
29. Tchernof A, Despres JP, Belanger A, et al. Reduced testosterone and adrenal C19 steroid levels in obese men. Metabolism 1995;44:513–9.
30. Schneider G, Kirschner MA, Berkowitz R, et al. Increased estrogen production in obese men. J Clin Endocrinol Metab 1979;48:633–8.
31. Goyal HO, Robateau A, Braden TD, et al. Neonatal estrogen exposure of male rats alters reproductive functions at adulthood. Biol Reprod 2003;68: 2081–91.
32. Akingbemi BT. Estrogen regulation of testicular function. Reprod Biol Endocrinol 2005;3:51.
33. de Boer H, Verschoor L, Ruinemans-Koerts J, et al. Letrozole normalizes serum testosterone in severely obese men with hypogonadotropic hypogonadism. Diabetes Obes Metab 2005;7:211–5.
34. Pavlovich CP, King P, Goldstein M, et al. Evidence of a treatable endocrinopathy in infertile men. J Urol 2001;165:837–41.
35. Kumanov P, Nandipati K, Tomova A, et al. Inhibin B is a better marker of spermatogenesis than other hormones in the evaluation of male factor infertility. Fertil Steril 2006;86:332–8.

36. Winters SJ, Wang C, Abdelrahaman E, et al. Inhibin-B levels in healthy young adult men and prepubertal boys: is obesity the cause for the contemporary decline in sperm count because of fewer Sertoli cells? J Androl 2006;27:560–4.
37. Cortet-Rudelli C, Pigny P, Decanter C, et al. Obesity and serum luteinizing hormone level have an independent and opposite effect on the serum inhibin B level in patients with polycystic ovary syndrome. Fertil Steril 2002;77:281–7.
38. De Pergola G, Maldera S, Tartagni M, et al. Inhibitory effect of obesity on gonadotropin, estradiol, and inhibin B levels in fertile women. Obesity (Silver Spring) 2006;14:1954–60.
39. Stellato RK, Feldman HA, Hamdy O, et al. Testosterone, sex hormone-binding globulin, and the development of type 2 diabetes in middle-aged men: prospective results from the Massachusetts male aging study. Diabetes Care 2000;23:490–4.
40. Luboshitzky R, Lavie L, Shen-Orr Z, et al. Altered luteinizing hormone and testosterone secretion in middle-aged obese men with obstructive sleep apnea. Obes Res 2005;13:780–6.
41. Luboshitzky R, Zabari Z, Shen-Orr Z, et al. Disruption of the nocturnal testosterone rhythm by sleep fragmentation in normal men. J Clin Endocrinol Metab 2001;86:1134–9.
42. Blank DM, Clark RV, Heymsfield SB, et al. Endogenous opioids and hypogonadism in human obesity. Brain Res Bull 1994;34:571–4.
43. Farooqi IS, Wangensteen T, Collins S, et al. Clinical and molecular genetic spectrum of congenital deficiency of the leptin receptor. N Engl J Med 2007;356:237–47.
44. Galtier-Dereure F, Pujol P, Dewailly D, et al. Choice of stimulation in polycystic ovarian syndrome: the influence of obesity. Hum Reprod 1997;12(Suppl 1):88–96.
45. Lobo RA, Gysler M, March CM, et al. Clinical and laboratory predictors of clomiphene response. Fertil Steril 1982;37:168–74.
46. Azziz R. Reproductive endocrinologic alterations in female asymptomatic obesity. Fertil Steril 1989;52:703–25.
47. Abbott DH, Dumesic DA, Franks S. Developmental origin of polycystic ovary syndrome—a hypothesis. J Endocrinol 2002;174:1–5.
48. Eisner JR, Dumesic DA, Kemnitz JW, et al. Timing of prenatal androgen excess determines differential impairment in insulin secretion and action in adult female rhesus monkeys. J Clin Endocrinol Metab 2000;85:1206–10.
49. Rexrode KM, Carey VJ, Hennekens CH, et al. Abdominal adiposity and coronary heart disease in women. JAMA 1998;280:1843–8.
50. Poretsky L, Cataldo NA, Rosenwaks Z, et al. The insulin-related ovarian regulatory system in health and disease. Endocr Rev 1999;20:535–82.
51. Agarwal A, Gupta S, Sharma RK. Role of oxidative stress in female reproduction. Reprod Biol Endocrinol 2005;3:28–49.
52. Agarwal SK, Vogel K, Weitsman SR, et al. Leptin antagonizes the insulin-like growth factor-I augmentation of steroidogenesis in granulosa and theca cells of the human ovary. J Clin Endocrinol Metab 1999;84:1072–6.
53. Duggal PS, Van Der Hoek KH, Milner CR, et al. The in vivo and in vitro effects of exogenous leptin on ovulation in the rat. Endocrinology 2000;141:1971–6.
54. Gammon CM, Freeman M Jr, Xie W, et al. Regulation of gonadotropin-releasing hormone secretion by cannabinoids. Endocrinology 2005;146:4491–9.
55. Murphy LL, Steger RW, Smith MS, et al. Effects of D9-tetrahydrocannabinol,cannabinol and cannabidiol, alone and in combinations, on luteinizing hormone and

prolactin release and on hypothalamic neurotransmitters in the male rat. Neuroendocrinology 1990;52:316–21.
56. Murphy LL, Munoz RM, Adrian BA, et al. Function of cannabinoid receptors in the neuroendocrine regulation of hormone secretion. Neurobiol Dis 1998;5: 432–46.
57. Catalano PM. Management of obesity in pregnancy. Obstet Gynecol 2007;109: 419–33.
58. Yu CKH, Teoh TG, Robinson S. Obesity in pregnancy. BJOG 2006;113:1117–25.
59. Ramsay JE, Greer I, Sattar N. Obesity and reproduction. BMJ 2006;333: 1159–62.
60. Lashen H, Fear K, Sturdee DW. Obesity is associated with increased risk of first trimester and recurrent miscarriage: matched case–control study. Hum Reprod 2004;19:1644–6.
61. Fedorcsak P, Storeng R, Dale PO, et al. Obesity is a risk factor for early pregnancy loss after IVF or ICSI. Acta Obstet Gynecol Scand 2000;79:43–8.
62. Wang JX, Davies MJ, Norman RJ. Polycystic ovarian syndrome and the risk of spontaneous abortion following assisted reproductive technology treatment. Hum Reprod 2001;16:2606–9.
63. Heijnen EMEW, Eijkemans MJC, Hughes EG, et al. A meta-analysis of outcomes of conventional IVF in women with polycystic ovary syndrome. Hum Reprod Update 2006;12:13–21.
64. Craig LB, Ke RW, Kutteh WH. Increased prevalence of insulin resistance in women with a history of recurrent pregnancy loss. Fertil Steril 2002;78: 487–90.
65. Tian L, Shen H, Lu Q, et al. Insulin resistance increases the risk of spontaneous abortion after assisted reproduction technology treatment. J Clin Endocrinol Metab 2007;92:1430–3.
66. Cnattingius S, Bergstrom R, Lipworth L, et al. Prepregnancy weight and the risk of adverse pregnancy outcomes. N Engl J Med 1998;338:147–52.
67. Cedergren MI. Maternal morbid obesity and the risk of adverse pregnancy outcome. Obstet Gynecol 2004;103:219–24.
68. Watkins ML, Rasmussen SA, Honein MA, et al. Maternal obesity and risk for birth defects. Pediatrics 2003;111:1152–8.
69. Cedergren M, Kallen B. Maternal obesity and the risk for orofacial clefts in the offspring. Cleft Palate Craniofac J 2005;42:367–71.
70. Cedergren MI, Kallen BA. Maternal obesity and infant heart defects. Obes Res 2003;11:1065–71.
71. Callaway LK, Prins JB, Chang AM, et al. The prevalence and impact of overweight and obesity in an Australian obstetric population. Med J Aust 2006; 184:56–9.
72. Hendler I, Blackwell SC, Bujold E, et al. Suboptimal second-trimester ultrasonographic visualization of the fetal heart in obese women: should we repeat the examination? J Ultrasound Med 2005;24:1205–9.
73. Hendler I, Blackwell SC, Bujold E, et al. The impact of maternal obesity on midtrimester sonographic visualization of fetal cardiac and craniospinal structures. Int J Obes Relat Metab Disord 2004;28:1607–11.
74. Smith GCS, Shah I, Pell JP, et al. Maternal obesity in early pregnancy and risk of spontaneous and elective preterm deliveries: a retrospective cohort study. Am J Public Health 2007;97:157–62.
75. Dokras A, Baredziak L, Blaine J, et al. Obstetric outcomes after in vitro fertilization in obese and morbidly obese women. Obstet Gynecol 2006;108:61–9.

76. Kaukua J, Pekkarinen T, Sane T, et al. Sex hormones and sexual function in obese men losing weight. Obes Res 2003;11:689–94.
77. Bastounis EA, Karayiannakis AJ, Syrigos K, et al. Sex hormone changes in morbidly obese patients after vertical banded gastroplasty. Eur Surg Res 1998;30:43–7.
78. Despres J-P, Lemieux I, Prud'homme D. Treatment of obesity: need to focus on high risk abdominally obese patients. BMJ 2001;322:716–20.
79. Huber-Buchholz MM, Carey DGP, Norman RJ. Restoration of reproductive potential by lifestyle modification in obese polycystic ovary syndrome: role of insulin sensitivity and luteinizing hormone. J Clin Endocrinol Metab 1999;84:1470–4.
80. Moran LJ, Noakes M, Clifton PM, et al. Dietary composition in restoring reproductive and metabolic physiology in overweight women with polycystic ovary syndrome. J Clin Endocrinol Metab 2003;88:812–9.
81. Wadden TA, Berkowitz RI, Womble LG, et al. Randomized trial of lifestyle modification and pharmacotherapy for obesity. N Engl J Med 2005;353:2111–20.
82. Hoeger KM, Kochman L, Wixom N, et al. A randomized, 48-week, placebo controlled trial of intensive lifestyle modification and/or metformin therapy in overweight women with polycystic ovary syndrome: a pilot study. Fertil Steril 2004;82:421–9.
83. Tang T, Glanville J, Hayden CJ, et al. Combined lifestyle modification and metformin in obese patients with polycystic ovary syndrome. A randomized, placebo-controlled, double-blind multicentre study. Hum Reprod 2006;21:80–9.
84. Teitelman M, Grotegut CA, Williams NN, et al. The impact of bariatric surgery on menstrual patterns. Obes Surg 2006;16:1457–63.
85. Deitel M, Stone E, Kassam HA, et al. Gynecologic-obstetric changes after loss of massive excess weight following bariatric surgery. J Am Coll Nutr 1988;7:147–53.
86. Dixon JB, Dixon ME, O'Brien PE. Birth outcomes in obese women after laparoscopic adjustable gastric banding. Obstet Gynecol 2005;106:965–72.
87. Moll E, Bossuyt PMM, Korevaar JC, et al. Effect of clomifene citrate plus metformin and clomifene citrate plus placebo on induction of ovulation in women with newly diagnosed polycystic ovary syndrome: randomized double blind clinical trial. BMJ 2006;332:1485–90.
88. Al-Azemi M, Omu FE, Omu AE. The effect of obesity on the outcome of infertility management in women with polycystic ovary syndrome. Arch Gynecol Obstet 2004;270:205–10.
89. Legro RS, Myers ER, Barnhart HX, et al. The pregnancy in polycystic ovary syndrome study: baseline characteristics of the randomized cohort including racial effects. Fertil Steril 2006;86:914–33.
90. Beck JI, Boothroyd C, Proctor M, et al. Oral antioestrogens and medical adjuncts for subfertility associated with anovulation. Cochrane Database Syst Rev 2005;(1):CD002249.
91. Hammond MG, Halme JK, Talbert LM. Factors affecting the pregnancy rate in clomiphene citrate induction of ovulation. Obstet Gynecol 1983;62:196–202.
92. Imani B, Eijkemans MJC, te Velde ER, et al. Predictors of chances to conceive in ovulatory patients during clomiphene citrate induction of ovulation in normogonadotropic oligoamenorrheic infertility. J Clin Endocrinol Metab 1999;84:1617–22.
93. Legro RS. Pregnancy considerations in women with polycystic ovary syndrome. Clin Obstet Gynecol 2007;50:295–304.

94. Legro RS, Barnhart HX, Schlaff WD, et al. Clomiphene, metformin, or both for infertility in the polycystic ovary syndrome. N Engl J Med 2007;356:551–66.
95. Siebert TI, Kruger TF, Steyn DW, et al. Is the addition of metformin efficacious in the treatment of clomiphene citrate-resistant patients with polycystic ovary syndrome? A structured literature review. Fertil Steril 2006;86:1432–7.
96. Harborne LR, Sattar N, Norman JE, et al. Metformin and weight loss in obese women with polycystic ovary syndrome: comparison of doses. J Clin Endocrinol Metab 2005;90:4593–8.
97. Douchi T, Oki T, Yamasaki H, et al. Body fat patterning in polycystic ovary syndrome women as a predictor of the response to clomiphene. Acta Obstet Gynecol Scand 2004;83:838–41.
98. Mulders AGMGJ, Laven JSE, Eijkemans MJC, et al. Patient predictors for outcome of gonadotrophin ovulation induction in women with normogonadotrophic anovulatory infertility: a meta-analysis. Hum Reprod Update 2003;9:429–49.
99. Laven JS, Mulders AG, Visser JA, et al. Anti-Mullerian hormone serum concentrations in normoovulatory and anovulatory women of reproductive age. J Clin Endocrinol Metab 2004;89:318–23.
100. Balen AH, Platteau P, Andersen AN, et al. The influence of body weight on response to ovulation induction with gonadotrophins in 335 women with World Health Organization group II anovulatory infertility. BJOG 2006;113:1195–202.
101. Dechaud H, Anahory T, Reyftmann L, et al. Obesity does not adversely affect results in patients who are undergoing in vitro fertilization and embryo transfer. Eur J Obstet Gynecol Reprod Biol 2006;127:88–93.
102. Ku SY, Kim SD, Jee BC, et al. Clinical efficacy of body mass index as predictor of in vitro fertilization and embryo transfer outcomes. J Korean Med Sci 2006;21:300–3.
103. Fedorcsak P, Dale PO, Storeng R, et al. Impact of overweight and underweight on assisted reproduction treatment. Hum Reprod 2004;19:2523–8.
104. Thessaloniki ESHRE/ASRM-Sponsored PCOS Consensus Workshop Group. Consensus on infertility treatment related to polycystic ovary syndrome. Fertil Steril 2008;89(3):505–22.

Obesity and Sexuality in Women

Mitul B. Shah, MD

KEYWORDS

• Obesity • Sexuality • Sexual health • Women
• Female sexual dysfunction • Reproductive health

There has been an alarming progressive worldwide increase in the prevalence of obesity according to many surveys dating back to the 1980s. Approximately 30% of the adult population in the United States is classified as obese.[1] The International Obesity Task Force estimates that at present 1.1 billion adults are overweight; of these, 312 million are obese.[2] Obesity also has been linked with a large number of general health diseases (ie, diabetes, hypertension, cardiovascular disease, osteoarthritis, certain malignancies, abnormal pulmonary functions, hyperlipidemia), mental health difficulties (depression and anxiety), and poor sexual health.

General health was defined by the World Health Organization in 1946 as "a state of complete physical, mental, and social well-being and not merely the absence of disease or infirmity."[3]

Mental health also has been defined, most recently in the 1999 report of the Surgeon General of the United States, as "a state of successful performance of mental function, resulting in productive activities, fulfilling relationships with other people, and the ability to adapt to change and to cope with adversity. Mental health is indispensable to personal well being, family and interpersonal relationships and contribution to community or society."[3]

There have been many definitions of sexual health during the past 30 years. Some, like the definitions quoted previously, have been from the World Health Organization and some from the Surgeon General. The 2001 definition from the Surgeon General is particularly relevant here:

> *Sexual health is inextricably bound to both physical and mental health. Just as physical and mental health can contribute to sexual dysfunction and diseases, those dysfunctions and diseases can contribute to physical and mental health problems. Sexual health is not limited to the absence of disease or dysfunction, nor is its importance confined to the reproductive years. It includes the ability to understand and weigh the risks, responsibilities, outcomes and impacts of sexual actions and to practice abstinence when appropriate. It includes the freedom from sexual abuse and discrimination and the ability to integrate their sexuality into their lives, derive pleasure from it, and reproduce if they so choose.*[3]

Department of Obstetrics and Gynecology and Women's Health, Saint Louis University, 6420 Clayton Road, Suite 290, Saint Louis, Missouri, USA
E-mail address: mshah11@slu.edu

Obstet Gynecol Clin N Am 36 (2009) 347–360
doi:10.1016/j.ogc.2009.04.004 **obgyn.theclinics.com**
0889-8545/09/$ – see front matter

Sexual health is an important and integral part of a person's life. It is intimately entwined with an individual's general health and mental health. In addition to the general and mental health components, sexual health specifically includes many facets. Two main categories are sexual functioning and reproductive health, as outlined in **Box 1**. This article details the potential impact of obesity on the components of sexual health highlighted in **Box 1**.

Sexual dysfunction is a prevalent condition and is an important public health concern. Laumann and colleagues[4] surveyed 1749 women and 1410 men between the ages of 18 and 59 years and identified some form of sexual dysfunction in 43% of women and in 31% of men. With the introduction of sildenafil, there has been a major focus on male sexual dysfunction (ie, erectile dysfunction) during the last 10 years. Female sexual dysfunction (FSD), however, has been found to be more prevalent, more difficult to define, and more complex to treat.

To understand the categories of FSD, one first must understand the female sexual response cycle. The original concept of the human sexual response cycle was based on the work of Masters and Johnson[5] who observed 100 white middle-class couples and described a linear model of sexual function for both men and women. The four phases of human sexual response in this model—desire, arousal/excitement leading to plateau, orgasm, and resolution—are shown in **Fig. 1**.

This model reflects the male sexual response cycle more accurately than the female sexual response cycle. The female sexual response has overlapping phases rather than a linear progression and is highly dependent on psychological and social factors such as partner intimacy, emotional well-being, and family life.

Specifically, a woman's sexual desire need not precede arousal, nor does a woman necessarily have to have spontaneous innate desire. She only requires the willingness to be receptive, which can be motivated by many reasons. These motivations can include the wish to increase intimacy with her partner, to increase her own sense of well-being (feeling attractive, appreciated, loved, desired), or to please her partner. Some women may experience spontaneous desire, and it is predictably increased in a new relationship.

Box 1
Components of sexual health

1. Sexual functioning
   - Female sexual dysfunction
   - Physical impairment
   - Self-acceptance, self-esteem, and body image
   - Maintenance of interpersonal relationships
2. Reproductive health
   - Family planning
   - Childbearing
     - Pregnancy
     - Infertility
   - Menopause

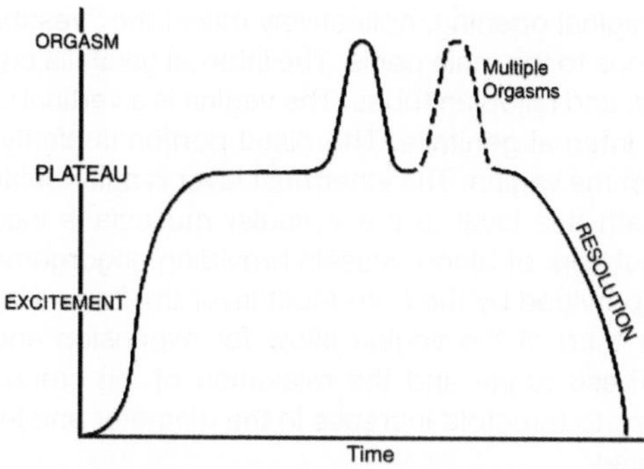

Fig. 1. Sexual response cycle defined by Masters and Johnson. (*From* Masters WH, Johnson VE. Human sexual response. Boston: Little Brown & Company; 1966. Obstet Gynecol Clin North Am 2008;35:170; with permission.)

If a women is willing to be receptive or possesses spontaneous innate desire, she will be able to respond to the appropriate sexual stimuli. In addition, there must be sufficient time available without distraction so she can remain focused; then sexual excitement and arousal can intensify to plateau and lead to orgasm and resolution.[6] As exemplified in the circular diagram created by Basson, with positive reinforcements the circular female sexual response cycle will be successful (**Fig. 2**).

It also is important to understand the anatomy of female sexual function.[7] The female genitalia are differentiated into external and internal structures. Each organ plays an important role in the female sexual response cycle. The outermost genital structure is the vulva, composed of the labia majora and labia minora. The labia majora cover and protect the labia minora. The labia minora cover and protect the clitoris,

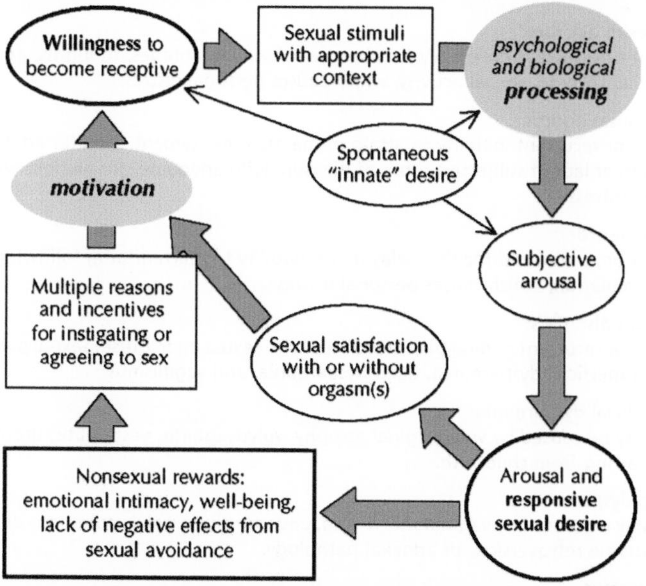

Fig. 2. Female sexual response cycle by Basson showing responsive desire as well as innate spontaneous desire. (*From* Basson R. Women's sexual dysfunction: revised and expanded definitions. Can Med Assoc J 2005;172:1328; with permission.)

urethral orifice, and vaginal opening, collectively called the "vestibule." The clitoris is erectile tissue analogous to the male penis. The internal genitalia consist of the vagina, cervix, uterus, ovaries, and fallopian tubes. The vagina is a vertical cylinder connecting the external with the internal genitalia. The distal portion is highly innervated. Three layers form the walls of the vagina. The innermost layer is aglandular epithelial mucous membrane. Underneath this layer is the vascular muscularis incorporating smooth muscle and a large network of blood vessels providing engorgement during arousal. Structural support is provided by the outermost layer the fibrosa layer. Multiple rugae throughout the lower third of the vagina allow for expansion and frictional tension during intercourse. These rugae and the relaxation of the smooth muscle layer of the vagina allow a two- to threefold increase in the diameter and length of the vaginal canal during intercourse.

With the understanding of female sexual response and the anatomy of female sexual function, one can examine FSD.

Female sexual difficulties are defined as dysfunctions if they are persistent, pervasive, and cause personal distress. FSD is divided into four categories: as described in **Box 2**.[8]

The effect of obesity on female sexual function remains unclear. A number of studies have explored the relationship between obesity and FSD. Specifically, Esposito and colleagues[9] studied 108 otherwise healthy women and administered the Female Sexual Function Index (FSFI) questionnaire and calculated the women's body mass index (BMI). The FSFI is a brief, validated 19-item questionnaire used to collect information on the four categories of sexual dysfunction.[10] This instrument has been

Box 2
Definitions of female sexual dysfunction

1. Sexual desire disorder:
   Persistent or recurrent deficiency (or absence) of sexual fantasies, thoughts, and/or desire for, or receptivity to, sexual activity, which causes personal distress.
2. Sexual arousal disorder:
   Persistent or recurrent inability to attain or maintain excitement, manifested by lack of lubrication or lack of subjective sense of pleasure with adequate stimulation, which causes personal distress.
3. Orgasmic disorder:
   Persistent or recurrent difficulty, delay in, or inability to reach orgasm following sufficient sexual stimulation, which causes personal distress.
4. Sexual pain disorders:
   Persistent or recurrent genital pain associated with sexual intercourse. Sexual pain disorders include: superficial dyspareunia, deep dyspareunia, and vaginismus.

   Superficial dyspareunia:
   May be caused by vulvovaginal atrophy, vulvovaginitis, vestibulitis, urethritis, or scarring from childbirth.

   Deep dyspareunia:
   May be caused by vaginal shortening, endometriosis, pelvic adhesions or relaxation, uterine retroversion, or adnexal pathology.

   Vaginismus:
   Is recurrent or persistent involuntary muscle spasm of the outer third of the vagina that interferes with vaginal penetration.

standardized, is easy to administer and score, and provides normal values for the general population. A value of 23 or less indicates overall FSD. The questionnaire is divided into six domains, and a lower score in any one of these domains further categorizes FSD into one of the four dysfunctions defined previously. Esposito found 52 women who had FSD (defined as an FSFI score less than 23) and 66 matched controls (defined as a FSFI score greater than 23). In women who had FSD, a strong inverse correlation was found between the patient's BMI and FSFI score ($P = .0001$) (**Fig. 3**).

Specifically, the higher the BMI, the lower the FSFI score. Therefore, the more obese a woman is, the greater is the likelihood that she will have a form of FSD. Correlations also were made between the six domains of the FSFI (desire, arousal, lubrication, orgasm, satisfaction, and pain) and BMI. Again there were strong inverse correlations with BMI and arousal ($P < .001$), lubrication ($P < .001$), orgasm ($P < .001$), and satisfaction ($P < .001$), but no significant correlation was found between BMI and desire ($P = .08$) or pain ($P = .3$). Of note, in the control group (ie, the women who did not have FSD) no correlation was found between BMI and FSFI ($P = .09$).

Esposito and colleagues[11] also investigated the association of metabolic syndrome and FSD, using the FSFI as previously. The metabolic syndrome was defined as abdominal adiposity, low serum high-density lipoprotein, hypertriglyceridemia, elevated blood pressure, and abnormal glucose homeostasis. The FSFI questionnaire was administered to 120 women who had metabolic syndrome and 80 matched controls. Compared with the control group, the women who had metabolic syndrome had overall lower FSFI scores (23.2 ± 5.4 versus 30.1 ± 4.7; $P < .001$) and lower scores on the six individual domains, all of which except desire were statistically significant ($P < .01$) (**Fig. 4**).

Much research has been done in the bariatric surgery field in examining FSD in patients preoperatively and re-examining them postoperatively with the hypothesis that FSD would improve in the postoperative period. These surgical procedures include Roux-en-Y gastric bypass and laparoscopic adjustable gastric banding.

It is well known that morbidly obese patients experience poor body image and low self-esteem. Because sexuality is intimately linked with these traits, it is no surprise that morbidly obese patients report impaired sexual quality of life. The advent of bariatric surgery as a viable treatment option for these patients has provided an

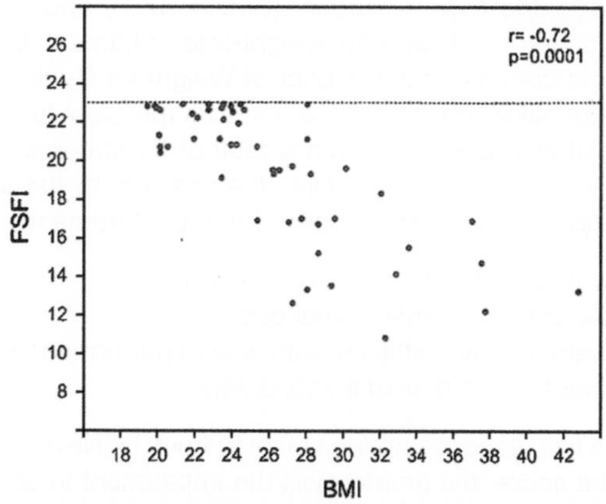

Fig. 3. Inverse correlation between BMI and FSFI in a population of women who have FSD. The horizontal line indicates the cutoff of 23 below which a diagnosis of FSD is currently made. (*From* Esposito K, Ciotola M, Giugliono F, et al. Association of body weight with sexual function in women. Int J Impot Res 2007;19:355; with permission.)

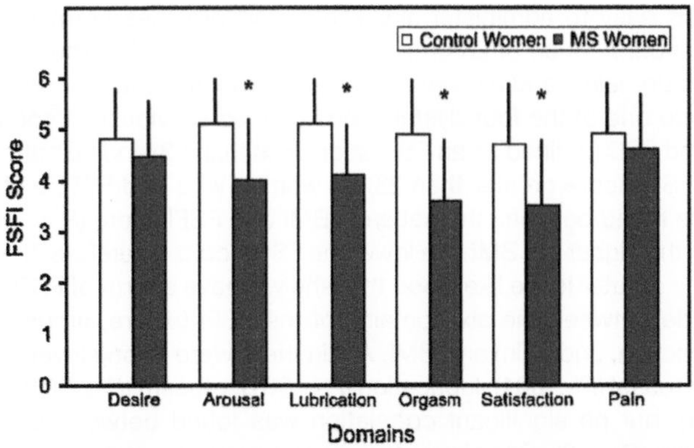

Fig. 4. Comparison of FSD individual domains of the FSFI scores in women with metabolic syndrome and matched controls. *, statistically significant ($P < .01$). (*From* Esposito K, Ciotola M, Marfella R, et al. The metabolic syndrome: a cause of sexual dysfunction in women. Int J Impot Res 2005;17:225; with permission.)

opportunity to assess sexual quality of life before and after surgery. Camps and colleagues[12] surveyed 94 patients and their partners. The questionnaires addressed body image and frequency of intercourse. There was an improvement postoperatively in the patients' body image, in their partners' assessment of the patients' attractiveness, and in frequency of intercourse (**Fig. 5**A, B).

One may theorize that obesity may pose a physical barrier to intercourse. If a woman is physically unable to perform intercourse, of course FSD is likely to follow. Camps and colleagues[12] also addressed sexual difficulties (ie, physical difficulty in engaging in sexual intercourse secondary to abdominal girth or poor physical condition) in their questionnaires. These investigators found that after bariatric surgery the difficultly engaging in intercourse lessens as a result of the postoperative decrease in abdominal girth.

Kolotkin and colleagues[13] also studied the effect of obesity on sexual quality of life in a large number of obese patients. Five hundred participants (277 women and 223 men) in a weight-loss program (BMI = 41.3), 372 patients (312 women and 60 men) being evaluated for gastric bypass surgery (BMI = 47.1), and 286 obese controls (211 women and 75 men) not seeking weight-loss treatment (BMI = 43.6) were surveyed. Participants completed the Impact of Weight on Quality of Life-Lite questionnaire. The questionnaire consists of five domains (physical function, self-esteem, sexual life, public distress, and work) with a total of 31 statements that begin with the phrase "Because of my weight ..." Only the answers to the sexual life domain were used in this study. This domain consisted of four statements:

1. Because of my weight I do not enjoy sexual activity.
2. Because of my weight I have little sexual desire.
3. Because of my weight I have difficulty with sexual performance.
4. Because of my weight I avoid sexual encounters.

Each question has five response options ranging from 1 ("Never true") to 5 ("Always true"). The higher the score, the greater was the impairment in sexual quality of life. The results indicate that higher BMI is associated with greater impairments in sexual quality of life (**Table 1**) and that sexual quality of life is more impaired in obese women than in obese men (**Table 2**). Furthermore, gastric bypass candidates reported more impairment than other obese individuals.

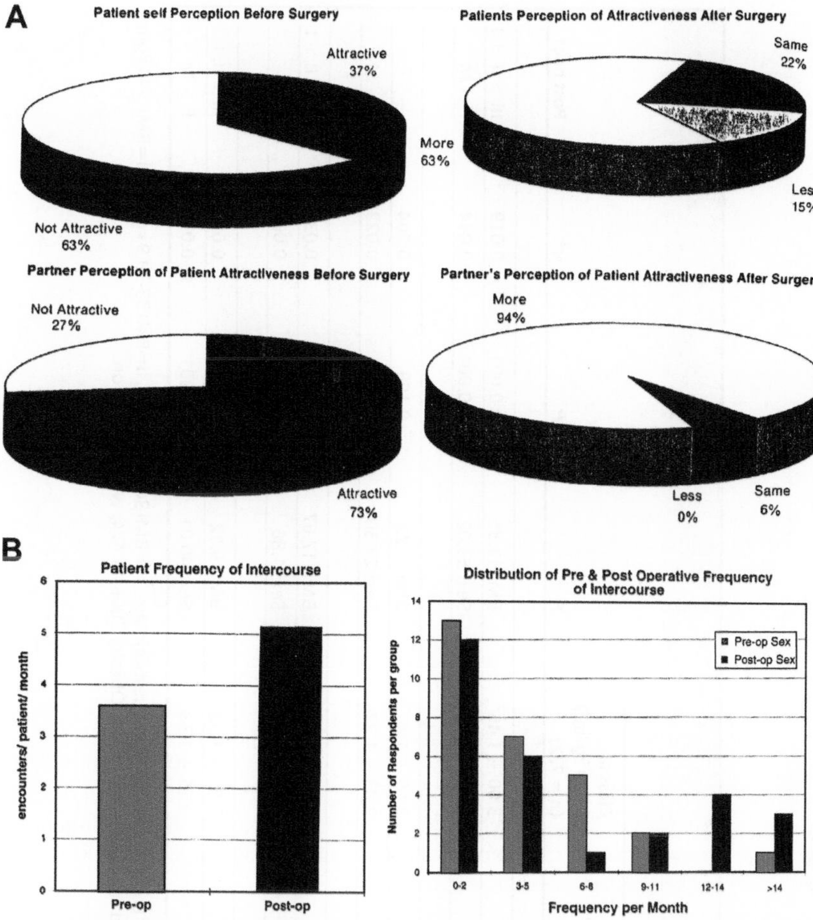

Fig. 5. (*A*) Patient's body image and partner's assessment of patient's attractiveness improved following bariatric surgery. (*B*) Frequency of intercourse before and after bariatric surgery. (*From* Camps M, Zervos E, Goode S, et al. Impact of bariatric surgery on body image perception and sexuality in morbidly obese patients and their partners. Obes Surg 1996;6:358; with permission.)

Dziurowicz-Kozlowska and colleagues[14] evaluated health-related quality of life after bariatric surgery in 61 patients who had undergone either gastric bypass or laparoscopic gastric banding in the last 3 to 6 months. Group I (n = 33; BMI 49.90) was tested before the operation. Group II (n = 17; BMI 34.26) was tested 6 months after the operation. They were administered the Nottingham Health Profile developed in Europe. It has 38 short questions related to six dimensions of health-related quality of life: energy, pain, emotional reactions, sleep, social isolation, and physical immobility. The second part of the instrument is related to seven spheres of life: paid employment, ability to perform jobs around the house, social life, home life, sex life, interests and hobbies, and holidays. Results indicated improvement in energy ($P < .0001$), pain ($P < .001$), and physical mobility ($P < .0001$) following bariatric surgery. Improvements also were noted in paid employment ($P < .05$), ability to perform jobs around the house (domestic work) ($P < .001$), social life ($P < .05$), sex life ($P < .05$), and holidays ($P < .01$) (**Table 3**).

Table 1
Sexual quality of life based on BMI category[a]

	BMI Category*						
	Class I (30–34.9 kg/m^2) (n = 159)	Class II (35–39.9 kg/m^2) (n = 277)	Class III (> 40 kg/m^2) (n = 722)	F	P	η^2	Post hoc*
Do not enjoy sexual activity							
Women	2.34 ± 1.36	2.59 ± 1.33	3.00 ± 1.46	BMI 11.35	< 0.001	0.019	III > II > 1
Men	1.68 ± 1.02	1.93 ± 1.14	2.11 ± 1.36	Sex: 53.02	< 0.001	0.044	F > M
Have little sexual desire							
Women	2.89 ± 1.32	2.72 ± 1.31	3.09 ± 1.41	BMI: 2.22	0.109	0.004	—
Men	2.29 ± 1.22	2.41 ± 1.23	2.43 ± 1.27	Sex: 27.50	<0.001	0.023	F > M
Difficulty with sexual performance							
Women	2.31 ± 1.37	2.55 ± 1.36	3.08 ± 1.41	BMI: 17.67	<0.001	0.030	III > II > I
Men	2.17 ± 1.05	2.58 ± 1.25	2.78 ± 1.40	Sex: 1.86	0.173	0.002	—
Avoid sexual encounters							
Women	2.67 ± 1.46	2.72 ± 1.43	3.02 ± 1.52	BMI: 6.12	0.002	0.011	III > II, I
Men	1.8 ± 0.98	2.15 ± 1.12	2.35 ± 1.38	Sex: 40.01	<0.001	0.034	F > M

[a] Assessed using the IWQol-Lite Impact of Weight on Quality of Life-Lite (IWQol-Lite) questionnaire. * I=BMI 30-34.9 kg/m^2, II=BMI 35-39.9 kg/m^2, III=BMI >40 kg/m^2.
Data from Kolotkin R, Binks M, Crosby R, et al. Obesity and sexual quality of life. Obesity 2006;14:474; with permission.

Table 2
Sexual quality of life in women versus men[a]

	Group	Never/ Rarely True (%)	Sometimes True (%)	Usually/Always True (%)
Do not enjoy sexual activity				
Women	Combined	43.4	23.9	32.8
	Residential program	63.9	19.1	17.0
	Gastric bypass	20.8	27.9	51.3
	Obese controls	49.8	24.2	26.1
Men	Combined	71.2	14.2	14.5
	Residential program	80.7	9.4	9.9
	Gastric bypass	35.0	26.7	38.3
	Obese controls	72.0	18.7	9.3
Have little sexual desire				
Women	Combined	38.8	23.6	37.6
	Residential program	45.5	23.8	30.7
	Gastric bypass	22.4	25.6	51.9
	Obese controls	54.0	20.4	25.6
Men	Combined	56.1	19.8	24.0
	Residential program	54.3	22.0	23.8
	Gastric bypass	38.3	21.7	40.0
	Obese controls	76.0	12.0	12.0
Difficulty with sexual performance				
Women	Combined	43.5	22.0	34.5
	Residential program	61.4	18.1	20.6
	Gastric bypass	20.8	24.0	55.1
	Obese controls	53.6	24.2	22.3
Men	Combined	50.6	22.3	27.1
	Residential program	53.4	22.0	24.7
	Gastric bypass	26.7	21.7	51.7
	Obese controls	61.3	24.0	14.7
Avoid sexual encounters				
Women	Combined	45.3	17.6	37.1
	Residential program	49.5	18.1	32.5
	Gastric bypass	32.7	17.0	50.3
	Obese controls	58.3	18.0	23.7
Men	Combined	64.5	17.3	18.2
	Residential program	63.7	17.9	18.4
	Gastric bypass	45.0	25.0	30.0
	Obese controls	82.7	9.3	8.0

[a] Assessed using the IWQol-Lite Impact of Weight on Quality of Life-Lite (IWQol-Lite) questionnaire.

Data from Kolotkin R, Binks M, Crosby R, et al. Obesity and sexual quality of life. Obesity 2006;14:475; with permission.

Obesity also causes serious psychological difficulties. Specifically, obese patients tend to have a negative body image, low self-esteem and self-acceptance, and difficulty with interpersonal relationships. Two studies described earlier elicited these factors in their results. In the study by Camps and colleagues,[12] patients noted they had an improvement in body image, felt more attractive, and were less likely to undress in darkness in front of their partners after bariatric surgery. In the study by Dziurowicz and colleatgues,[14] participants reported an improvement in paid

Table 3
Improvement in health-related quality of life after bariatric surgery

Main Nottingham Health Profile Dimensions	Group I (n = 33) Mean ± SD		Group II (n = 17) Mean ± SD		Test t^a	Test *P*
Energy	70.71 ± 38.87		17.65 ± 31.44		4.94	.0000
Pain	39.39 ± 33.67		5.88 ± 12.59		3.90	.0003
Emotional reactions	37.37 ± 30.78		26.80 ± 28.34		1.18	.2434
Sleep	30.30 ± 34.68		32.94 ± 32.36		0.26	.7956
Social isolation	24.85 ± 24.51		14.12 ± 25.26		1.45	.1532
Physical mobility	43.18 ± 21.44		14.17 ± 14.81		4.94	.0000
Does your current health state cause problems in such spheres as	**Group I (n = 33)**		**Group II (n = 17)**		**Chi-Square**	
	Yes n (%)	**No n (%)**	**Yes n (%)**	**No n (%)**	χ^{2b}	***P***
Paid employment	18 (54.54)	15 (45.45)	3 (17.65)	14 (2.35)	6.27	.0123
Jobs around the house	21 (63.64)	12 (36.36)	2 (11.76)	15 (8.24)	12.15	.0005
Social life	18 (54.54)	15 (45.45)	4 (23.53)	13 (76.47)	4.38	.0364
Home life	10 (30.30)	23 (69.70)	3 (17.65)	14 (82.35)	0.93	.3338
Sex life	22 (66.67)	11 (69.70)	5 (29.41)	12 (70.59)	6.27	.0123
Interests and hobbies	13 (66.67)	20 (60.61)	3 (17.65)	14 (82.35)	2.44	.1184
Holidays	20 (60.61)	13 (39.39)	2 (39.39)	15 (88.24)	10.86	.0010

[a] t_{crit} (48) = 2.01 ($P < .05$).
[b] χ^2_{crit} (1) = 3.84 ($P < .05$).

Data from Dziurowicz-Kozlowska A, Lisik W, Wierzbick M, et al. Health related quality of life after the surgical treatment of obesity. J Physiol Pharmacol 2005;56 (Supp 6):130–1; with permission.

employment, social life, sex life, and holidays after bariatric surgery, indicating an improvement in interpersonal relationships as well.

Female sexual health is improved and psychological difficulties (body image, self-esteem, and interpersonal relationships) are strengthened following bariatric surgery. It also was pointed out that physical impairment does play a role in obesity and sexuality. Specifically, a decrease in obesity improves sexual health and decreases physical impairment.

These studies have highlighted an association between obesity and FSD. In particular, obesity seems to be risk factor for women to develop sexual dysfunction. When treatment options (ie, diet and exercise, medications, or bariatric surgery) are being considered, it is important to include an assessment of sexual health in the overall care of the obese patient.

The first step in this endeavor is to ask a question that could elicit a sexual health complaint. In taking a sexual health history, there are many ways to ask a question, phrased either directly or more generally. For example, one could ask, "Do you have problems with sex?" or "Many women who are struggling with their weight also have sexual problems, how about you?" In a study by Sadovsky and colleagues,[15] the more general style (second question above) had a higher response rate, especially with older women. Once a complaint is elicited, the FSFI questionnaire may be administered to identify the problem and also may be used to monitor progress if multiple dysfunctions are found.

It is also imperative to have the patient fully clothed and to avoid being judgmental. Once identified, FSD usually is best treated by a team approach. Particularly in an obese patient, the focus should be on achieving weight loss, which thereby might improve FSD. The team usually consists of the physician, nutritionist, exercise physiologist, psychologist, and physical therapist. An individualized program of diet and exercise with clear-cut goals should be developed for each patient with the help of a nutritionist and exercise physiologist. In addition to the physician's screening for other medical disorders, referrals may also be necessary for psychotherapy for improvement in body image and self-esteem. Last, physical therapy referrals may be appropriate specifically to strengthen pelvic floor muscles to improve sexual function.

The second important facet of sexual health that may be affected by obesity is reproductive health: family planning, childbearing, and menopause.

The presence of comorbid risk factors can limit the contraceptive options for obese women. Obese women are at risk for developing diabetes mellitus, hypertension, heart attacks, strokes, and deep vein thrombosis or pulmonary embolism. These medical disorders may preclude the use of using estrogen-containing contraceptives as a method of family planning. Therefore, obese women are candidates for contraceptives containing only progestin (injectable progestin i.e. depot medroxyprogesterone acetate, progestin only pill, progestin implant, or levonorgestrel intrauterine system) or non-hormonal methods (copper implantable uterine device, condoms, sponge, or diaphragm).

Even after controlling for comorbid risk factors, contraception for obese patients poses a challenge. It is imperative to discuss family planning in the context of pregnancies potentially complicated by comorbidities. The effectiveness of different methods of contraception in obese patients has been studied. Oral contraceptive pills, particularly combination oral contraceptive pills (COCs) have been found to have decreased effectiveness in obese women because of increased metabolism in the periphery by adipocytes.[16–19] Like COCs, the progestin-only pill has been found to have decreased efficacy.[17] Obesity is not an absolute contraindication to the use of COCs or the progestin-only pill, because they are more effective than barrier contraception alone. On the other hand, obese patients have an even higher incidence (a two- to fivefold increased risk) of venous thromboembolism than their lean counterparts taking COCs. Because of this elevated risk, COCs are contraindicated in patients who have a BMI greater than 35.[18] The contraceptive patch and progestin implant have been found to be less effective because of decreased absorption.[16,17] The injectable progestin (depot medroxyprogesterone acetate, DMPA) and vaginal ring have been found to be effective.[17,19] The vaginal ring, as a combined hormonal contraceptive, does carry a higher risk of venous thromboembolism, but the risk is lower than with COCs because there is less systemic absorption. The copper implantable uterine device and levonorgestrel intrauterine system have been found to very effective, with minimal effects of weight gain, and are the primary choices for these patients.[16–18] When considering permanent sterilization, these patients are at particularly high risk for surgical complications from laparoscopic procedures.[16,18] They are excellent candidates for hysteroscopic selective tubal occlusion with microinserts as an alternative to permanent sterilization, with comparable results.[18]

Obese patients are high risk when seeking pregnancy. They are at risk for many complications of pregnancy, including but not limited to miscarriage and stillbirth. These pregnancy-related topics are discussed in detail elsewhere in this issue. In addition, the obese patient is highly likely to be infertile. Obese women are at increased risk for infertility because of comorbid risk factors such as diabetes, hypertension, and polycystic ovarian syndrome. Even after controlling for these comorbidities, obese patients remain at higher risk for infertility, mainly because of anovulation.

The cause of anovulation in the obese patient is complex and involves alteration of hormones and proteins. Specifically, peripheral estrogen is increased by the conversion of estrone in the adipocytes, leading to an increased negative feedback on gonadotropin secretion.[20] Increased levels of insulin lead to increased androgen levels.[20] Last, obese patients have elevated levels of leptin, a protein that interferes with follicular development in the ovaries.[20] All these alterations result in anovulation leading to infertility. It has been shown that minimal weight loss can improve reproductive function significantly.[21] Treatment of obesity via a weight-loss program, diet, and exercise will improve menstrual function by minimizing the occurrence of anovulatory cycles and thus increasing the likelihood of spontaneous pregnancy. In fact, for obese patients who have BMI greater than 35, weight loss is the first line of intervention for ovulation induction, before pharmacologic induction agents.[22]

Hormone replacement therapy (ie, estrogen) often is contraindicated in postmenopausal obese women because of the previously mentioned comorbid risk factors. They may be offered alternative interventions such as herbal therapy, selective serotonin reuptake inhibitors, or conservative management only. In addition, BMI is known to increase in midlife (at 50–59 years). The cause of this increase is the decrease in metabolic rate (2% per decade), increased central obesity, and decreased physical activity. Body weight is unaffected by menopause itself. Therefore, women who were not classified as obese at a younger age may become obese in the postmenopausal years, and treatment will be required not only for menopausal syndrome but for obesity as well.

Counseling about reproductive health is imperative, as highlighted earlier. The obese patient must be urged to address family planning despite the reduced number of options for contraception, because unintended pregnancy carries high risks for both the woman and the baby. Weight loss should be the main treatment option during preconceptional counseling in the obese patient. The obese patient also is likely to be infertile because of to anovulation; again, weight loss should be the main treatment option to achieve spontaneous pregnancy. The management of menopausal syndrome in the obese patient is significantly limited, but there are some alternatives to traditional therapy, as outlined earlier.

In conclusion, sexual health is an important part of an individual's overall health. This article has presented the definitions and classifications of FSD. It has emphasized the importance of obtaining a sexual health assessment and has described the tools that can be used for this assessment. The relationship between obesity and FSD has been demonstrated in the literature. One may theorize that there is an increased prevalence of FSD in obese patients, but confirmation with further studies is needed. Because of the recently modified understanding of the female sexual response cycle, additional studies also need to explore whether obesity has an impact on the circular female sexual response cycle. The major impact of obesity on reproductive health over a women's entire life span (family-planning years, reproductive years, and menopause years) also has been described. Therefore, the treatment of obesity as a major health concern will have a positive effect on women's sexual health, with an improvement in FSD and a decrease in risk factors related to contraception, pregnancy, infertility, and menopause.

REFERENCES

1. Assimakopoulos K, Panayiotopoulos S, Iconomou G, et al. Assessing sexual function in obese women preparing for bariatric surgery. Obes Surg 2006;16: 1087–91.
2. Esposito K, Giugliano F, Ciotola M, et al. Obesity and sexual dysfunction, male and female. Int J Impot Res 2008;20:358–65.
3. Edwards W, Coleman E. Defining sexual health: a descriptive overview. Arch Sex Behav 2004;33:189–95.
4. Laumann EO, Paik A, Rosen RC. Sexual dysfunction in the United States: prevalence and predictors. JAMA 1999;281:537–44.
5. Kammerer-Doak D, Rogers R. Female sexual function and dysfunction. Obstet Gynecol Clin North Am 2008;35:169–83.
6. Basson R. Women's sexual dysfunction: revised and expanded definitions. Can Med Assoc J 2005;172:1327–33.
7. Miller H, Hunt J. Female sexual dysfunction: review of the disorder and evidence for available treatment alternatives. J Pharm Pract 2003;16:200–6.
8. Basson R, Berman J, Burnett A, et al. Report of the international consensus development conference on female sexual dysfunction: definitions and classifications. J Urol 2000;163:888–93.
9. Esposito K, Ciotola M, Giugliono F, et al. Association of body weight with sexual function in women. Int J Impot Res 2007;19:353–7.
10. Rosen R, Brown C, Heiman J, et al. The Female Sexual Function Index (FSFI): a multidimensional self report instrument for the assessment of female sexual function. J Sex Marital Ther 2000;26:191–208.
11. Esposito K, Ciotola M, Marfella R, et al. The metabolic syndrome: a cause of sexual dysfunction in women. Int J Impot Res 2005;17:224–6.
12. Camps M, Zervos E, Goode S, et al. Impact of bariatric surgery on body image perception and sexuality in morbidly obese patients and their partners. Obes Surg 1996;6:356–60.
13. Kolotkin R, Binks M, Crosby R, et al. Obesity and sexual quality of life. Obesity 2006;14:472–9.

14. Dziurowicz-Kozlowska A, Lisik W, Wierzbick M, et al. Health related quality of life after the surgical treatment of obesity. J Physiol Pharmacol 2005;56 (Supp 6): 127–34.
15. Sadovsky R, Alam W, et al. Sexual problems among a specific population of minority women aged 40–80 years attending a primary care practice. J Sex Med 2006;3(5):795–803.
16. Grimes D, Shields W. Family planning for obese women: challenges and opportunities. Contraception 2004;72:1–4.
17. Teal S, Ginosar D. Contraception for women with chronic medical conditions. Obstet Gynecol Clin North Am 2007;34:113–26.
18. Mansour D. Implications of the growing obesity epidemic on contraception and reproductive health. J Fam Plann Reprod Health Care 2004;30(4):209–11.
19. Gordon L, Thakur N, Atlas M, et al. Clinical inquiries. What hormonal contraception is most effective for obese women? J Fam Pract 2007;56(6):471–3.
20. Metwally M, Li T, Ledger W, et al. The impact of obesity on female reproductive function. Obes Rev 2007;8:515–23.
21. Clark A, Thornley B, Tomlinson L, et al. Weight loss in obese infertile women results in improvement in reproductive outcome for all forms of fertility treatment. Hum Reprod 1998;13(6):1502–6.
22. Nelson SM, Fleming R. The preconceptional paradigm: obesity and infertility. Hum Reprod 2007;22(4):912–5.

Maternal and Child Obesity: The Causal Link

Emily Oken, MD, MPH

KEYWORDS

• Child • Obesity • Pregnancy • Weight gain • Maternal

As the prevalence of obesity has increased over the past few decades in the United States among adults and pregnant women, so has the proportion of children who are obese.[1] Children who are obese tend to become overweight adults,[2,3] and once present, obesity is notoriously difficult to treat. Longitudinal data indicate that rising obesity trends are apparent even among young infants (**Fig. 1**),[4] suggesting that influences occurring very early in life are contributing to the rise in childhood obesity.

The field of the Developmental Origins of Health and Disease posits that influences that occur during sensitive periods of development, such as the prenatal period, can have lifelong effects on health.[5] Before birth, the development of organs and systems is both profuse and plastic, and thus susceptible to perturbation. Numerous animal experiments dating back decades show that experiences during early life such as energy deficiency or excess, deficiencies of specific nutrients, or toxicant exposures can have long-lasting, sometimes irreversible, effects on offspring obesity and associated cardio-metabolic markers.[6] Evidence suggests that similar experiences also influence weight regulation and chronic disease risk among humans.

This article summarizes animal and human evidence linking maternal weight, weight gain during pregnancy, and related prenatal experiences with offspring obesity. Some possible pathways by which maternal weight status may influence child weight regulation, public health implications, and areas for future research are discussed.

CLASSIFICATION OF OBESITY

Most epidemiologic and clinical studies use self-reported or measured weight and height to calculate body mass index (BMI) and thereby define obesity. Whereas in adulthood obesity definitions are static (a BMI of at least 30 kg/m^2 indicates obesity, and BMI between 25.0 and 29.9 kg/m^2 indicates overweight[7]), among children body proportions, and therefore obesity thresholds, vary physiologically with age and

The author has no conflicts of interest to report.

Department of Ambulatory Care and Prevention, Harvard Medical School and Harvard Pilgrim Health Care, 133 Brookline Avenue, Boston, MA 02215, USA
E-mail address: emily_oken@hphc.org

Obstet Gynecol Clin N Am 36 (2009) 361–377
doi:10.1016/j.ogc.2009.03.007
obgyn.theclinics.com

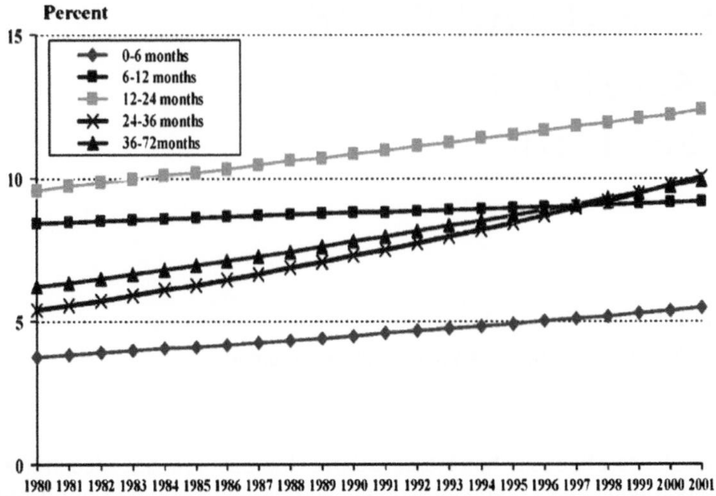

Fig. 1. Age-specific predicted prevalence of overweight from 1980 through 2001 among 120,680 children 0 to 71.9 months seen at 366,109 well-child care visits at a Massachusetts HMO, by age group. (*From* Kim J, Peterson KE, Scanlon KS, et al. Trends in overweight from 1980 through 2001 among preschool-aged children enrolled in a health maintenance organization. Obesity [Silver Spring] 2006;14:1107–12; with permission.)

sex. In the United States, childhood obesity is typically defined as a BMI at or above the 95th percentile for age and sex, and overweight as a BMI between the 85th and 94th percentile, based on growth charts created by the Centers for Disease Control and Prevention (CDC).[8] To calculate these percentiles, the CDC use as a reference population United States children measured in the 1970s, most of whom were not breastfed. Others, especially outside the United States, use World Health Organization growth charts, which used as a reference healthy breastfed children from several countries.[9] Although these different standards yield somewhat different estimates of obesity prevalence, escalating obesity trends are consistent regardless of the growth standard used.

The use of BMI affords many conveniences, as weight and height can be measured or can be reported on a questionnaire, recalled even over many years, or obtained from clinical records, all with reasonable accuracy. However, in addition to any inaccuracy or bias in reported height and weight, BMI may over- or underestimate the true proportion of individuals with excess body fat, since it does not directly assess adiposity. BMI tends to be less accurate among populations with greater variation in lean body mass, such as children who had been born small for gestational age and certain racial or ethnic groups.[10,11] In clinical practice, BMI remains the recommended method of screening for obesity among both adults and children aged 2 years and older.[7,12]

Some investigators have also used measurement of skinfold thicknesses to estimate regional or global body fat, although this technique requires training and is operator dependent.[13] Radiologic methods, such as ultrasound, MRI, and dual-energy x-ray absorptiometry scans, or plethysmography, measure body adiposity more directly, but are expensive and not portable. Bioelectrical impedance analysis overcomes many of the practical limitations of these methods, but equations for the calculation of body fat among children are still being validated.[14,15]

MATERNAL WEIGHT AND CHILD OBESITY

A mother's prepregnancy weight is directly associated with the intrauterine growth of her fetus.[16] Mothers who are overweight or obese entering pregnancy are likely to have infants with higher birth weight and increased risk for being large for gestational age or macrosomic.[16] Extensive research links greater size at birth with increased risk for obesity in later life.[17,18] Thus, we might expect that heavier mothers have heavier children. In fact, evidence now decades old confirms that obese children tend to have obese mothers.[19–21]

Initially these associations were mostly studied as evidence for a genetic underpinning of obesity risk.[22] More recently, investigators have considered whether the obese intrauterine environment itself programs higher body weight. Studies examining this question have consistently found that higher maternal weight entering pregnancy increases risk for obesity among offspring in childhood, adolescence, or adulthood (**Table 1**).[3,20,23–31] Escalating risks among heavier mothers provide evidence for a dose-effect.[23]

Limited evidence also links maternal prenatal weight with the cardio-metabolic complications of obesity among offspring. At birth, infants born to obese mothers have higher body fat,[32–35] reduced energy expenditure,[32] and a more atherogenic lipid profile.[36] These associations may persist, even after adjustment for offspring attained BMI. Maternal prepregnancy BMI predicts child blood pressure and risk for metabolic syndrome.[37,38] In a study of adult men born from 1924 to 1933 in Finland, higher maternal BMI during pregnancy was associated with increased risk of death from coronary heart disease.[39] However, among 627 adult men and women from China, higher maternal BMI recorded in early or late pregnancy was associated with lower offspring glucose and insulin measured at age 45 years.[40] As all of these Chinese mothers were quite thin, with the highest group having a BMI of greater than 22.3 kg/m^2, the relevance of these findings to modern United States populations is unclear.

GESTATIONAL WEIGHT GAIN AND CHILD OBESITY

A number of epidemiologic studies have found that higher maternal gestational weight gain is associated with higher child weight in childhood[21,27,41–46] and adolescence,[47,48] and consequent risk for obesity and elevated blood pressure. One found an association of higher gestational weight gain with increased risk for early-onset, but not late-onset, childhood obesity.[27] Additional preliminary studies have suggested that the direct association of higher weight gain with offspring obesity persists into adulthood.[49,50] However, the association of higher gestational weight gain with child adiposity has not been found in all studies.[23,29,51] In a study of 16 infants, maternal weight gain during pregnancy predicted infant weight and fat-free mass, but not fat mass.[52] Another study of 110 children reported an inverse correlation, although estimates were not adjusted for maternal weight or other factors.[53] Published studies that have reported an association of maternal gestational weight gain with risk for offspring obesity are summarized in **Table 2**.

Some preliminary studies have reported a U- or J-shaped association, with greater overweight risks also with the lowest maternal gains, especially in women with lower prepregnancy BMI.[49,54] However, in a recent study we observed an apparent U-shaped relationship between gestational weight gain and attained offspring weight in adolescence, which became linear after adjustment for maternal prepregnancy BMI (**Fig. 2**).[47] This shift derived from the fact that women who enter pregnancy at a higher weight tend to gain less weight during pregnancy, and highlights the importance of considering both prepregnancy weight and gestational weight gain. One study found

Table 1
Studies reporting associations of maternal or paternal prenatal BMI with offspring attained weight in childhood or adulthood

1st Author, Year	Population	Measure of Exposure	Adjusted Odds Ratio (95% CI) for Offspring Obesity
Whitaker, 2004[23]	8494 low-income US children—ages 2–4 y	Maternal 1st trimester BMI	(age 4 y)
		25–29.9 kg/m^2	1.75 (1.40, 2.18)
		30–39.9 kg/m^2	3.07 (2.48, 3.79)
		≥40 kg/m^2	4.31 (3.17, 5.87)
		(vs. 18.5–24.9 kg/m^2)	
Li, 2005[24]	2636 US children in the NLSY—ages 2–14 y	Maternal pre-pregnancy BMI	
		overweight	2.5 (1.8, 3.6)
		obesity	4.1 (2.6, 6.4)
Rielly, 2005[25]	8234 UK children in the ALSPAC study—age 7 y	BMI >30 kg/m^2 (vs. both parents <30)	
		Mother	4.25 (2.86, 6.32)
		Father	2.54 (1.72, 3.75)
		Both	10.44 (5.11, 21.32)
Li, 2007[27]	1739 US children of women in the NLSY—ages 2–12 y	Maternal pre-pregnancy BMI ≥30 (vs. <25 kg/m^2)	5.1 (2.9, 9.1)—early onset obesity 5.8 (2.6, 13.0)—late onset-obesity
Salsberry, 2007[28]	2212 pairs in NLSY child-mother file born 1980–1990—ages 12–13 y	Maternal pre-pregnancy BMI	
		25-29.9 kg/m^2	2.18 (1.51, 3.13)
		≥30 kg/m^2	4.28 (2.69, 6.83)
		(vs. <25 kg/m^2)	
Koupil, 2008[29]	1103 Swedish army conscripts—age 18 y	per 1 kg/m^2 maternal BMI	1.23 (1.16, 1.30)
Li, 2009[31]	2908 UK children born to parents in the 1958 British birth cohort—ages 9–18 y	1 SD increase in BMI at parent age 16 y	
		Mother	1.57 (1.26, 1.95)
		Father	1.45 (1.03, 2.05)

Abbreviations: ALSPAC, Avon Longitudinal Study of Parents and Children; NLSY, National Longitudinal Study of Youth; US, United States; UK, United Kingdom.

stronger associations among overweight and obese mothers,[41] some found somewhat stronger associations among underweight mothers,[44,54] one found an effect only among mothers currently normal weight but not overweight,[46] and others found no evidence for effect modification by maternal BMI.[42,47]

EVIDENCE FOR CAUSALITY

Overall, then, observational evidence is consistent in confirming that mothers who are heavier entering pregnancy, or with higher weight gain during pregnancy, have children who are more likely to be overweight. The question remains whether the intrauterine experience of infants born to mothers who are obese or gain excess weight during pregnancy programs long-term weight regulation and disease risk, or whether

Table 2
Published studies reporting associations of maternal gestational weight gain with risk for offspring obesity

1st Author, Year	Population	Measure of Exposure	Adjusted Odds Ratio (95% CI) for Offspring Obesity
Maffeis, 1994[51]	1363 Italian children—ages 4–12 y	Per 1 kg	1.01 (0.96, 1.05)
Oken, 2007[42]	1044 US children in Project Viva—age 3 y	Per 5 kg	1.52 (1.19, 1.94)
Moreira, 2007[45]	4845 Portuguese children—ages 6–12 y	≥16 kg vs. <9 kg	1.27 (1.01, 1.61)
Li, 2007[27]	1739 US children of women in the NLSY—ages 2–12 y	≥45 lbs vs. 25–35 lbs	1.7 (1.0, 2.9)—early-onset obesity 0.8 (0.3, 2.1)—late-onset obesity
Oken, 2008[47]	11,994 US adolescents in the Growing Up Today Study—ages 9-14 y	Per 5 lbs	1.09 (1.06, 1.13)
Wrotniak, 2008[44]	10,226 participants from the US Collaborative Perinatal Project (1959–1972)—age 7 y	Per 1 kg	1.03 (1.02, 1.05)
Kleiser, 2009[46]	13,450 German children—ages 3–17 y	>20 kg (vs. ≤20 kg)	
		Mother normal weight	2.81 (1.6, 5.0)
		Mother overweight	0.71 (0.3, 1.6)

Abbreviations: NLSY, National Longitudinal Study of Youth; US, United States.

maternal weight is solely a marker for other, shared causes of both maternal weight and child weight.

Shared genes certainly account for some of the similarity in maternal and offspring weight.[55] The extrauterine environment is also shared by mother and child and contributes to obesity risk.[56] For example, parents and children tend to have similar diet quality.[57] Even among individuals genetically predisposed to develop obesity, environment matters a great deal. Compared with Pima Indians just across the border in Mexico, Pima Indians living in the United States have dramatically higher rates of obesity (70% versus 13%) and type 2 diabetes (38% versus 7%).[58,59]

Infant feeding may also confound associations of maternal weight with child weight. Mothers who are obese and those who gain excessive weight during pregnancy tend to be less likely to initiate and maintain breastfeeding, likely for both psychologic and physiologic reasons.[60–63] While meta-analyses have found that longer breastfeeding duration is associated with lower attained weight in childhood, these associations have been modest,[64,65] and a recent randomized trial of breastfeeding promotion did not find any evidence that longer duration and exclusivity of breastfeeding was associated with lower weight at age 6.5 years.[66] In addition, associations of maternal

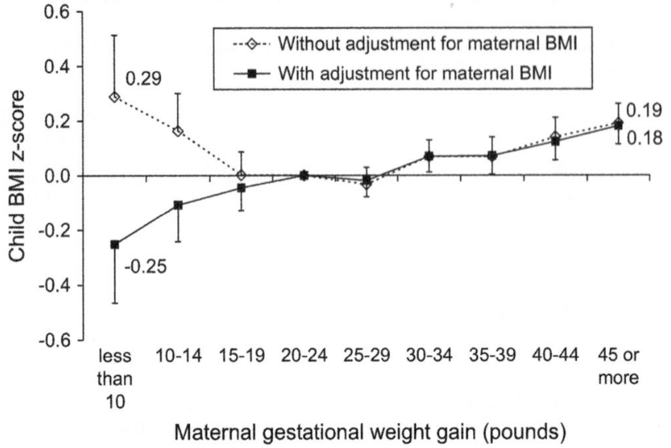

Fig. 2. Maternal gestational weight gain and child obesity prevalence among 11,994 mother–child pairs in the Growing Up Today Study. (*From* Oken E, Rifas-Shiman SL, Field AE, et al. Maternal gestational weight gain and offspring weight in adolescence. Obstet Gynecol 2008;112:999–1006; with permission.)

weight or gestational weight gain with child weight persist even after adjustment for breastfeeding.[42] Therefore, breastfeeding likely does not entirely mediate the association of higher maternal weight or weight gain with higher child weight.

Obese mothers may also have poorer feeding interactions with their infants, may feed their children too much, or may provide a poor quality diet to their children.[67,68] In animal and human studies, postnatal overfeeding or rapid infant weight gain is associated with higher weight, greater fat mass, and adverse cardio-metabolic changes, similar to the effects of maternal overnutrition during pregnancy.[69–73] These factors are more difficult to measure and thus account for in epidemiologic studies.

An optimal approach to isolating the role of intrauterine exposure would be to conduct a well-powered randomized clinical trial, in which women are randomized to usual care or to an effective weight change intervention before or during pregnancy, and follow children longitudinally. No previous randomized trials have been performed of an intervention delivered before pregnancy. In an undernourished population in Guatemala, a group randomized to receive a protein-energy supplement during pregnancy, lactation, and early childhood had greater size at birth, greater attained height, and lower plasma glucose compared with a group randomized to a no-protein or low-energy supplement, but the relevance of this study for overnourished populations is unclear.[74] Trials among overweight mothers to improve diet or other behaviors during pregnancy and thereby prevent excess gestational weight gain have generally been underpowered to examine infant outcomes.[75–78] In one intervention, women randomized to a high volume of exercise in mid and late pregnancy had infants with less body fat.[79] Gestational weight gain intervention trials that are adequately powered and with follow-up past birth have not yet been reported, although some are in progress.

Several observational studies that examined associations of maternal gestational obesity or weight gain with child weight have attempted to control for shared behaviors such as diet and physical activity, or confounders such as socioeconomic status, maternal smoking during pregnancy, and gestational diabetes, that may underlie maternal and child overweight risk.[23,41,42,44,45,47] Associations generally did not attenuate substantially after statistical adjustment for these factors. However, since these characteristics can be difficult to measure, it is hard to eliminate the role of shared behaviors in observational studies.

Some investigators have compared the association of mother's weight with that of the father's on child weight, as a way to highlight the role of the prenatal environment. Since each parent contributes 50% of the child's genetic makeup, if shared genes were the sole cause of shared obesity risk we might expect similar strength of association of maternal or paternal weight with child weight. The few studies with information about both parents have generally found that estimates for maternal weight are somewhat stronger than estimates for paternal weight.[25,27,30,80] However, nonpaternity may explain some of this difference. Recent analyses that accounted for possible nonpaternity have had conflicting findings. In an Australian population, maternal BMI remained a stronger predictor of child BMI at age 14 years versus paternal BMI,[81] whereas in a United Kingdom population, associations of maternal and paternal BMI with child BMI at age 7.5 years were similar.[82] The United Kingdom group did find stronger effects of maternal versus paternal BMI on offspring fat mass at age 9 to 10 years, even after accounting for nonpaternity, although effect sizes were modest.[83] However, maternal FTO genotype, a predictor of obesity not associated with other sociodemographic characteristics, did not predict child fat mass after accounting for the child's genotype. These authors concluded that developmental overnutrition related to greater maternal BMI is unlikely to have driven the recent obesity epidemic.[83] However, variation in this one gene likely explains a very small amount of obesity risk.

Another approach to accounting for shared genes and behaviors is to compare outcomes in siblings with discordant intrauterine exposures; for example, siblings whose mother experienced different gestational weight gain, or interpregnancy weight gain or loss. Most extant studies included outcomes only at birth.[84,85] In a study of 90 women with at least two pregnancies complicated by gestational diabetes mellitus, maternal overweight was associated with offspring birth weight on a between-mother but not within-mother analysis, whereas gestational weight gain was associated with birth weight even on within-mother analysis.[86] However, the influence of gestational diabetes mellitus may have overwhelmed that of weight. In another study, investigators examined the prevalence of obesity in 172 children, aged 2 to 18 years, born to obese mothers with substantial weight loss after biliopancreatic bypass surgery, compared with 45 same-age siblings who were born before maternal surgery.[87] After maternal surgery, the prevalence of obesity among offspring decreased by 52%, and severe obesity by 45%.

Thus, many pathways may explain observed associations of high maternal prepregnancy weight and gestational weight gain with child obesity (**Fig. 3**).[88] While some of the risk is certainly mediated by shared genes and behaviors, the preponderance of human evidence suggests these exposures directly program offspring obesity risk.

EVIDENCE FROM ANIMAL STUDIES

A number of animal studies have been performed examining maternal gestational nutrition and offspring obesity.[89] Advantages of animal studies include the ability to compare genetically identical individuals, to isolate specific time periods of exposure (prepregnancy, pregnancy, or lactation), and to evaluate the role of offspring diet and physical activity. However, animals are not people—they may have different physiology and different sensitive periods for exposures.

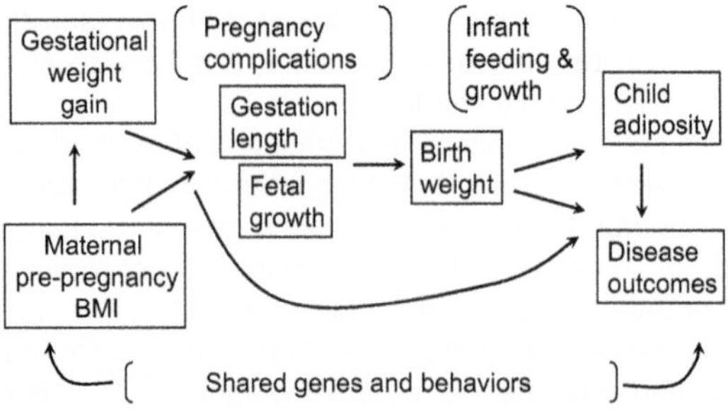

Fig. 3. Pathways linking maternal weight and weight gain with child outcomes. (*From* Oken E. 2006 maternal weight and gestational weight gain as predictors of long-term offspring growth and health. Presentation at the Workshop on the Impact of Pregnancy Weight on Maternal and Child Health. May 30, 2006, Washington, DC; with permission.)

Investigators have fed rodent dams obesogenic diets during the preconception period, pregnancy, or lactation. Results from these experimental protocols confirm that maternal peripartum overnutrition programs lifelong offspring overweight and excess adiposity.[90–95] Results were similar in a series of studies among sheep.[96,97] Excess offspring weight is especially likely among those genetically predisposed to obesity or who also are overfed postnatally.[90] A high-fat diet during pregnancy may program offspring obesity even if the mothers themselves do not become overweight, suggesting that maternal diet may influence offspring phenotype even in the absence of maternal phenotype.[92] Experiments have isolated pregnancy as a critical period of exposure, as maternal diet before conception or during lactation only, or unhealthy offspring diet commencing only after weaning, do not confer similar risks.[68,98,99]

Animal studies also help detail the metabolic sequelae of maternal overnutrition. Higher attained weight among offspring of overfed mothers is accompanied by increased fat mass, fat cell hypertrophy, reduced muscle mass, higher glucose, insulin, leptin, and triglyceride levels, lower adiponectin secretion, and elevated blood pressure associated with altered cardiovascular structure and function.[91,92,94,96–102] Some of the same obesity-related sequelae have been seen in human children born to mothers who are obese or experience excess gestational gain.[36,37,42]

MECHANISMS

How might excess maternal weight or weight gain during pregnancy have a persistent influence on offspring weight and related cardio-metabolic risk? Maternal overnutrition appears to influence several aspects of offspring physiology, including appetite, metabolism, and activity levels (**Fig. 4**).[103] Offspring of overfed rat dams have reduced energy expenditure[91,92] and a greater taste for junk food,[93] as do human children of obese mothers.[32,104] Lambs of overfed ewes have changes in the central appetite regulatory system, altered gene expression in adipose tissue, and increased expression of leptin.[96,97,105]

Maternal nutrition may influence the development of fetal cells and organs. For example, maternal overnutrition may result in fetal overnutrition and thereby increased fetal adipose tissue deposition.[106] Since adipocyte number appears to be set in the first years of life,[107] excess fat formed in early life may result in lifelong excess

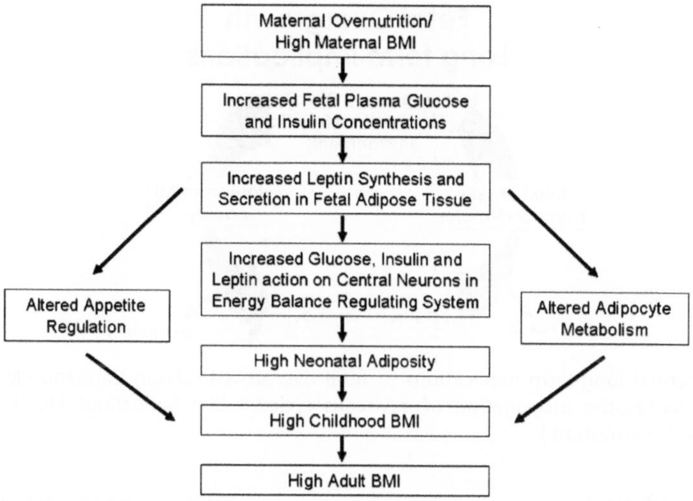

Fig. 4. Potential pathways explaining the relationship between maternal nutrition and offspring obesity. (*From* McMillen IC, Edwards LJ, Duffield J, et al. Regulation of leptin synthesis and secretion before birth: implications for the early programming of adult obesity. Reproduction 2006;131(3):415–27; with permission.)

adiposity. Maternal overnutrition may also influence the fetal epigenome, thereby influencing expression of genes that direct the accumulation of body fat or related metabolism.[95,99,108]

Analogous to the circumstances of diabetes during pregnancy, obese women or women with excess gestational gains may have increased circulating levels of glucose and other nutrients. Infants of mothers with diabetes during pregnancy are larger and have higher body fat at birth and during childhood and adolescence, have higher blood pressure, and are at increased risk for developing diabetes themselves.[109–113] Although these associations have not been replicated in populations with milder diabetes,[26,114] sibling studies[115] and an extensive animal literature[116] provide strong evidence that intrauterine exposure to maternal diabetes conveys risk for later overweight. Fetal hyperglycemia results in hyperinsulinemia and elevated leptin, which influences appetite regulation in the brain even prenatally.[103]

CLINICAL AND PUBLIC HEALTH IMPLICATIONS

Obesity in childhood and adolescence is associated with both short- and long-term adverse outcomes, including both physical and psychosocial consequences[117–120] and shortened lifespan.[121–123] Increasing trends of maternal weight and gestational weight gain may be propagating an intergenerational "vicious cycle" of obesity, as heavier mothers give birth to heavier daughters, who are then even more likely to be obese and diabetic entering their own pregnancies (**Fig. 5**).[106]

Encouraging women to attain a healthy weight before conception is an obvious goal, though a difficult one to attain. The postpartum period is also a window of opportunity for interventions to encourage healthy maternal weight entering subsequent pregnancies. Clearly, avoiding excess weight gain during pregnancy is crucial. However, the optimal amount of gestational weight gain remains uncertain, especially among obese women. Birth outcomes do appear to be improved with somewhat lower weight gains

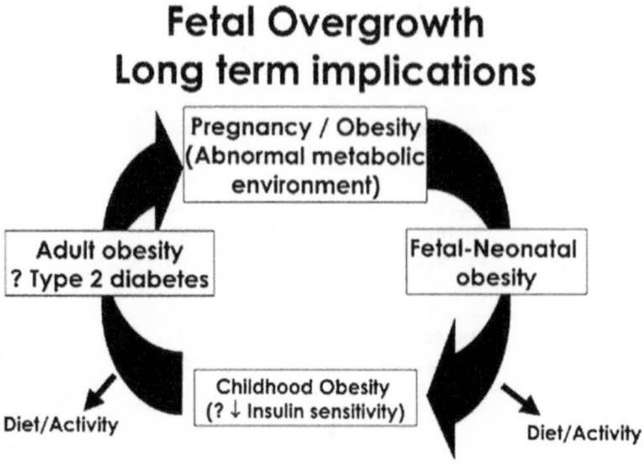

Fig. 5. Potential long-term implications of fetal overgrowth. (*From* Catalano PM. Obesity and pregnancy—the propagation of a viscous cycle? J Clin Endocrinol Metab 2003;88: 3505–6; with permission.)

than current guidelines recommend, especially among obese mothers,[124] but data on longer-term offspring outcomes and the risk–benefit balance of lower gains are scant. As infants with lower birth weights are at elevated risk for adverse neurologic development as well as later hypertension, type 2 diabetes, and cardiovascular disease,[11,17,125,126] efforts to reduce gestational weight gains should be carefully evaluated for their effects on offspring longer-term health. In 2009, the Institute of Medicine will release revised gestational weight gain guidelines.

Healthy behaviors after birth are also important. Whereas postnatal overfeeding magnifies the adverse metabolic effects of exposure to adverse intrauterine nutrition, an appropriate diet can block these effects.[98,127,128] Thus, efforts to promote breastfeeding, appropriate maternal feeding behaviors, healthful postweaning diet, and physical activity in childhood are critical.

Several intervention studies targeted at preventing excess gestational weight gain are planned, and should provide useful information in years to come about how best to improve health outcomes for mothers and their children. Additional research is also needed regarding how to help women achieve healthy weights entering pregnancy and how to prevent excess weight gain in infancy. Efforts to interrupt the intergenerational cycle of excess weight gain and obesity are not only important but also economical, as a single intervention could benefit the child, the mother, her future pregnancies, and subsequent generations.

REFERENCES

1. Ogden CL, Carroll MD, Curtin LR, et al. Prevalence of overweight and obesity in the United States, 1999–2004. JAMA 2006;295(13):1549–55.
2. Freedman DS, Khan LK, Serdula MK, et al. The relation of childhood BMI to adult adiposity: the Bogalusa Heart Study. Pediatrics 2005;115(1):22–7.
3. Whitaker RC, Wright JA, Pepe MS, et al. Predicting obesity in young adulthood from childhood and parental obesity. N Engl J Med 1997;337(13):869–73.
4. Kim J, Peterson KE, Scanlon KS, et al. Trends in overweight from 1980 through 2001 among preschool-aged children enrolled in a health maintenance organization. Obesity (Silver Spring) 2006;14(7):1107–12.
5. Gluckman P, Hanson M. Developmental origins of health and disease. New York: Cambridge University Press; 2006.

6. Taylor PD, Poston L. Developmental programming of obesity in mammals. Exp Physiol 2007;92(2):287–98.
7. National Heart Lung and Blood Institute. Clinical Guidelines on The Identification, Evaluation, and Treatment of Overweight and Obesity in Adults: National Institutes of Health, US Department of Health and Human Services. 1998. Publication Number 98-4083. Available at: http://www.nhlbi.nih.gov/guidelines/obesity/ob_gdlns.htm.
8. National Center for Health Statistics. CDC growth charts, United States. Available at: http://www.cdc.gov/growthcharts. 2000. Accessed February 16, 2009.
9. World Health Organization. The WHO child growth standards. Available at: http://www.who.int/childgrowth/en. 2006. Accessed February 19, 2009.
10. Xu YQ, Ji CY. Report on childhood obesity in China (7). Comparison of NCHS and WGOC. Biomed Environ Sci 2008;21(4):271–9.
11. Hediger ML, Overpeck MD, Kuczmarski RJ, et al. Muscularity and fatness of infants and young children born small- or large-for-gestational-age. Pediatrics 1998;102(5):E60.
12. Whitlock EP, Williams SB, Gold R, et al. Screening and interventions for childhood overweight: a summary of evidence for the US Preventive Services Task Force. Pediatrics 2005;116(1):e125–44.
13. Watts K, Naylor LH, Davis EA, et al. Do skinfolds accurately assess changes in body fat in obese children and adolescents? Med Sci Sports Exerc 2006;38(3):439–44.
14. Williams J, Wake M, Campbell M. Comparing estimates of body fat in children using published bioelectrical impedance analysis equations. Int J Pediatr Obes 2007;2(3):174–9.
15. Wright CM, Sherriff A, Ward SC, et al. Development of bioelectrical impedance-derived indices of fat and fat-free mass for assessment of nutritional status in childhood. Eur J Clin Nutr 2008;62(2):210–7.
16. Institute of MedicineIn: Nutrition during pregnancy, vol. 1. Washington, DC: National Academy Press; 1990.
17. Oken E, Gillman MW. Fetal origins of obesity. Obes Res 2003;11(4):496–506.
18. Parsons TJ, Power C, Logan S, et al. Childhood predictors of adult obesity. Int J Obes Relat Metab Disord 1999;23(Suppl 8):S1–107.
19. Guillaume M, Lapidus L, Beckers F, et al. Familial trends of obesity through three generations. Int J Obes Relat Metab Disord 1995;19(Suppl 3):S5–9.
20. Lake JK, Power C, Cole TJ. Child to adult body mass index in the 1958 British birth cohort: associations with parental obesity. Arch Dis Child 1997;77(5):376–81.
21. Fisch RO, Bilek MK, Ulstrom R. Obesity and leanness at birth and their relationship to body habitus in later childhood. Pediatrics 1975;56(4):521–8.
22. Stunkard AJ, Sorensen TI, Hanis C, et al. An adoption study of human obesity. N Engl J Med 1986;314(4):193–8.
23. Whitaker RC. Predicting preschooler obesity at birth: the role of maternal obesity in early pregnancy. Pediatrics 2004;114(1):e29–36.
24. Li C, Kaur H, Choi WS, et al. Additive interactions of maternal prepregnancy BMI and breast-feeding on childhood overweight. Obes Res 2005;13(2):362–71.
25. Reilly JJ, Armstrong J, Dorosty AR, et al. Early life risk factors for obesity in childhood: cohort study. BMJ 2005;330(7504):1357.
26. Jeffery AN, Metcalf BS, Hosking J, et al. Little evidence for early programming of weight and insulin resistance for contemporary children: EarlyBird Diabetes Study report 19. Pediatrics 2006;118(3):1118–23.

27. Li C, Goran MI, Kaur H, et al. Developmental trajectories of overweight during childhood: role of early life factors. Obesity (Silver Spring) 2007;15(3):760–71.
28. Salsberry PJ, Reagan PB. Taking the long view: the prenatal environment and early adolescent overweight. Res Nurs Health 2007;30(3):297–307.
29. Koupil I, Toivanen P. Social and early-life determinants of overweight and obesity in 18-year-old Swedish men. Int J Obes (Lond) 2008;32(1):73–81.
30. Moschonis G, Grammatikaki E, Manios Y. Perinatal predictors of overweight at infancy and preschool childhood: the GENESIS study. Int J Obes (Lond) 2008;32(1):39–47.
31. Li L, Law C, Lo Conte R, et al. Intergenerational influences on childhood body mass index: the effect of parental body mass index trajectories. Am J Clin Nutr 2009;89(2):551–7.
32. Rising R, Lifshitz F. Lower energy expenditures in infants from obese biological mothers. Nutr J 2008;7:15.
33. Bernstein IM, Goran MI, Amini SB, et al. Differential growth of fetal tissues during the second half of pregnancy. Am J Obstet Gynecol 1997;176(1 Pt 1):28–32.
34. Neggers Y, Goldenberg RL, Cliver SP, et al. The relationship between maternal and neonatal anthropometric measurements in term newborns. Obstet Gynecol 1995;85(2):192–6.
35. Harvey NC, Poole JR, Javaid MK, et al. Parental determinants of neonatal body composition. J Clin Endocrinol Metab 2007;92(2):523–6.
36. Merzouk H, Meghelli-Bouchenak M, Loukidi B, et al. Impaired serum lipids and lipoproteins in fetal macrosomia related to maternal obesity. Biol Neonate 2000; 77(1):17–24.
37. Boney CM, Verma A, Tucker R, et al. Metabolic syndrome in childhood: association with birth weight, maternal obesity, and gestational diabetes mellitus. Pediatrics 2005;115(3):e290–6.
38. Lawlor DA, Najman JM, Sterne J, et al. Associations of parental, birth, and early life characteristics with systolic blood pressure at 5 years of age: findings from the Mater-University study of pregnancy and its outcomes. Circulation 2004; 110(16):2417–23.
39. Forsen T, Eriksson JG, Tuomilehto J, et al. Mother's weight in pregnancy and coronary heart disease in a cohort of Finnish men. BMJ 1997;315(7112):837–40.
40. Mi J, Law C, Zhang KL, et al. Effects of infant birthweight and maternal body mass index in pregnancy on components of the insulin resistance syndrome in China. Ann Intern Med 2000;132(4):253–60.
41. Olson CM, Strawderman MS, Dennison BA. Maternal weight gain during pregnancy and at age 3 years. Matern Child Health J, in press.
42. Oken E, Taveras EM, Kleinman KP, et al. Gestational weight gain and child adiposity at age 3 years. Am J Obstet Gynecol 2007;196(4):322.e1–8.
43. Vohr BR, McGarvey ST, Tucker R. Effects of maternal gestational diabetes on offspring adiposity at 4–7 years of age. Diabetes Care 1999;22(8):1284–91.
44. Wrotniak BH, Shults J, Butts S, et al. Gestational weight gain and risk of overweight in the offspring at age 7 y in a multicenter, multiethnic cohort study. Am J Clin Nutr 2008;87(6):1818–24.
45. Moreira P, Padez C, Mourao-Carvalhal I, et al. Maternal weight gain during pregnancy and overweight in Portuguese children. Int J Obes (Lond) 2007;31(4): 608–14.
46. Kleiser C, Schaffrath Rosario A, Mensink GB, et al. Potential determinants of obesity among children and adolescents in Germany: results from the cross-sectional KiGGS Study. BMC Public Health 2009;9:46.

47. Oken E, Rifas-Shiman SL, Field AE, et al. Maternal gestational weight gain and offspring weight in adolescence. Obstet Gynecol 2008;112(5):999–1006.
48. Seidman DS. Excessive maternal weight gain during pregnancy and being overweight at 17 years of age [abstract]. Pediatr Res 1996;39:112A.
49. Stuebe A, Michels K. Gestational weight gain and obesity at age 18 in the daughter [abstract]. Am J Obstet Gynecol 2006;195(6):S228.
50. Schack-Nielsen L, ME, Michaelsen KF, et al. High maternal pregnancy weight gain is associated with an increased risk of obesity in childhood and adulthood independent of maternal BMI [abstract]. Pediatr Res 2005;58(5):1020.
51. Maffeis C, Micciolo R, Must A, et al. Parental and perinatal factors associated with childhood obesity in north-east Italy. Int J Obes Relat Metab Disord 1994; 18(5):301–5.
52. Catalano PM, Drago NM, Amini SB. Maternal carbohydrate metabolism and its relationship to fetal growth and body composition. Am J Obstet Gynecol 1995;172(5):1464–70.
53. Esposito-Del Puente A, Scalfi L, De Filippo E, et al. Familial and environmental influences on body composition and body fat distribution in childhood in southern Italy. Int J Obes Relat Metab Disord 1994;18(9):596–601.
54. Sharma AJ, Cogswell ME, Grummer-Strawn LM. The association between pregnancy weight gain is associated with an increased risk of obesity in childhood and adulthood independent of maternal BMI [abstract]. Pediatr Res 2005; 58(5):1038.
55. Rankinen T, Zuberi A, Chagnon YC, et al. The human obesity gene map: the 2005 update. Obesity (Silver Spring) 2006;14(4):529–644.
56. Nelson MC, Gordon-Larsen P, North KE, et al. Body mass index gain, fast food, and physical activity: effects of shared environments over time. Obesity (Silver Spring) 2006;14(4):701–9.
57. Oliveria SA, Ellison RC, Moore LL, et al. Parent-child relationships in nutrient intake: the Framingham Children's Study. Am J Clin Nutr 1992;56(3):593–8.
58. Schulz LO, Bennett PH, Ravussin E, et al. Effects of traditional and western environments on prevalence of type 2 diabetes in Pima Indians in Mexico and the U.S. Diabetes Care 2006;29(8):1866–71.
59. Ravussin E, Valencia ME, Esparza J, et al. Effects of a traditional lifestyle on obesity in Pima Indians. Diabetes Care 1994;17(9):1067–74.
60. Gunderson EP. Breastfeeding after gestational diabetes pregnancy: subsequent obesity and type 2 diabetes in women and their offspring. Diabetes Care 2007; 30(Suppl 2):S161–8.
61. Li R, Jewell S, Grummer-Strawn L. Maternal obesity and breast-feeding practices. Am J Clin Nutr 2003;77(4):931–6.
62. Hilson JA, Rasmussen KM, Kjolhede CL. Excessive weight gain during pregnancy is associated with earlier termination of breast-feeding among White women. J Nutr 2006;136(1):140–6.
63. Hilson JA, Rasmussen KM, Kjolhede CL. High prepregnant body mass index is associated with poor lactation outcomes among white, rural women independent of psychosocial and demographic correlates. J Hum Lact 2004;20(1): 18–29.
64. Harder T, Bergmann R, Kallischnigg G, et al. Duration of breastfeeding and risk of overweight: a meta-analysis. Am J Epidemiol 2005;162(5):397–403.
65. Owen CG, Martin RM, Whincup PH, et al. The effect of breastfeeding on mean body mass index throughout life: a quantitative review of published and unpublished observational evidence. Am J Clin Nutr 2005;82(6):1298–307.

66. Kramer MS, Matush L, Vanilovich I, et al. Effects of prolonged and exclusive breastfeeding on child height, weight, adiposity, and blood pressure at age 6.5 y: evidence from a large randomized trial. Am J Clin Nutr 2007;86(6):1717–21.
67. Rising R, Lifshitz F. Relationship between maternal obesity and infant feeding-interactions. Nutr J 2005;4:17.
68. Robinson S, Marriott L, Poole J, et al. Dietary patterns in infancy: the importance of maternal and family influences on feeding practice. Br J Nutr 2007;98(5):1029–37.
69. Widdowson EM, McCance RA. Some effects of accelerating growth. I. General somatic development. Proc R Soc Lond B Biol Sci 1960;152:188–206.
70. Plagemann A, Harder T, Rake A, et al. Perinatal elevation of hypothalamic insulin, acquired malformation of hypothalamic galaninergic neurons, and syndrome x-like alterations in adulthood of neonatally overfed rats. Brain Res 1999;836(1–2):146–55.
71. Lewis DS, Bertrand HA, McMahan CA, et al. Preweaning food intake influences the adiposity of young adult baboons. J Clin Invest 1986;78(4):899–905.
72. Belfort MB, Rifas-Shiman SL, Rich-Edwards J, et al. Size at birth, infant growth, and blood pressure at three years of age. J Pediatr 2007;151(6):670–4.
73. Stettler N, Zemel BS, Kumanyika S, et al. Infant weight gain and childhood overweight status in a multicenter, cohort study. Pediatrics 2002;109(2):194–9.
74. Habicht JP, Yarbrough C, Lechtig A, et al. Relationship of birthweight, maternal nutrition and infant mortality. Nutr Rep Int 1973;7(5):533–46.
75. Wolff S, Legarth J, Vangsgaard K, et al. A randomized trial of the effects of dietary counseling on gestational weight gain and glucose metabolism in obese pregnant women. Int J Obes (Lond) 2008;32(3):495–501.
76. Polley BA, Wing RR, Sims CJ. Randomized controlled trial to prevent excessive weight gain in pregnant women. Int J Obes Relat Metab Disord 2002;26(11):1494–502.
77. Artal R, Catanzaro RB, Gavard JA, et al. A lifestyle intervention of weight-gain restriction: diet and exercise in obese women with gestational diabetes mellitus. Appl Physiol Nutr Metab 2007;32(3):596–601.
78. Kinnunen TI, Pasanen M, Aittasalo M, et al. Preventing excessive weight gain during pregnancy—a controlled trial in primary health care. Eur J Clin Nutr 2007;61(7):884–91.
79. Clapp JF 3rd, Kim H, Burciu B, et al. Continuing regular exercise during pregnancy: effect of exercise volume on fetoplacental growth. Am J Obstet Gynecol 2002;186(1):142–7.
80. Danielzik S, Langnase K, Mast M, et al. Impact of parental BMI on the manifestation of overweight 5–7 year old children. Eur J Nutr 2002;41(3):132–8.
81. Lawlor DA, Smith GD, O'Callaghan M, et al. Epidemiologic evidence for the fetal overnutrition hypothesis: findings from the Mater-University study of pregnancy and its outcomes. Am J Epidemiol 2007;165(4):418–24.
82. Davey Smith G, Steer C, Leary S, et al. Is there an intrauterine influence on obesity? Evidence from parent child associations in the Avon Longitudinal Study of Parents and Children (ALSPAC). Arch Dis Child 2007;92(10):876–80.
83. Lawlor DA, Timpson NJ, Harbord RM, et al. Exploring the developmental overnutrition hypothesis using parental-offspring associations and FTO as an instrumental variable. PLoS Med 2008;5(3):e33.
84. Maggard MA, Yermilov I, Li Z, et al. Pregnancy and fertility following bariatric surgery: a systematic review. JAMA 2008;300(19):2286–96.

85. Villamor E, Cnattingius S. Interpregnancy weight change and risk of adverse pregnancy outcomes: a population-based study. Lancet 2006;368(9542): 1164–70.
86. Hutcheon JA, Platt RW, Meltzer SJ, et al. Is birth weight modified during pregnancy? Using sibling differences to understand the impact of blood glucose, obesity, and maternal weight gain in gestational diabetes. Am J Obstet Gynecol 2006;195(2):488–94.
87. Kral JG, Biron S, Simard S, et al. Large maternal weight loss from obesity surgery prevents transmission of obesity to children who were followed for 2 to 18 years. Pediatrics 2006;118(6):e1644–9.
88. Hayes M, Abrams B, Davidson EC, et al, editors. Influence of pregnancy weight on maternal and child health. Washington, DC: National Academies Press; 2007.
89. Nathanielsz PW, Poston L, Taylor PD. In utero exposure to maternal obesity and diabetes: animal models that identify and characterize implications for future health. Obstet Gynecol Clin North Am 2007;34(2):201–12, vii–viii.
90. Levin BE, Govek E. Gestational obesity accentuates obesity in obesity-prone progeny. Am J Physiol 1998;275(4 Pt 2):R1374–9.
91. Shankar K, Harrell A, Liu X, et al. Maternal obesity at conception programs obesity in the offspring. Am J Physiol Regul Integr Comp Physiol 2008;294(2): R528–38.
92. Samuelsson AM, Matthews PA, Argenton M, et al. Diet-induced obesity in female mice leads to offspring hyperphagia, adiposity, hypertension, and insulin resistance: a novel murine model of developmental programming. Hypertension 2008;51(2):383–92.
93. Bayol SA, Farrington SJ, Stickland NC. A maternal 'junk food' diet in pregnancy and lactation promotes an exacerbated taste for 'junk food' and a greater propensity for obesity in rat offspring. Br J Nutr 2007;98(4):843–51.
94. Bayol SA, Simbi BH, Bertrand JA, et al. Offspring from mothers fed a 'junk food' diet in pregnancy and lactation exhibit exacerbated adiposity that is more pronounced in females. J Physiol 2008;586(13):3219–30.
95. Bayol SA, Simbi BH, Stickland NC. A maternal cafeteria diet during gestation and lactation promotes adiposity and impairs skeletal muscle development and metabolism in rat offspring at weaning. J Physiol 2005;567(Pt 3):951–61.
96. Muhlhausler BS, Adam CL, Findlay PA, et al. Increased maternal nutrition alters development of the appetite-regulating network in the brain. FASEB J 2006; 20(8):1257–9.
97. Muhlhausler BS, Duffield JA, McMillen IC. Increased maternal nutrition increases leptin expression in perirenal and subcutaneous adipose tissue in the postnatal lamb. Endocrinology 2007;148(12):6157–63.
98. Howie GJ, Sloboda DM, Kamal T, et al. Maternal nutritional history predicts obesity in adult offspring independent of postnatal diet. J Physiol 2009;587 (Pt 4):905–15.
99. Wu Q, Suzuki M. Parental obesity and overweight affect the body-fat accumulation in the offspring: the possible effect of a high-fat diet through epigenetic inheritance. Obes Rev 2006;7(2):201–8.
100. Armitage JA, Lakasing L, Taylor PD, et al. Developmental programming of aortic and renal structure in offspring of rats fed fat-rich diets in pregnancy. J Physiol 2005;565(Pt 1):171–84.
101. Parente LB, Aguila MB, Mandarim-de-Lacerda CA. Deleterious effects of high-fat diet on perinatal and postweaning periods in adult rat offspring. Clin Nutr 2008;27(4):623–34.

102. Srinivasan M, Katewa SD, Palaniyappan A, et al. Maternal high-fat diet consumption results in fetal malprogramming predisposing to the onset of metabolic syndrome-like phenotype in adulthood. Am J Physiol Endocrinol Metab 2006;291(4):E792–9.
103. McMillen IC, Edwards LJ, Duffield J, et al. Regulation of leptin synthesis and secretion before birth: implications for the early programming of adult obesity. Reproduction 2006;131(3):415–27.
104. Wardle J, Guthrie C, Sanderson S, et al. Food and activity preferences in children of lean and obese parents. Int J Obes Relat Metab Disord 2001;25(7):971–7.
105. Muhlhausler BS, Duffield JA, McMillen IC. Increased maternal nutrition stimulates peroxisome proliferator activated receptor-gamma, adiponectin, and leptin messenger ribonucleic acid expression in adipose tissue before birth. Endocrinology 2007;148(2):878–85.
106. Catalano PM. Obesity and pregnancy—the propagation of a viscous cycle? J Clin Endocrinol Metab 2003;88(8):3505–6.
107. Spalding KL, Arner E, Westermark PO, et al. Dynamics of fat cell turnover in humans. Nature 2008;453(7196):783–7.
108. Aagaard-Tillery KM, Grove K, Bishop J, et al. Developmental origins of disease and determinants of chromatin structure: maternal diet modifies the primate fetal epigenome. J Mol Endocrinol 2008;41(2):91–102.
109. Plagemann A, Harder T, Kohlhoff R, et al. Overweight and obesity in infants of mothers with long-term insulin-dependent diabetes or gestational diabetes. Int J Obes Relat Metab Disord 1997;21(6):451–6.
110. Silverman BL, Rizzo TA, Cho NH, et al. Long-term effects of the intrauterine environment. The Northwestern University Diabetes in Pregnancy Center. Diabetes Care 1998;21(Suppl 2):B142–9.
111. Gillman MW, Rifas-Shiman S, Berkey CS, et al. Maternal gestational diabetes, birth weight, and adolescent obesity. Pediatrics 2003;111(3):e221–6.
112. Wright CS, Rifas-Shiman SL, Rich-Edwards JW, et al. Intrauterine exposure to gestational diabetes, child adiposity, and blood pressure. Am J Hypertens 2009;22(2):215–20.
113. Bunt JC, Tataranni PA, Salbe AD. Intrauterine exposure to diabetes is a determinant of hemoglobin A(1)c and systolic blood pressure in Pima Indian children. J Clin Endocrinol Metab 2005;90(6):3225–9.
114. Whitaker RC, Pepe MS, Seidel KD, et al. Gestational diabetes and the risk of offspring obesity. Pediatrics 1998;101(2):E9.
115. Dabelea D, Hanson RL, Lindsay RS, et al. Intrauterine exposure to diabetes conveys risks for type 2 diabetes and obesity: a study of discordant sibships. Diabetes 2000;49(12):2208–11.
116. Merzouk H, Madani S, Chabane Sari D, et al. Time course of changes in serum glucose, insulin, lipids and tissue lipase activities in macrosomic offspring of rats with streptozotocin-induced diabetes. Clin Sci (Lond) 2000;98(1):21–30.
117. Mattsson N, Ronnemaa T, Juonala M, et al. Childhood predictors of the metabolic syndrome in adulthood. The Cardiovascular Risk in Young Finns Study. Ann Med 2008;40(7):542–52.
118. Gardner DS, Hosking J, Metcalf BS, et al. Contribution of early weight gain to childhood overweight and metabolic health: a longitudinal study (EarlyBird 36). Pediatrics 2009;123(1):e67–73.
119. Zeller MH, Modi AC. Predictors of health-related quality of life in obese youth. Obesity (Silver Spring) 2006;14(1):122–30.

120. Slyper AH. Childhood obesity, adipose tissue distribution, and the pediatric practitioner. Pediatrics 1998;102(1):e4.
121. Olshansky SJ, Passaro DJ, Hershow RC, et al. A potential decline in life expectancy in the United States in the 21st century. N Engl J Med 2005;352(11): 1138–45.
122. Hoffmans MD, Kromhout D, de Lezenne Coulander C. The impact of body mass index of 78,612 18-year old Dutch men on 32-year mortality from all causes. J Clin Epidemiol 1988;41(8):749–56.
123. Must A, Jacques PF, Dallal GE, et al. Long-term morbidity and mortality of overweight adolescents. A follow-up of the Harvard Growth Study of 1922 to 1935. N Engl J Med 1992;327(19):1350–5.
124. Oken E. Excess gestational weight gain amplifies risks among obese mothers. Epidemiology 2009;20(1):82–3.
125. Curhan GC, Chertow GM, Willett WC, et al. Birth weight and adult hypertension and obesity in women. Circulation 1996;94(6):1310–5.
126. Curhan GC, Willett WC, Rimm EB, et al. Birth weight and adult hypertension, diabetes mellitus, and obesity in US men. Circulation 1996;94(12):3246–50.
127. Armitage JA, Khan IY, Taylor PD, et al. Developmental programming of the metabolic syndrome by maternal nutritional imbalance: how strong is the evidence from experimental models in mammals? J Physiol 2004;561(Pt 2):355–77.
128. Srinivasan M, Aalinkeel R, Song F, et al. Maternal hyperinsulinemia predisposes rat fetuses for hyperinsulinemia, and adult-onset obesity and maternal mild food restriction reverses this phenotype. Am J Physiol Endocrinol Metab 2006;290(1): E129–34.

Obesity in Minority Women: Calories, Commerce, and Culture

Sharon T. Phelan, MD, FACOG

KEYWORDS

- Obesity • Minority women • Obesity prevalence
- Social networks

Obesity is now prevalent and spreading quickly among individuals in the United States. The rate of increasing prevalence of obesity has been particularly stunning over the past 20 years as illustrated in the CDC map graphs (**Fig. 1**).[1] As a result, obesity qualifies as a national epidemic, impacting all socioeconomic groups. This epidemic disproportionately affects lower-socioeconomic populations. These include rural and urban African American, Native American, and Latino populations and many rural white populations. Women in these groups are especially impacted.

Traditionally, obesity has been viewed as an individual weakness with a lack of an internal locus of control.[2] This view contends that more will power and exercise (pushing away from the table) will solve the problem. When over 33% of the population in the United States is overweight and an additional 34% is obese, there is more at work than just poor decision making by individuals. Entire populations are now facing the medical and social complications of obesity. A striking example of this transition is the United States' Native American population. In the 1950s medical providers believed these populations were genetically protected from cardiovascular disease and diabetes.[3] When native populations required medical care it was usually for infectious concerns, trauma, and issues related to malnutrition. In 1967 malnutrition was still being documented among Native American children.[3,4] In 1955 their infant mortality rate of 62.7/1000 live births was primarily from infectious and nutritional concerns. By 1991, it was 8/1000.[3] Now diabetes and cardiovascular disease are the primary health concerns in the Native American populations.[5] In fact, cardiovascular disease is the leading cause of death (18%) within the Native American population compared with 10% in the non-native population in individuals over 45 years of age.[3] This represents a 6- to 10-fold increase from 1987 to 1996.[5]

What has changed? In the 1950s, the diet was barely at a subsistence level for most because of large calorie expenditures for hunting, farming, and ranching. Now, with more ready access to nutrition, including surplus programs, and major shifts in daily

Department of Obstetrics and Gynecology, School of Medicine, University of New Mexico, 2211 Lomas Boulevard, NE, MSC10 5580, Albuquerque, NM 87131, USA
E-mail address: stphelan@salud.unm.edu

Obstet Gynecol Clin N Am 36 (2009) 379–392
doi:10.1016/j.ogc.2009.04.003

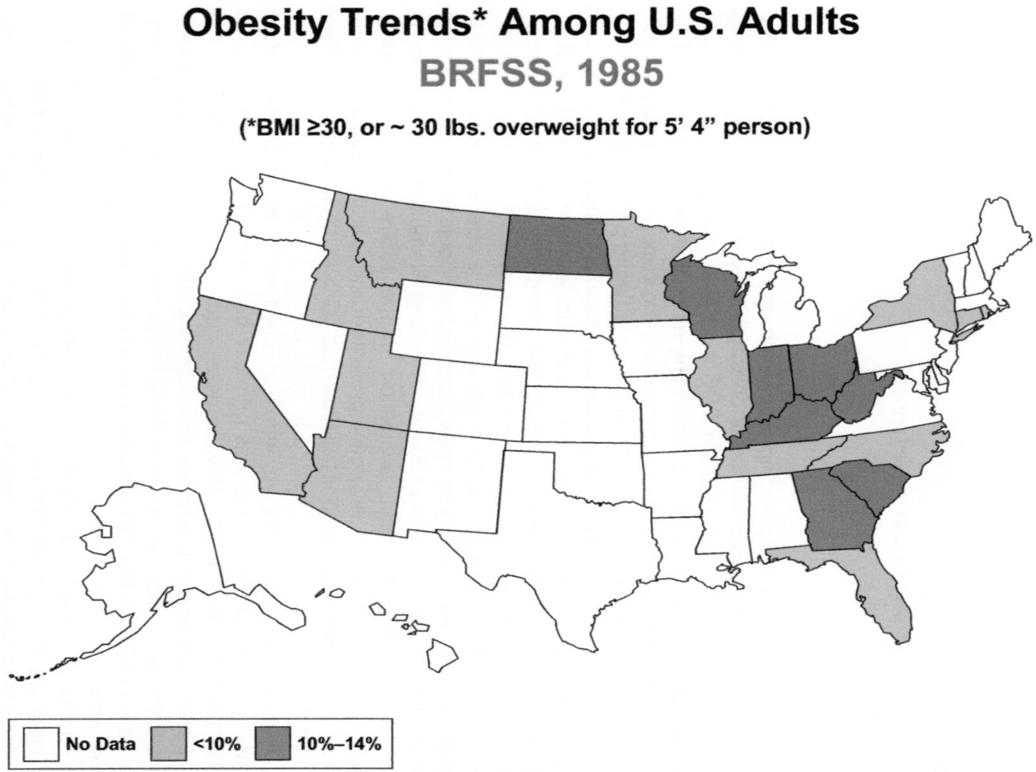

Fig. 1. Obesity Trends among United States Adults from 1985 to 2005. (*From* Center for Disease Control and Prevention. Behavioral Risk Factor Surveillance System (BRFSS). Department of Health and Human Services. Obesity Trends among U.S. adults from 1985–2005. Available at: http://www.cdc.gov/nccdphp/dnpa/obesity/trend/maps). Accessed April 24, 2009.

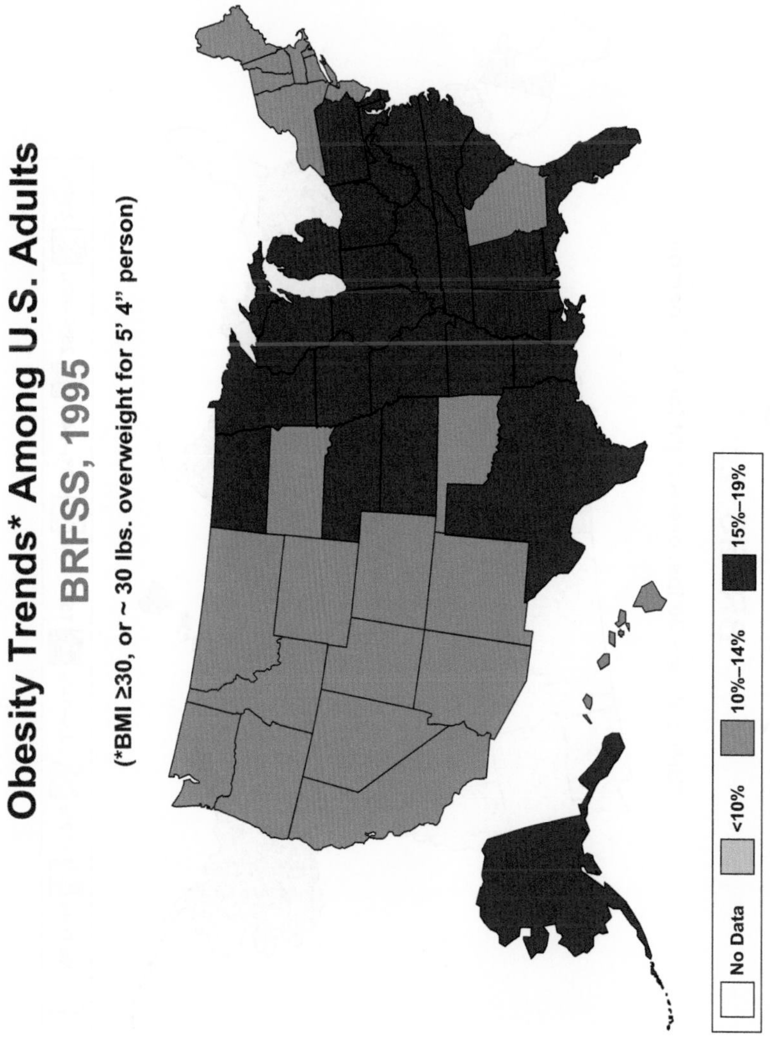

Fig. 1. *(continued)*

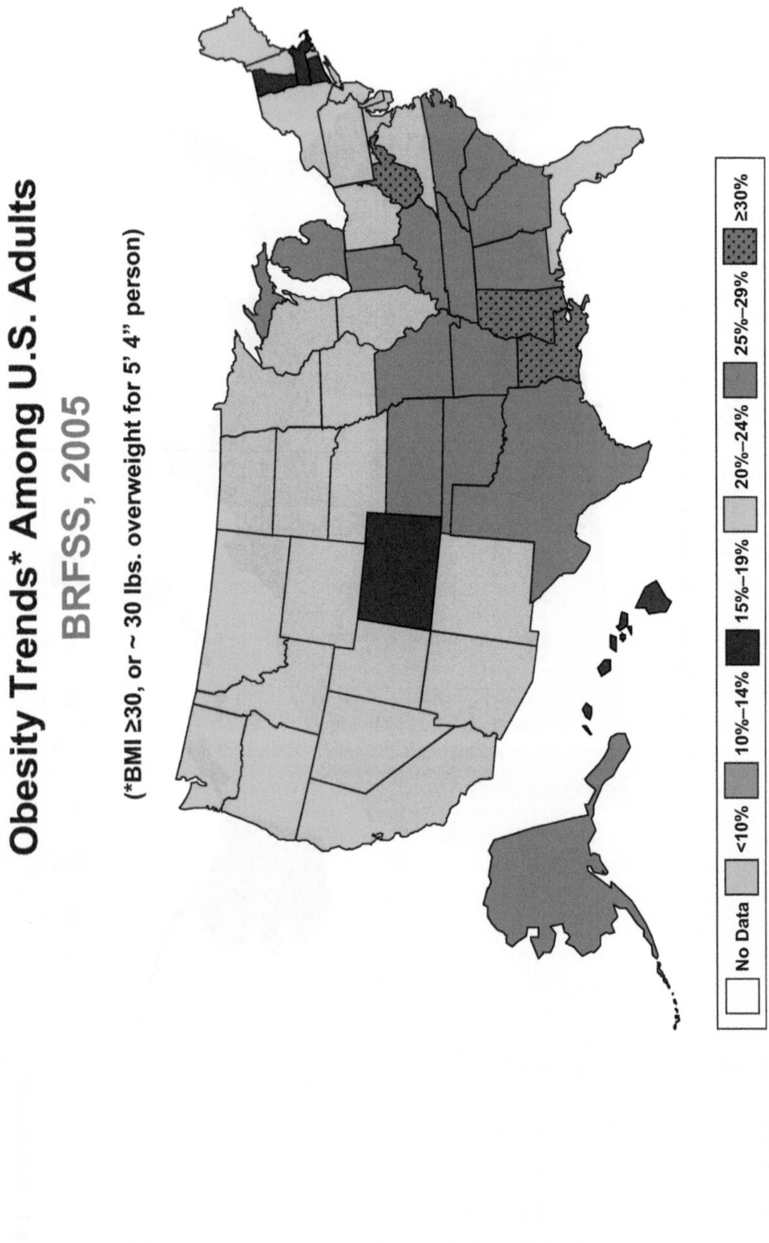

Fig. 1. *(continued)*

activity and calorie expenditure, obesity has become normal for many tribes. In 2002, over 40% of 5-year-old Native American children were overweight and 25% were obese. This is increasing at approximately 4% to 5% each decade.[6,7] Medical providers in these communities now understand that obesity is not only an individual concern but also a community problem.

MORBIDITIES OF OBESITY IN MINORITY POPULATIONS

It is well known that obesity contributes to the development of many comorbidities including hypertension, diabetes, cardiovascular disease, and certain cancers. Obesity is a major contributor to Type II diabetes and hypertension. Both African American women and Mexican American women have higher rates of these comorbidities than white women. However obesity-related hypertension occurs at higher rates among African Americans and obesity-related diabetes occurs at higher rates among Mexican Americans.[8] Data indicate that obesity is a greater risk factor for breast cancer than the use of hormone replacement therapy.[9] In addition, women experience numerous reproductive complications including infertility, increased risk of spontaneous abortion, twin pregnancies, and complicated pregnancies.[10] Prevalence of obesity in pregnancy is increasing, especially among African Americans. In 2001 35% of pregnant African Americans weighed over 200 pounds at delivery with 7.3% weighing between 251 to 300 pounds and 2.7% over 300 pounds.[11] Complications are directly related to increasing obesity. Women over 300 pounds had the highest adjusted-odds ratio for gestational diabetes (OR 5.2), preeclampsia (OR 5.0), cesarean delivery (OR 2.7), macrosomic infant (OR 4.2) or neonate admitted to newborn intensive care unit (NBICU)(OR 1.9).[12] Despite the initial thought that increased-weight gain in adolescent African Americans during pregnancy would improve infant birth weight, it does not.[13] Neonates of obese black mothers have an elevated risk of mortality throughout the neonatal period as compared with obese white women.[14] Within the Native American female population over 49% were obese when they became pregnant and almost half of the population had excessive weight gain during the pregnancy.[15] Obese native women with excessive weight gain had a high prevalence of preeclampsia (14.6%) than obese women with low (3.7%) or acceptable (6.3%) weight gain.[15] Thus, minority women are particularly impacted by the obesity epidemic.

PREVALENCE IN MINORITY POPULATIONS

A 2008 study in Chicago[16] found the prevalence of obesity in children aged 2 to 12 years ranged from 11.8% for non-Hispanic whites to 34% for Latinos and 56% for blacks. The prevalence of obesity has been increasing over the past decade in adults (**Table 1**) and children (**Table 2**) for all ethnic and racial populations. All groups have an increasing prevalence of obesity except for the adolescent Mexican American population. This group has had a decrease in obesity for both males and females. It is unclear how the recent influx of immigrants from Mexico and Central America are impacting the prevalence in this age group. The overall increasing prevalence in obesity has occurred because of a nutritional transition. This transition is caused by a shift in nutritional concerns from malnutrition, and even starvation, to overweight and obesity as a predominant nutritional pattern within a group. The transition is based on large shifts in diet structure related to changing economic, social, and cultural factors. Such a transition often has unintended consequences, such as changes in morbidity and mortality patterns, reductions in physical activity, and increased caloric intake. In the case of minority populations, the result is increased prevalence of

Table 1
Prevalence of overweight and obesity among adult women in the United States (≥20 years old) by ethnic/racial groups

	Overweight BMI>25 (%)			Obesity BMI>30 (%)			Severe Obesity BMI>40 (%)		
Racial/Ethnic Group	**1988–1994**	**1999–2000**	**2003–2004**	**1988–1994**	**1999–2000**	**2003–2004**	**1988–1994**	**1999–2000**	**2003–2004**
White, nonHispanic	47.2	57.5	58.0	23.3	30.6	30.2	3.4	4.9	5.8
Mexican American	69.6	71.8	75.4	36.1	40.1	42.3	4.8	5.5	7.8
Black, nonHispanic	68.5	78.0	81.6	39.1	50.8	53.9	7.9	5.8	14.7
Native American	NA	NA	NA	—	—	—	—	—	—

Data from Flegal KM, Carroll MD, Odgen CL, et al. CDC National Center for Health Statistics, National Health and Nutrition Examination Survey. Prevalence and trends in obesity among US adults 1999–2000. JAMA 2002;268:1723–7; and Ogden CL, Carroll MD, Curtin LR, et al. Prevalence of overweight and obesity in the United States, 1999–2004. JAMA 2006;295(13):1549–55.

Table 2
Percentage of overweight/obesity in children and adolescents in the United States 2003 to 2004

	Ages 2–5 (%)		Ages 6–11 (%)		Ages 12–19 (%)	
Racial/Ethnic Group	**Males**	**Females**	**Males**	**Females**	**Males**	**Females**
White Non-Hispanic	13	10	18.5	16.9	19.1	15.4
Mexican American	23.2	15.1	23.5	19.4	18.3	14.1
Black (non-Hispanic	9.7	6.3	17.5	26.5	18.5	25.4
Native American	24.2	24.1	29.9	26.1	27.5	26.3

Data from Ogden CL, Carroll MD, Curtin LR, et al. Prevalence of overweight and obesity in the United States 1999–2004. JAMA 2006;295(13):1549–55. Zephier E, Himes JH, Story M, et al. Increasing prevalence of overweight and obesity in northern plains American Indian children. Arch Pediatr Adolesc Med 2006;160:34–9.

obesity as traditional foods and activities are replaced with high-sugar, and high-fat convenience foods and a more sedentary lifestyle.[3]

The obesity epidemic is a combination of influences including changes in caloric intake and expenditure (calories), cost and ease of acquiring food along with pressures from the marketplace and media (commerce) and the community response to the increasing prevalence of obesity and sedentary lifestyle (culture). This article outlines the influence of each and some of the strategies that have been attempted in the most vulnerable populations.

Calories

In the early 20th century poorer socioeconomic groups and many minority groups often depended on an agricultural culture for food. This type of environment resulted in production of low-fat foods (wild game), complex carbohydrates (fresh vegetables and fruit) and not a great deal of preprocessed food.[3] Portion size was smaller than it is today, especially when compared with the calories expended during hunting, gathering, and farming. This type of environment promotes the development of thrifty genes, able to optimize the metabolic conversion and use of calories.[17] These genes are very effective in converting extra calories to adipose for later access, and have been selected for within these populations for generations. The human species has no limit to the ability to store fat and extra fat stores do not impact an individual's perception of hunger. This storage ability was essential in populations where reliable access to food was uncertain.

Today less of our food comes from hunting, gathering, or farming and is more likely to be commercially preprocessed with high-fat content (cheese, whole milk, peanut butter) and high simple-calorie content (from the use of sugar and fructose from corn syrup) Portion sizes have increased, both in restaurants and at home. Researchers have indicated that acculturation of immigrants often deteriorates their traditional diet. In Latinos, the less acculturated eat more fruit, rice, beans, and less sugar and sugar- sweetened beverages than their more acculturated peers.[18] The prevalence of obesity among immigrants living in the United States for at least 15 years approaches that of adults born in the United States.[19]

Physical activity levels have decreased dramatically. The availability of affordable, high-caloric foods means that individuals do not have to expend as many calories for food acquisition. Fewer individuals are involved in activities such as farming, herding, and hunting. These activities have not been replaced with other physical activities that involve walking, running or other cardiovascular activities. Instead, we engage in sedentary activities like watching television. African American households have some of the highest rates of television watching, often over 75 h/wk.[20] Television is a safe electronic baby sitter, but increases an appetite for preprocessed foods because of the increasingly frequent and lengthy advertisements.[3,21] There are more advertisements for candy and carbonated soft drinks in black prime-time shows in comparison to general prime time.[20]

Many individuals in inner-city settings or rural environments may not have a safe environment to walk or exercise. On reservations, packs of dogs, snakes, or lack of trails and roads may discourage walking. In the inner city, concerns about crime and personal safety will prevent many individuals from walking, jogging, or other physical activities. To make matters worse, schools have even decreased their physical education classes because of budgetary constraints.[21,22]

Commerce

The cost of certain foods may be a major barrier to a healthy diet. This is problematic on several levels. The government spends large amounts on agricultural subsidies: wheat, corn, rice, soybeans, and livestock raised on these grains. These subsidies have decreased the price over the past 25 years for fats, sugars, and carbonated beverages. In contrast, the prices of fresh fruits and vegetables have increased by 50%, forcing many to go without if they cannot raise their own. Farm subsidies help explain why fast foods are so economical compared with more healthy fresh fruits and vegetables. This lack of affordable, healthy food has resulted in an increase of 300 kcal/d per person from 1985 to 2000 after having remained constant for the previous 75 years.[23] This, along with the increased portion sizes at fast-food restaurants, contributes greatly to our obesity.[24]

Many fresh foods require refrigeration for storage and have a limited shelf life. In isolated rural settings, individuals may not have ready access to electricity, and hence refrigeration. Their meats must be canned or dried, both processes resulting in meat that is high in fat (SPAM) or salt (jerky). Fruits are often canned in syrup or dried (commonly sweetened with fructose). Vegetables are canned, with salt, or sweetened and may be creamed (eg, creamed corn).

The greater problem is what is stocked in the grocery stores in these inner-city or rural communities. The profit margin is greatest with snack foods, bakery goods (packaged cakes, muffins, and cookies), soft drinks, and candy. In an effort to be healthier, stores may carry fruit juices, but these are typically fortified with sweeteners for taste. Cereal may be available, but is commonly a presweetened, processed product that is marketed to children. These are relatively inexpensive, have a long shelf life and are more profitable. Canned foods are less popular and typically have a lower profit margin. The canned foods available are typically high in calories, such as baked beans, canned stew, and pasta products. Fresh fruits, vegetables, and meats are very limited in their availability, if available at all. Many individuals who reside in these communities do not have access to reliable transportation to access more fully stocked traditional grocery stores. In short, these convenience stores find it too expensive to stock fresh food and what may be available is often poor quality at high prices.[6,17]

The Women, Infant and Children (WIC) program was initiated in the 1970s and was based on nutritional needs identified in the 1950s to 1960s. At that time malnutrition/undernutrition with inadequate calories and protein was endemic among these rural and inner-city populations. For that reason, the focus of the WIC program was to provide high-calorie loads along with protein sources. The program stressed cheese, whole milk, peanut butter, canned fruit, cereal, and infant formula. The Food

Distribution Program on Indian Reservations and food banks typically depend greatly on surplus foods that include solid cheeses, cereals, cooking oils, butter, canned meats, and peanut butter. The result is that poorer families have food sources that are high in calories and fat.

The introduction and resulting popularity of fast food and fast-food restaurants has made the consumption of high-density, inexpensive food even easier. The dollar menus that have become popular in many chains allow families to treat themselves to eating a meal out. Using the dollar menu at McDonalds, a person can buy a McDouble cheeseburger (390 kcal), small fries (230 kcal), a hot fudge sundae (330 kcal) and a small soft drink (150 kcal) (nutritional information from McDonald's Restaurants revised August 2008). In short, for less than $5.00 one can purchase 1200 calories, or more than half the daily requirements for a woman. All you can eat buffet restaurants are often inexpensive and encourage over eating so one will get their money's worth. These buffets stress fried foods, heavy sauces, and great amount of starches. These are cheaper to make and promote feeling full sooner, thus maintaining profit margins for the restaurant. For families with limited financial resources, a dinner out needs to be at a restaurant which offers the most for the money, with the most often being a sense of emotional and caloric fulfillment. These buffet restaurants, and the one dollar menus at many fast food chain restaurants, are popular, especially if they are located close to home. The demand for fast food depends greatly on the demand for convenience, which includes the ease of the consumer to access the product. The increasing number of fast-food restaurants in poorer communities directly increases the quantity of fast food consumed by the community.[25] The increase in fast-food restaurants is a double-edged sword for inner-city and rural communities. Although there is the negative impact of an increasingly poor diet, the restaurants bring jobs, possible career advancement, and new developments to a community. Fast-food restaurants are seen as helping to create a sense of community, providing young people with job opportunities and fighting poverty.[26] In turn, these same communities are the ones often ignored by grocery chains and other businesses.[26] Many inner-city residents may not like fast food at all. However, this may be the only source of food at an affordable price.

Menus for school lunches commonly use ingredients that are subsidized commodities which can be cheaper to purchase for poor school districts. Children are more likely to eat foods that they are familiar with and eat at home or are similar to the foods purchased at popular fast food restaurants. These include fried breaded meats (chicken fingers), french fries, canned fruit in heavy syrup, and so forth. Macaroni and cheese may be considered a vegetable, or the entrée, and ketchup may be considered a vegetable. This is not what is recommended in the United States Department of Agriculture food pyramid. Milk is commonly whole milk rather than 1% or nonfat. To help financially, many schools have brought in vending machines for staff and student use. These are typically stocked with candy and soft drinks. There are movements to decrease or prohibit this activity, but it is unclear how poorer schools will replace this source of funding for projects and supplies.

Given our current economic difficulties, there is a risk of increasing obesity. As financial situations get more problematic more individuals turn to food banks and subsidized food programs including school lunch programs. As already noted these are often calorie and fat laden since they are based on 1960 to 1970 studies. Families turn to less expensive foods. A 10% increase in the number of people in poverty will result in a 6% increase in the prevalence of obesity in our country.[27] Unlike conditions during the Great Depression, calorie-dense food is plentiful, cheap, and easier to access.

Poverty only accounts for some of the obesity epidemic. In fact, over the past 30 years, it is not the poor who have experienced the largest gains in obesity prevalence. Among black women, there was a 27% increase in the middle income group compared with a 14% increase for the poor.[28] A 2005 study looked at weight change as it related to race and education in a sample of women in midlife. It has often been assumed that the obesity problem in the African American population is caused by low economic status. In fact, the mean BMI between blacks and whites at the lowest level of education were similar at 31. However, at the highest level of education (college graduate) African Americans had a mean BMI of 31.5 compared with whites at 27.8.[29]

Culture

Recent studies are supporting what many health care workers in rural communities and inner-city communities have suspected for years. The obesity epidemic is more than simply a lack of individual responsibility. Social networks within a community exert powerful influences over individual behavior.[30] These influences are evident at many levels.

Minority group family structures are often matriarchal in nature. Many great grandmothers still remember times when malnutrition and infection caused many deaths, especially among the young. For this reason, they often promote the concept that big babies or children are healthier. In their experience, these were the children that survived. Over the past few decades the perception of ideal birth weight has gradually shifted from a healthy 7- to 8-pound newborn to a 9- to 10-pound newborn. Community standards have shifted from a normal-weight child being seen as healthy to being seen as skinny, underfed, and sickly.[4] The overweight child is now seen as healthy and described as thick, big boned, or carrying baby fat.[4] Studies have shown that parents on the reservation are losing the ability to correctly identity an at-risk obese child. This increases the risk for heart disease, diabetes, cancer, and hypertension. Only 15% of obese children are correctly identified by family members and these children have a BMI greater than 99%.[4] Among African American children, even when a parent correctly identifies their child as obese they do not relate this to the risk factors for comorbidities.[31]

Within an extended family or community many, if not all, celebrations or other group activities revolve around food. These foods may be traditional for that culture, but the expectation is that everyone partakes in large quantities or risks insulting family, friends or the culture itself.[32] Since many traditional foods of minority groups used in celebrations have high-fat and sugar content (eg, fried foods, cakes or pastries) this adds to the community contribution to individual obesity.

Many traditional communities do not promote either the idea of exercise or provide safe opportunities to exercise. The concept of exercise for the sake of physical activity is not embraced by many traditional or urban communities. The woman who does exercise is seen as placing her desires above her family's and breaking with tradition. It is rare for her to receive support for such activities and in fact she may be looked at with suspicion.[32] Women will feel guilty or worry about the safety of the family when she is gone from the home engaging in physical activity. A women's safety, even when just walking, is not certain. Packs of dogs, snakes, and poor drivers may endanger the rural woman while gangs and gun violence may worry the urban woman.[22,32]

Community and tribal leaders need to develop a culture that supports and encourages healthier life choices. This can be done through community activities that promote group identity with healthier diets and activities. These communities must provide programs that allow and encourage women to have increased physical activity in a safe environment. These could include walking trails, exercise groups, child care, and classes on traditional cooking that decrease the emphasis on fat, sugar, and preprocessed foods. These programs must be compatible with the role expectations of their family, community, and social networks and encourage physical activity.[2]

During pregnancy women are at greatest risk of excessive weight gain. Part of this tendency is physiologic. Pregnant women tend to crave more carbohydrates during pregnancy and this is a time in an individual's life when new fat cells can be formed. Physiologic impacts may pale in comparison to the influences and beliefs of a woman's social network. Lack of large weight gain in some is seen as starving the baby. Commonly, pregnant women are given extra food to feed the baby. Traditional Latino culture teaches young pregnant women that a craving must be satisfied because the baby needs it. This belief, coupled with the common cravings for carbohydrates, can lead to unhealthy weight gain.

INTERVENTION

Many women report dieting in the past or are currently dieting. Low-income women frequently use maladaptive strategies, such as diet pills and purging.[33] Statistically these diet efforts are not successful because the individual's motivation is typically to change appearance only. This, in turn, may promote a rebound of more weight regained than lost. Many minority individuals or individuals who are socioeconomically challenged have more tolerance, or open acceptance of, a larger figure. They see diets as something rich people do.[32] Instead, a more successful approach for many groups is to stress decreasing the risk of comorbidities, not ultimate weight. Many Native American, African American, and Latina women have, or know someone with, hypertension, diabetes, heart disease, and the complications associated with these diseases. By decreasing this complication they increase their life span, and as a result, have more time with family and grandchildren. The focus on health may encourage more family and community support to provide time and resources to change behavior.[32] A health-promotion approach to obesity encourages self esteem and common goals among members of the group, fostering pride in group identity, ethnic identity, and traditions. Many of these traditions include diets that are healthier with less preprocessed and sweetened food and more grains, vegetables, and meat.

Intervention must acknowledge and incorporate the influences that peers and family have on food choices, amount of intake, physical activity, and weight management.[21] "Most social groups use group focused strategies to effectively build (or coerce) members to adopt common behavior and behave on behalf of the good of the group."[2] Harnessing these preexisting social networks and emphasizing group pride or loyalty to promote change is more effective for the individual and the group. Group-focused strategies build on these influential relationships (**Box 1**). As social animals, we are influenced by the social norms of the groups that are important to use. Groups (tribes, churches, communities, clubs, and gangs) stress social cohesiveness to establish strong group identity and allegiance.[2] Intervention programs need to tap into these resources within the community.

The Pathway program has been used on some reservations.[34] This approach embraces the concept that community and individual change is best accomplished through education and opportunities. These programs are school based and involve

- Culturally appropriate classroom curriculum to promote healthy eating and increased activity
- Physical activity components to increase energy expenditure during physical education
- A food service intervention to decrease fat in school menus

Box 1
Factors that relate to physical activity

Socio-cultural environment	Physical environment and policy
Social support–promoters • Partner or family member(s) provide support • Church, family gatherings, cultural events provide support for decreased intake and provide physical activity	*Work environment–promoters* • Active co-workers • Supportive employers
Social support–barriers • Lack of support for chores and child care leaving little time/energy • Balance of household and society roles while incorporating activity • Community does not value physical activity • Fear of pressure about breaking community norms regarding activity	*Work environment–barriers* • Lack of work related programs • Brief lunch hour – too short for activity • Lack of support for physical activity at the work site. • Overweight/obese co-workers
Cultural characteristics • Strong emphasis on family is top priority • Acceptance of larger body types • Demands of traditional activities • Social norm to eat large portions of high-fat foods • Lack of facilities and programs	*Community environment–barriers* • Lack of safe places to walk • Weather • Lack of access to affordable and convenient facilities • Dangers – dogs, snakes, gangs, dangerous roads, fear of home invasion while gone.

Data from Thompson JL, Allen P, Cunningham-Sabo L, et al. Environmental, policy and cultural factors related to physical activity in sedentary American Indian women. Women Health 2002;36:59–74.

A family program that includes several school-based family events to promote decreased fat in meals and increase exercise

Some communities will require programs that increase the availability of fresh fruits, vegetables, and meats along with other healthy foods. To sustain the availability, the demand must also increase to motivate grocers to continue to provide cost-effective quality food.[17]

Knowledge can be powerful, especially at times when women are vulnerable, such as during pregnancy. A study done in 2007 in Texas[35] found that greater nutritional knowledge is associated with lower 1-year postpartum weight retention in low-income women. Another study found that intervention with nutritional education had a positive impact on more appropriate pregnancy weight gain.[36]

In summary, a successful intervention in any population to prevent or treat obesity requires an understanding of the influence of calories, commerce and culture for that particular group of people. One must provide healthy foods, promote their use, and get community leaders to support the change before the motivated individual can successfully achieve a healthier weight.

REFERENCES

1. Center for Disease Control and Prevention. Risk Factor Surveillance System (BRFSS). Obesity trends among U.S. adults from 1985–2005. Available at: www.cdc.gov/nccdphp/dnpa/obesity/trend/maps. Accessed April 24, 2009.
2. Teufel-Shone NI. Promising strategies for obesity prevention and treatment within American Indian communities. J Transcult Nurs 2006;17(3):224–9.
3. Compher C. The nutrition transition in American Indians. J Transcult Nurs 2006; 17(3):217–23.
4. Adams AK, Quinn RA, Prince RJ. Low recognition of childhood overweight and disease risk among Native-American caregivers. Obes Res 2005;13(1):146–52.
5. Doshi SR, Jiles R. Health behaviors among American Indian/Alaska Native women, 1998–2000 BRFSS. J Womens Health (Larchmt) 2006;15(8):919–27.
6. Zephier E, Himes JH, Story M, et al. Increasing prevalence of overweight and obesity in northern plains American Indian children. Arch Pediatr Adolesc Med 2006;160:34–9.
7. Story M, Stevens J, Evans M, et al. Weight loss attempts and attitudes toward body size, eating, and physical activity in American Indian children: relationship to weight status and gender. Obes Res 2001;9(6):356.
8. Cossrow N, Falkner B. Race/ethnic issues in obesity and obesity-related comorbidities. J Clin Endocrinol Metab 2004;89(6):2590–4.
9. Huang Z, Hankinson SE, Colditz GA, et al. Dual effect of weight and weight gain on breast cancer risk. JAMA 1997;278(17):1407–11.
10. Ramos GA, Caughey AB. Interrelationship between ethnicity and obesity on obstetric outcomes. Am J Obstet Gynecol 2005;193(3 Pt 2):1089–93.
11. Ehrenberg HM, Dierker L, Milluzzi C, et al. Prevalence of maternal obesity in an urban center. Am J Obstet Gynecol 2002;187(5):1189–93.
12. Rosenberg TJ, Garbers S, Chavkin W, et al. Prepregnancy weight and adverse perinatal outcomes in an ethnically diverse population. Obstet Gynecol 2003; 102(5 Pt 1):1022–7.
13. Nielsen JN, O'Brien KO, Witter FR, et al. High gestational weight gain does not improve birth weight in a cohort of African American adolescents. Am J Clin Nutr 2006;84(1):183–9.
14. Salihu HM, Alio AP, Wilson RE. Obesity and extreme obesity: new insights into the black-white disparity in neonatal mortality. Obstet Gynecol 2008;11(6):1410–6.
15. Brennand EA, Dannenbaum D, Willows ND. Pregnancy outcomes of First Nations women in relation to pregravid weight and pregnancy weight gain. J Obstet Gynaecol Can 2005;27(10):936–44.
16. Margellos-Anast H, Shah AM, Whitman S. Prevalence of obesity among children in six Chicago communities: findings from a health survey. Public Health Rep 2008;123(2):117–25.
17. Curran S, Gittelsohn J, Anliker J, et al. Process evaluation of a store-based environmental obesity intervention on two American Indian reservations. Health Educ Res 2005;20(6):719–29.
18. Ayala GX, Baquero B, Klinger S. A systematic review of the relationship between acculturation and diet among Latinos in the United States: implications for future research. J Am Diet Assoc 2008;108(8):1330–44.

19. Goel MS, McCarthy EP, Phillips RS, et al. Obesity among U.S. immigrant subgroups by duration of residence. JAMA 2004;292(23):2860–7.
20. Tirodkar MA, Jain A. Food messages on African American television shows. Am J Public Health 2003;93(3):439–41.
21. Gray A, Smith C. Fitness, dietary intake and body mass index in urban Native American youth. J Am Diet Assoc 2003;103:1022–7.
22. Bennett GG, McNeill LH, Wolin KY, et al. Safe to walk? Neighborhood safety and physical activity among public housing residents. PLoS Med 2008;5(1):e15.
23. Ludwig DS, Pollack HA. Obesity and the economy: from crisis to opportunity. JAMA 2009;301(5):533–5.
24. Nielsen SJ, Popkin BM. Patterns and trends in food portion sizes, 1977–1998. JAMA 2003;289(4):450–3.
25. Jekanowski MD, Binkley JK, Eales J. Convenience accessibility and the demand for fast food. J Agr Resource Econ 2001;26:58–74.
26. Morland K, Wing S, Roux AD, et al. Neighborhood characteristics associated with the location of food stores and food service places. Am J Prev Med 2002;22:23–9.
27. Drewnowski A, Darmon N. The economics of obesity: dietary energy density and energy cost. Am J Clin Nutr 2005;82:265S–73S.
28. Chang VW, Lauderdale DS. Income disparities in body mass index and obesity in the United States, 1971–2002. Arch Intern Med 2005;165(18):2122–8.
29. Lewis TT, Everson-Rose SA, Sternfeld B, et al. Race education and weight change in a biracial sample of women at midlife. Arch Intern Med 2005;165(5):545–51.
30. Christakis NA, Fowler JH. The spread of obesity in a large social network over 32 years. N Engl J Med 2007;357:370–9.
31. Young-Hyman D, Herman LJ, Scott DL, et al. Caregivers perception of children's obesity-related health risks: a study of African American families. Obes Res 2000;8:241–8.
32. Thompson JL, Allen P, Cunningham-Sabo L, et al. Environmental, policy and cultural factors related to physical activity in sedentary American Indian women. Women Health 2002;36:59–74.
33. Breitkopf CR, Berenson AB. Correlates of weight loss behaviors among low-income African-American, Caucasian, and Latina women. Obstet Gynecol 2004;103(2):231–9.
34. Steckler A, Ethelbah B, Martin CJ, et al. Pathways process evaluation results: a school-based prevention trial to promote healthful diet and physical activity in American Indian third, fourth and fifth grade students. Prev Med 2003;37:S80–90.
35. Nuss H, Freeland-Graves J, Clarke K, et al. Greater nutrition knowledge is associated with lower 1–year postpartum weight retention in low-income women. J Am Diet Assoc 2007;107(10):1801–6.
36. Asbee SM, Jenkins TR, Butler JR, et al. Preventing excessive weight gain during pregnancy through dietary and lifestyle counseling: a randomized controlled trial. Obstet Gynecol 2009;113(2 Pt 1):305–12.

Index

Note: Page numbers of article titles are in **boldface** type.

Obstet Gynecol Clin N Am 36 (2009) 393–399
doi:10.1016/S0889-8545(09)00053-9
0889-8545/09/$ – see front matter

W

Printed and bound by CPI Group (UK) Ltd, Croydon, CR0 4YY
03/10/2024
01040464-0019